Global Chi

Advocacy

On the Front Lines

EDITORS

Stephen Berman, MD, FAAP
Professor of Pediatrics and Public Health
Director, Colorado Center for Global Health
Children's Hospital Colorado Endowed Chair of General Pediatrics
University of Colorado School of Medicine
Colorado School of Public Health
Children's Hospital Colorado
Aurora, CO

Judith S. Palfrey, MD, FAAP
T. Berry Brazelton Professor of Pediatrics
Harvard Medical School
Senior Associate in Medicine
Boston Children's Hospital
Boston, MA

Zulfiqar Bhutta, MBBS, FRCP, FRCPCH, FAAP(Hon), PhD
Division of Women & Child Health, The Aga Khan University
Karachi, Pakistan
Programme for Global Paediatric Research at the Hospital for Sick Children
Toronto, Canada

Adenike O. Grange, MBChB, DCH, FMCPAED, FWACP, FAAP(Hon)
Former Minister of Health
Federal Republic of Nigeria

American Academy of Pediatrics
DEDICATED TO THE HEALTH OF ALL CHILDREN™

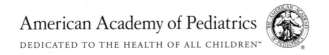

American Academy of Pediatrics Department of Marketing and Publications

Maureen DeRosa, MPA, Director, Department of Marketing and Publications

Mark Grimes, Director, Division of Product Development

Martha Cook, MS, Senior Product Development Editor

Eileen Glasstetter, MS, Manager, Product Development

Carrie Peters, Editorial Assistant

Sandi King, MS, Director, Division of Publishing and Production Services

Theresa Wiener, Manager, Publications Production and Manufacturing

Jason Crase, Manager, Editorial Services

Linda Diamond, Manager, Art Direction and Production

Julia Lee, Director, Division of Marketing and Sales

Linda Smessaert, MSIMC, Manager, Clinical and Professional Publications Marketing

Library of Congress Control Number: 2013932240
ISBN: 978-58110-780-7
eISBN: 978-1-58110-829-3
MA0664

Cover photo © 2008 Arturo Sanabria, courtesy of Photoshare

The recommendations in this publication do not indicate an exclusive course of treatment or serve as a standard of medical care. Variations, taking into account individual circumstances, may be appropriate.

This book has been developed by the American Academy of Pediatrics. The authors, editors, and contributors are expert authorities in the field of pediatrics. No commercial involvement of any kind has been solicited or accepted in the development of the content of this publication.

Statements and opinions expressed are those of the authors and not necessarily those of the American Academy of Pediatrics.

Products are mentioned for informational purposes only. Inclusion in this publication does not imply endorsement by the American Academy of Pediatrics.

The publishers have made every effort to trace the copyright holders for borrowed material. If they have inadvertently overlooked any, they will be pleased to make the necessary arrangements at first opportunity.

Contributors

Bronwen Anders, MD, FAAP
Professor, Department of Pediatrics
University of California, San Diego
San Diego, CA

Jon Kim Andrus, MD
Deputy Director
Pan American Health Organization/
 World Health Organization
Professor of Global Health
The George Washington University
 School of Public Health and
 Health Sciences
Washington, DC
Associate Adjunct Professor
University of California San
 Francisco School of Medicine
San Francisco, CA
Associate Adjunct Professor
Johns Hopkins University
 Bloomberg School of
 Public Health
Baltimore, MD

MaryCatherine Arbour, MD, MPH
Associate Physician for Research
Division of Global Health Equity
Department of Medicine, Brigham
 and Women's Hospital
Boston, MA

Edwin J. Asturias, MD
Associate Professor of Pediatrics
 and Public Health
Director for Latin America
Center for Global Health
University of Colorado School of
 Medicine and Colorado School
 of Public Health
Aurora, CO

**Louise A. Baur, AM, MBBS(Hons),
 BSc(Med), PhD, FRACP**
Professor, Discipline of Paediatrics
 and Child, University of Sydney
Professor, Sydney School of Public
 Health, University of Sydney
Head, Weight Management Services,
 The Children's Hospital at
 Westmead
Westmead, New South Wales,
 Australia

Juan Pablo Beca, MD
Professor, Facultad de Medicina
Director, Centro de Bioetica
Clinica Alemana-Universidad
 del Desarrollo
Santiago, Chile

Paula Bedregal, MD, MPH, PhD
Associate Professor, School of
 Medicine
P. Catholic University of Chile
Santiago, Chile

Ann Behrmann, MD, FAAP
Assistant Clinical Professor of
 Pediatrics
University of Wisconsin School of
 Medicine and Public Health
Pediatrician, Group Health
 Cooperative of South Central
 Wisconsin
Madison, WI

Warren L. Berggren, MD, MPH, DrPH
Board Member
Colorado Haiti Project
Louisville, CO

Elizabeth Bocaletti, MD, MPH
Regional Health Advisor
Save the Children
Antigua, Guatemala

Jaime Burrows, MD, PhD
Facultad de Medicina
Centro de Bioetica
Clinica Alemana-Universidad del Desarrollo
Santiago, Chile

Harry Campbell, MD
Professor of Genetic Epidemiology and Public Health
Director, Centre for Population Health Sciences
University of Edinburgh
Edinburgh, Scotland
Formerly Medical Officer
Programme for Control of Acute Respiratory Infections
World Health Organization
Geneva, Switzerland

Chok Wan Chan, MBBS(HK), MMed(PAED)(SINGAPORE), DCH(LOND), FRCP(EDIN), FRCP(IREL)
Past President, International Pediatric Association
Professor, Chinese University of Hong Kong
President, Hong Kong Society of Child Neurology and Developmental Paediatrics
Hong Kong

Louis Z. Cooper, MD, FAAP
Professor Emeritus of Pediatrics
Columbia University
New York, NY

Hoosen Coovida, MBBS, FCP, MSc, PhD
Director, Maternal Adolescent and Child Health
University of the Witwatersrand
Johannesburg, South Africa
Commissioner, National Planning Commission
The Presidency, Republic of South Africa

Miguel Cordero Vega, MS
Research Fellow
School of Social and Community Medicine
University of Bristol
Bristol, UK

Jai K. Das, MBBS, MD, MBA
Division of Women & Child Health
The Aga Khan University
Karachi, Pakistan

Stéphane Doyon, BA
Nutrition Advocacy Advisor
Médecins Sans Frontières
Paris, France

Burris Duncan, MD, FAAP
Professor Emeritus, Pediatrics
University of Arizona College of Medicine
Tucson, AZ

T. Jacob John, MD
Formerly Professor and Head of the Department of Clinical Virology

Past President of the Indian
  Academy of Pediatrics
Founder Member, Rotary
  International PolioPlus
  Committee
Past President of the Rotary Club
  of Vellore
Christian Medical College, Vellore
Tamil Nadu, India

Juliana Kain, MPH
Biochemist
Associate Professor
Institute of Nutrition and Food
  Technology (INTA)
University of Chile
Santiago, Chile

William J. Keenan, MD, FAAP
Professor of Pediatrics
Saint Louis University
Executive Director
International Pediatric Association
St. Louis, MO

Kate J. Kerber, MPH
Senior Specialist Implementation
Saving Newborn Lives, Save the
  Children
Cape Town, South Africa

Mary Kinney, MSc
Specialist Data & Communications
Saving Newborn Lives, Save the
  Children
Cape Town, South Africa

Jonathan Klein, MD, MPH, FAAP
Director, Julius B. Richmond
  Center of Excellence
Associate Executive Director
American Academy of Pediatrics
Elk Grove Village, IL

Mark W. Kline, MD, FAAP
J.S. Abercrombie Professor and
  Chairman
Ralph D. Feigin Chair
Department of Pediatrics
Baylor College of Medicine
Physician-in-Chief
Texas Children's Hospital
Houston, TX

**Mirzada Kurbasic, MD, MSCR,
  FAAP**
Professor, Department of Pediatrics
University of Louisville
Louisville, KY

Claudio F. Lanata, MD, MPH
Senior Researcher
Instituto de Investigacion
  Nutricional
Science Director
US Naval Medical Research
  Unit No. 6
Professor, School of Medicine
Universidad Peruana de Ciencias
  Aplicadas
Lima, Peru
Associate, Department of
  International Health
Johns Hopkins University
  Bloomberg School of
  Public Health
Baltimore, MD
Honorary Professor
London School of Hygiene and
  Tropical Medicine
University of London
London, UK

Joy Lawn, MBBS,
 MRCP(Paeds), MPH, PhD
Professor
Director of MARCH Center,
 London School of Hygiene
 and Tropical Medicine
Director of Global Evidence
 and Policy
Saving Newborn Lives, Save the
 Children
Cape Town, South Africa

Cherry Chun-Yiu Li, MSc
Project Assistant
Ipsos Health Care
Hong Kong

Emmalita M. Manalac, MD,
 MPH, FPPS
Independent Consultant for
 Child Health
Philippines

Anna Maria Mandalakas, MD,
 FAAP
Associate Professor, Department
 of Pediatrics
Baylor College of Medicine
Director, Global Tuberculosis and
 Mycobacteriology Program
Texas Children's Hospital
Houston, TX

Susan Mercado, MD, MPH
World Health Organization
Western Pacific Regional Office
Tobacco Free Initiative
Manila, Philippines

Helia Molina, MD, MPH
Assistant Professor of Public
 Health, School of Medicine
P. Catholic University of Chile
Santiago, Chile

Charles Mwansambo, MBChB,
 BSc, DCH, MRCP, FRCPCH(UK)
Secretary for Health
Malawi Ministry of Health
Lilongwe, Malawi

Susan Niermeyer, MD, MPH, FAAP
Professor of Pediatrics and Public
 Health
Codirector, Division of Maternal
 and Child Health
Center for Global Health
University of Colorado School of
 Medicine
Colorado School of Public Health
Children's Hospital Colorado
Aurora, CO

Isaac Odame, MD
Global Sickle Cell Disease Network
The Hospital for Sick Children
Department of Pediatrics
Faculty of Medicine
University of Toronto
Toronto, Canada

Walter Orenstein, MD, FAAP
Associate Director, Emory Vaccine
 Center
Professor of Medicine, Pediatrics,
 and Global Health
Emory University
Atlanta, GA

Antonio Pio, MD
Former Manager of the Acute
 Respiratory Infections Program
World Health Organization
Geneva, Switzerland
Senior Consultant in Public Health
 and Respiratory Diseases
Mar del Plata, Argentina

James Rarick, MPH
World Health Organization
Western Pacific Regional Office
Tobacco Free Initiative
Manila, Philippines

Julio Cesar Reina, MD
Professor, Department of Pediatrics
Escuela de Medicina
Universidad del Valle
Cali, Colombia

Desmond K. Runyan, MD, DrPH, FAAP
Jack and Viki Thompson Professor
of Pediatrics
Executive Director, Kempe Center
The University of Colorado School
of Medicine
Aurora, CO

Katherine Seib, MSPH
Epidemiologist
Rollins School of Public Health
Emory University
Atlanta, GA

Susan Shepherd, MD, FAAP
Médecins Sans Frontières
Paris, France

Jonathan M. Spector, MD, FAAP
Returned Volunteer, Médecins
Sans Frontières
Research Scientist
Harvard School of Public Health
Cambridge, MA

Donna M. Staton, MD, MPH, FAAP
Affiliate to Department of Pediatrics
University of Massachusetts School
of Medicine
Worcester, MA

Boyd Swinburn, MBChB, MD(Otago), FRACP
Professor of Population Nutrition
and Global Health
School of Population Health
University of Aukland
Aukland, New Zealand

Ricardo Uauy, MD, PhD
Professor Nutrition INTA
(University of Chile)
Pediatrics (Catholic University
of Chile)
Chile, South America

Peter Waiswa, MBChB, MPH, PhD
Lecturer, Department of Health
Policy, Planning and Management
Makerere University School of
Public Health
Kampala, Uganda
Postdoctoral Fellow, Division of
Global Health, Karolinska
Institutet
Solna, Sweden

Kerri Wazny, MA
Research Project Coordinator
Programme for Global Paediatric
Research at the Hospital for
Sick Children
Toronto, Canada

Zonghan Zhu, MD
Professor
Capital Institute of Pediatrics
Chairman
Pediatrician Society of Chinese
Medical Doctors Association
Beijing, China

Table of Contents

Preface

Advocacy is a core component of practicing pediatrics and caring for children. Being an advocate fulfills its definition: to give voice to those who can't speak for themselves. As pediatricians we bring all the tools of science, intergenerational professionalism, and multidisciplinary partnerships and perspectives to advocate for children. Deciding to become a pediatrician means committing to becoming a child advocate, working at the grassroots level, promoting health, providing care, and implementing child health-targeted policies. A child advocate actively works to create change that helps children to have a better future. It is essential that pediatricians have strong advocacy training to develop needed skills and competency during the undergraduate and postgraduate medical education levels. Advocacy should be an obligatory component of the curricula in all pediatric residence programs. Pediatricians should not be put off by a fear of partisan political involvement or concerns about infringing on the responsibilities of parents.

This book provides young pediatricians with a view into how successful advocates from around the world have worked in their communities to improve the lives of children. It is the first book of its kind and can motivate and inspire pediatricians to define problems, identify solutions, and develop partnerships to implement positive changes in their communities. The International Pediatric Association (IPA) and its regional, national, and pediatric specialty member societies are proud that the authors and the American Academy of Pediatrics will release this book at the IPA meeting in Melbourne, Australia, in August 2013. We believe it will become essential reading for anyone interested in a career in pediatrics.

Sergio Augusto Cabral, MD
President, International Pediatric Association

Foreword

Act and Advocate: The Front Lines of Global Child Health Advocacy

It is 2004, fully 8 years after the advent of the miraculous, lifesaving HIV cocktail. It is not available in most places in the developing world, but in the public clinic at l'Hopital Saint Therese in Hinche, Haiti, treatment has finally come. The first patients, adults and children, are being enrolled on antiretroviral therapy. Two young teenagers sit, crying, clutching each other, afraid to be talking about their illness. Their chief complaint? "Mama'n mouri, papa'n mouri, yo kite'nou an ak maladi sa-a": "Our mother died, our father died, and they left us with this disease," says the older brother. Freddy and Orcelia were seeking not just a pill, a treatment, but care, protection, love, and understanding. They were hungry, homeless, orphans, not in school—and yes, in addition, they had HIV. Freddy and Orcelia's story might just be about access to HIV treatment; however, it is more for those of us fortunate to work with an organization, Partners In Health (and its Haitian sister organization, Zanmi Lasante), that for 25 years has learned that to improve the health of the poor and vulnerable, we must address all complexities of this chief complaint—from providing food to psychosocial support, addressing mental and physical health needs. Over the course of multiple visits—first to the animal shed in which they lived, later to a more secure house—and by enrolling them in school, clothing them, and helping them to cope with the multitude of challenges they faced, Zanmi Lasante physicians, nurses, psychologists, social workers, and community health workers became advocates for Freddy and Orcelia. We call this strategy *accompaniment*—working together with affected people and their communities to act directly to ameliorate suffering. Though Freddy and Orcelia are still poor, they are alive and healthy today, have finished school, and are able, as young adults, to work and support themselves. Critical to the strategy of Partners In Health is amplifying the voices of those like Freddy and Orcelia through advocacy on local and global scales. Local leaders as well as international financial institutions focusing attention on such stories helps us to fight to improve not only the health but the social determinants of the lives of children. The story of Freddy and Orcelia, one of social and economic vulnerability that leaves disease and disability in its wake, is a common one. Thus, addressing social determinants as we act to address the burden of diseases like AIDS does more to change the trajectory of children's lives like Freddy and Orcelia than any pill or cocktail could ever do alone.

At Partners In Health we believe that health is an entrée for the struggle for human rights—a platform for action and from which to do advocacy. Developing countries bear 90% of the global burden of disease armed with only 20% of the world's gross domestic product and 12% of the world's health expenditures to combat this burden. Africa is particularly hard-hit, bearing fully one-quarter of the world's disease burden with 3% of the global health workforce, who are paid less than 1% of global health expenditures. With such paltry resources available in these settings, how can people get the health services they need? The answer is that they do not. As a result, life expectancy in Lesotho is 35.1 years (compared with 76.7 years in Cuba); in Malawi, 600 women die in childbirth for every 100,000 live births (as compared with 2 in Sweden); and in Chad, 170 children per 1,000 die before their fifth birthday (compared with 8 per 1,000 in the United States), and neonatal and infant mortality statistics differ even more between the developed and developing world.

Yet change is afoot. In 2000, the United Nations hosted its 189 member-states for the Millennium Summit, during which various challenges facing the world were broadly addressed, including poverty, environmental threats, and human rights abuses and violations. From this summit, the Millennium Development Goals (MDGs) were drafted and unanimously approved by UN member-states. The 8 MDGs address the major facets of development, linking social and economic determinants with health and well-being. To achieve the MDGs it is estimated that health spending would need to reach US $60 per capita. While challenges in meeting the MDGs remain, there are examples such as Rwanda, where the government has increased its own per capita spending on health and harnessed external financing and partners toward the achievement of the MDGs, and child mortality has been halved in less than 5 years. Similarly, the global fight for AIDS treatment access has been a lesson in action and advocacy. Advocacy by people living with AIDS and those in solidarity with them has resulted in the flow of billions of dollars for AIDS treatment from rich countries in the global North to poorer ones in the global South. The global action needed to implement treatment once drugs were available laid bare weaknesses of the massively under-resourced public health sector. Action in the AIDS epidemic lead to even more advocacy around health systems strengthening, rooted in the lived experience that demonstrated that a lion's share of people presenting to clinic, especially in rural areas, come because they are sick, not because they want to know their HIV status. Today, few doubt that health systems strengthening is the real issue in the provision of care, not just providing access to a vertical program. This loop of praxis—practice, action, reflection—is fundamental to the work of Partners In Health and underpins all of the advocacy work we have done for 25 years.

This book on global child health advocacy is a welcome addition to the literature in global health. It comes at a critically important time when children's health is on the agenda of large international organizations such as WHO, the United Nations Children's Fund, the World Bank, and the Global Fund to Fight AIDS, Tuberculosis and Malaria. All countries agree that achievement of the MDGs is within reach and that meeting the child health goals is fundamental to a just and healthy world. The stories in the book are written by inspiring and successful child advocates who are our teachers, mentors, students, and mentees. Their accumulated wisdom will encourage child health practitioners all around the world—those who are already acting to address health inequities to advocate for social change. The arc of history has shown that human rights can only be advanced through active engagement with and for the people most affected by their lack. This book will equip those standing with children everywhere to become advocates for and with children so that children everywhere can achieve their potential as world citizens.

Mirebalais, Haiti
March 25, 2013

Joia S. Mukherjee, MD, MPH
Chief Medical Officer, Partners In Health
Associate Professor, Global Health and Social Medicine,
    Harvard Medical School
Boston, MA

Paul E. Farmer, MD, PhD
Founder, Partners In Health
Kolokotrones University Professor, Harvard Medical School
Boston, MA

Acknowledgments

A commitment to child advocacy has been at the core of pediatrics since the discipline of pediatrics emerged within the medical community. The American Academy of Pediatrics (AAP) was established in the early 20th century to provide a strong and unified voice to support the need for government programs to care and feed poor, vulnerable children. During this same time in Europe, Janusz Korczak, a Polish pediatrician, became an eloquent advocate for the rights of children. Subsequently, in countries throughout the world, pediatricians and other child advocates have worked hard to make meaningful differences in the lives of children living in their communities. Today pediatric societies and residency training programs around the world recognize the power of effective child advocacy to transform communities, save the lives of millions of newborns and children, and promote the health and welfare of many more. Advances in communication technology have empowered people who were isolated and powerless to communicate their plight or improve their lives.

Today, when many pediatricians join in efforts to transform their communities and speak out for children, a movement is created and change happens. This book is to encourage pediatricians and other health professionals who care for children to join this movement. Everyone has an important part to play in successful child advocacy. We will only move the needle enough to reach the Millennium Development Goals and improve the health and welfare of the world's children when all of us become involved. We can become involved as individuals or through our children's schools, professional societies, community-based organizations, or governmental organizations. This book provides insights into the many ways to become involved in successful advocacy.

This book was made possible by the encouragement and support of the AAP and the International Pediatric Association (IPA). We would like to recognize the assistance of Errol R. Alden, MD, FAAP, AAP executive director/CEO; Jonathan Klein, MD, MPH, FAAP, AAP associate executive director/director, Julius B. Richmond Center of Excellence; AAP International Affairs; as well as the AAP Section on International Child Health, especially the members of the International Community Access to Child Health (I-CATCH) committee who have worked so hard to make this program successful. We also appreciate the support of William J. Keenan, MD, FAAP, executive director of the IPA, as well as the president of the IPA,

Sergio Augusto Cabral, MD, and members of the IPA executive committee. Finishing the book on time would not have been possible without the organization, energy, and competence of Martha Cook, MS, AAP senior product development editor.

The American Academy of Pediatrics would like to acknowledge and thank the Pan American Health Organization/World Health Organization Regional Office for the Americas for their generous contribution in the production of this publication.

One of the most rewarding aspects of this endeavor has been the opportunity for us to work together and with the chapter authors. We have great admiration and respect for their advocacy efforts and accomplishments. We hope that you will be as inspired and moved to action as we have been in reading their chapters.

Stephen Berman, MD, FAAP

Judith S. Palfrey, MD, FAAP

Zulfiqar Bhutta, MBBS, FRCP, FRCPCH, FAAP(Hon), PhD

Adenike O. Grange, MBChB, DCH, FMCPAED, FWACP, FAAP(Hon)

Section 1

Overview of Global Child Health Advocacy

Chapter 1

Advocacy on the Front Lines

Judith S. Palfrey, MD, FAAP
Stephen Berman, MD, FAAP

This book is unabashedly about advocacy. It is a call to action for child health clinicians around the globe to band together, learn from one another, and use advocacy tools and skills that are effective in improving child health and well-being.

A group of the world's most successful child health advocates have graciously written the book's chapters, sharing what they have experienced on the front lines with the larger child health community. These are people who have looked beyond problems to envision solutions. With key information and data, they have convincingly made their cases and spurred action. These advocates have had the courage and ability to work with allies and opponents; they have changed fundamental conditions for children. They have never forgotten that children and families are in the center of their concern.

What Is Advocacy?

Advocacy is the call for change and the drive for excellence. Advocacy can and should be practiced at all levels. Any time a pediatrician suggests an improvement in office routines or adds a new resource or joins a public health campaign, that is clinical advocacy. When a child health team chooses to focus its efforts on improving care for a particular group of children (eg, malnourished children, teen parents, child soldiers, HIV-affected children, youth with disabilities), that is advocacy. When child health providers enter the fray and join with parents and others to call for system reforms, that is advocacy. And when professionals take a long, serious look at how they are spending their time, talent, and energy as individuals or a coordinated group, that is advocacy.

How Is Advocacy Accomplished?

Advocacy works through a cycle of dynamic relationships among data gathering, action, and monitoring (Figure 1-1).

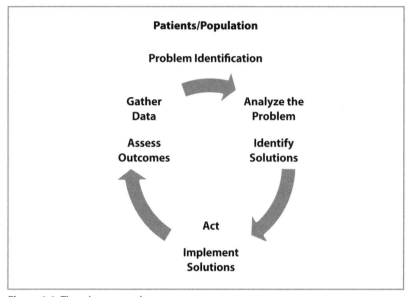

Figure 1-1. The advocacy cycle.

Problem identification is the initial step in the advocacy cycle and is informed by boots-on-the-ground work with children and families in clinical and community settings. The authors tell their stories in this book by describing how they selected the area of their greatest concern for action. Some were motivated by children they cared for who died needlessly. Others chose their advocacy focus because of a deep concern for social justice. Still others wanted their research findings to make a difference at the bedside or in the community. No matter their motivation, in each case they saw that to have an effect, they must specify a concrete problem, develop a systematic social strategy, and throw themselves into the sometimes messy work of getting started.

Advocates demonstrate how, in each case, they *analyzed their selected problem* by establishing what was already known about the population and problem locally, regionally, nationally, and internationally using literature searches and relevant databases available from governmental agencies, nongovernmental agencies, academic institutions, or international organizations such as the World Health Organization, United Nations

Children's Fund, and World Bank. Since the early 1990s, the availability of high-quality data at the country level on the Internet has made this work increasingly possible. For local data, advocates often need to probe more deeply at the community level with surveys and focus groups.

To *identify solutions,* advocates searched for evidence about successes in other parts of their country or the global arena. They recognized that successful solutions are very community specific—what has worked in one region or country may not be appropriate in another community. Nonetheless, in each community, the following questions can be helpful in choosing and tailoring the solution: 1) Is the intervention politically and culturally feasible? 2) Are there sufficient resources, funding, and people to implement the solution? 3) Is the solution ethical? Will the planned intervention affect vulnerable and disadvantaged populations fairly and equitably?

Advocacy *action* almost always involves team and coalition building, whether it is to roll out a program in the clinic, community, or an entire region or country. Authors tell how they developed these teams and coalitions by calling on community leaders, other child advocates, business leaders, religious organizations, professional societies, hospitals, academic centers, and community service programs. Team and coalition building is hard but rewarding work.

After pulling together the team, a key advocacy action is raising the public visibility of the problem to elicit an even broader constituency for action. Child health advocates have learned that communicating stories of affected children and families is a very effective way to pressure elected officials to improve health care for children. Getting an issue on the public radar sometimes requires aggressive, decisive action. The advocate authors demonstrate that it is valuable to appeal to the full range of the political spectrum, keeping children's issues above extreme partisan and political spheres as much as possible.

The real creativity of advocacy comes in the *implementation of solutions.* Advocates discover that a road map with a clear end point is enormously helpful for this implementation. To get to the "last mile" of the journey, each of the advocates planned their interventions with the end in mind.

The *actions* in child health advocacy on a global level occur as a 3-step process. Researchers and innovators conceive of new ways to address old problems with a new vaccine, antibiotic, nutritional supplement, or primary care model. They launch a project to test their idea and if possible, prove that their idea was effective and feasible. With proof-of-concept data in hand, they advocate adoption of a community, regional, or national program that incorporates their intervention. Finally, a third critical step is the wholesale adoption of the practice and faithful implementation by large numbers of day-to-day child health advocates who dare to make a change in their local environment in the pursuit of excellence for children. At each of these stages, the rules and rewards of advocacy are the same.

Advocacy as an Essential Component of Child Health Care

Combined with research, clinical care, and teaching, advocacy moves forward the child health agenda. Four Ps define how advocacy is best integrated into daily child health practice.

Personal experience often determines the population or issue for which a child health clinician decides to advocate. Experiences with a family member or patient can galvanize a resolve to make a change in the way a particular problem is handled.

Persistence is required in advocacy efforts through zigs and zags, near success, and heart-stopping failures. Forming teams and coalitions and keeping them going is a formidable task. Advocates must patiently persist through rough patches as they work to change health practices and policies at any level. Inertia and bureaucracy are powerful forces that can only be counteracted by slow, steady, unremitting pressure.

Passion is essential for effective advocacy. Effective advocates feel so personally connected to an issue that the passion itself can sustain them. This is especially true for child health practitioners living in low-resource countries who have several jobs and little free time to spend with their families. Child health practitioners should know themselves well enough to recognize that a particular passion is real and long lasting.

Finally, advocates must be *principled.* This means having a strong sense of integrity, credibility, fairness, and responsibility. Having integrity means committing to gain a complete and unbiased understanding of the issue, acknowledging what is known and not known. Having credibility means that advocates serve the best interests of children rather than special interests. Being fair means advocating policy recommendations based on a uniform standard of care for all children, not on different standards influenced by ethnicity or race, family income, insurance status, or other socio-demographic factors. Being responsible means recognizing that an advocacy effort could have unintended consequences that are detrimental to other populations or the public good.

The advocates featured in this book have lived by the 4 Ps. They have started us on our way, but there is still much to be done. As long as babies are being born too early; any of their births are unattended by persons who can resuscitate them; any child contracts a vaccine-preventable illness, HIV, or malaria; any child goes to bed hungry; and any child cannot get access to quality health care, our advocacy job is not done. We can do better by children. We can keep them safe from injury. We can promote their healthy lifestyles. We can coordinate our work with our colleagues in education, social welfare, and other child-oriented fields to help them reach their potential.

We sincerely hope that this book will provide inspiration and guidance to child health clinicians around the globe to keep advocating for our children's health and well-being.

Chapter 2

Caring for Our Children as One World Community

Chok Wan Chan, MBBS(HK), MMed(PAED)(SINGAPORE), DCH(LOND), FRCP(EDIN), FRCP(IREL)

Introduction

During the 20th century, the countries of the world began to recognize the interdependence of all human societies. Despite disagreements, sovereignty challenges, and wars, the world's nations created mechanisms for working globally. With the initiation of institutions such as the United Nations, the World Health Organization (WHO), and the United Nations Children's Fund (UNICEF), processes were put into place for child health advocacy at a global level.

The importance to the world of having healthy children and the understanding of how to promote child health have evolved over time as world bodies have considered the definition of *health*. In the first half of the 20th century health was generally considered to be the absence of disease. In 1946, the framers of the WHO constitution modified this view with an expansive definition of health as "a state of complete physical, mental and social well-being and not merely the absence of disease or infirmity."[1]

This new conceptual framework acknowledged the importance of social as well as biologic determinants of health. In 2004, the Institute of Medicine broadened the definition of child health, stating that it is the extent to which children are "able or enabled to develop and realize their potential."[2] This adds a major functional characteristic to the notion of children's state of health and well-being and calls on the larger community to enhance the opportunities for children to grow, develop, and thrive.

While much of the initial focus on child health centered on children aged 0 to 5 years, recent global efforts have expanded the scope of child health to include young people up to at least the age of 18 years. The current view stresses the continuum of care from parents to newborn, then to babies, children, and adolescents, who begin the cycle anew as the healthy parents of the next generation.

Throughout the second half of the last century, WHO and UNICEF developed programs to improve children's health status, especially in the lowest resource settings. Over the past 2 to 3 decades, other global organizations such as the GAVI Alliance; Global Fund to Fight AIDS, Tuberculosis and Malaria; and World Bank have joined in global child health advocacy efforts. Such advocacy is now at an explosive stage with the coordinated call for the attainment of the Millennium Development Goals (MDGs) for children.

Child health providers have been key actors in this global advocacy. Child health clinicians and researchers have documented the deplorable situation of children's health status in many parts of the world. Child health providers have helped develop and implement effective and affordable tools and strategies to combat excessive child mortality and morbidity.[3,4]

The UN Convention on the Rights of the Child

A major step for children and their health came in 1989, when the UN General Assembly adopted the Convention on the Rights of the Child.[5] The convention has since been ratified by all but 3 countries (the United States, Somalia, and the South Sudan). Countries who have ratified the convention and become parties to it agree to report to the Committee on the Rights of the Child on their progress toward improving the status of children in their nation.[6]

The convention declares basic, universal, and forward-looking principles as follows:

1. *Nondiscrimination (article 2)*
   "Irrespective of the child's or his or her parent's or legal guardian's race, color, sex, language, religion, political or other opinion, national, ethnic or social origin, property, disability, birth or other status."

2. *Best interests of the child (article 3)*
   This principle relates to decisions by courts of law, administrative authorities, legislative bodies, and public and private social-welfare institutions.

3. *The views of the child (article 12)*
   Children should be free to have opinions in all matters affecting them, *"in accordance with the age and maturity of the child."*

4. *The right to life, survival, and development (article 6)*
   The right-to-life article includes formulations about the rights to survival and development, which should be ensured "to the maximum extent possible."

5. Optimum care to children with developmental needs depends on
   - Social justice
   - Evidence-based practice
   - Professional readiness
   - Resource availability
   - Government support and endorsement

The convention set the stage for ensuring that children would be a focus of international attention and that the health of infants, children, and adolescents would receive specific consideration. As a complement to the convention, the MDGs have provided a concrete set of child health outcomes for the world's nations to achieve.

The Millennium Development Goals

In September 2000, 189 heads of states adopted the UN Millennium Declaration and endorsed a framework for development. The plan was for countries and development partners to work together to reduce poverty and hunger and tackle ill health, lack of education, gender inequality, environmental degradation, and lack of access to clean water.

The 8 MDGs 2000–2015 were set to be reached by the year 2015.[7]

1. Eradicate extreme poverty and hunger.
2. Achieve universal primary education.
3. Promote gender equality and empower women.
4. Reduce child mortality by two-thirds by 2015.
5. Improve maternal health.
6. Combat HIV/AIDS, malaria, and other diseases.
7. Ensure environmental sustainability.
8. Develop a global partnership for development.

The power of these 8 MDGs comes from the establishment of 18 targets and 46 measurable indictors as objective criteria for evaluation. Six of the targets (1, 4, 5, 6, 7, and 8) and at least 23 indicators are relevant to child health, growth, and well-being. The framers of the MDGs took the conditions of each country in 1990 as a baseline and set aspirational but feasible end points to be achieved by 2015. The rigorous ongoing evaluation requires periodic reports from each country to gather information about achievement and progress. The process attempts to promote the highest level of effort by each country to meet the MDGs.

Millennium Development Goal 4 is the centerpiece of advocacy for child health practitioners. Goal 4 calls the world's nations to "Reduce by two-thirds, between 1990 and 2015, the under-five mortality rate." In 1990, the baseline year, the under-5 mortality rate ranged from 179 of 1,000 live births in the least developed countries to 10 of 1,000 live births in industrialized countries. In 2008, the range of under-5 mortality was 129 of 1,000 live births in the least developed countries to 6 of 1,000 live births in industrialized countries.[8]

In 2003, a group of child and public health professionals met in Bellagio, Italy, to deliberate on the most effective ways the world medical community could contribute to achieving MDG 4. The group produced a seminal series of articles for *The Lancet* addressing the question, "Where and why are 10 million children in the world dying?"[9] The authors showed that the vast majority of deaths of children younger than 5 years were from preventable or readily treatable conditions. They pointed out that in 2000, 4 million of the nearly 11 million under-5 deaths were babies who did not survive beyond the first month of life; countless millions of other children survived with impaired health and development; 0.5 million mothers died during pregnancy and child birth. Table 2-1 shows the most recent distribution of child deaths for 2010 with a similar pattern.

The Bellagio Study Group on Child Survival discussed major advances made in child health in the developed world with the deployment of inexpensive and straightforward interventions including healthy nutrition, immunizations, and antibiotics for common infections. It laid out a clear road map for the journey toward accomplishing the MDGs, with specific indications for differential approaches depending on the epidemiology in any given low-resource setting. Examples of these interventions are stabilization of newborn temperature, tetanus toxoid, antibiotics for premature rupture of membranes, breastfeeding, and antibiotics for sepsis and dysentery.

Beyond MDG 4, each of the other MDGs is also linked directly or indirectly to the reduction of child mortality. Millennium Development

Table 2-1. Causes of Death Among Children Aged 0 to 59 Months, 2010

Cause of Death	Percent of Total Deaths
Causes Death in Neonates	*40%*
Pneumonia, neonatal	4%
Preterm birth complications	14%
Intrapartum-related events	9%
Sepsis and meningitis, neonatal	5%
Congenital abnormalities	4%
Neonatal tetanus	1%
Other neonatal	2%
Causes Death in Children Beyond Newborn Period	*60%*
Diarrhea	10%
Malaria	7%
Injury	5%
AIDS	2%
Meningitis	2%
Measles	1%
Other non-neonatal	18%
Pneumonia	14%

Source: Liu L, Johnson HL, Cousens S, et al. Child Health Epidemiology Reference Group of the World Health Organization and UNICEF. Global, regional, and national causes of child mortality: an updated systematic analysis for 2010 with the time trends since 2000. *Lancet.* 2012;379(9832):2151–2161

Goal 5 (the improvement of maternal care) has specific ties with infant survival. Increasingly, planners are aligning strategies that address infant and maternal health with the recognition of interdependence. Millennium Development Goal 6 (combat HIV, malaria, and other infectious diseases) has strong clinical bearing on the achievement of MDG 4. In 2010, infectious diseases accounted for roughly 50% of under-5 mortality. The achievement of MDG 1 (the eradication of poverty and hunger), MDG 2 (education), MDG 3 (gender equity), and MDG 7 (environmental stability) each will contribute indirectly to improvement in child health outcomes. Millennium Development Goal 8 fosters global partnerships to build an effective, efficient, and sustainable system of supports to ensure the full achievement of the all the other MDGs.

The MDGs have helped to galvanize and organize worldwide advocacy by large global organizations, ministries of health, universities, professional organizations, nongovernmental organizations, missionary groups, and individuals. Since their adoption in 2000, there has been steady progress in decreasing child mortality, with the 2011 figure being 6.9 million.[10]

Unfortunately, the success in combatting child mortality is very uneven. While much of East Asia and Pacific, Europe and Central Asia, Latin America and the Caribbean, the Middle East, and North Africa are on track to meet the MDG target in 2015, targets in 2 geographic regions, sub-Saharan Africa and South Asia, are markedly behind progress toward MDG 4.

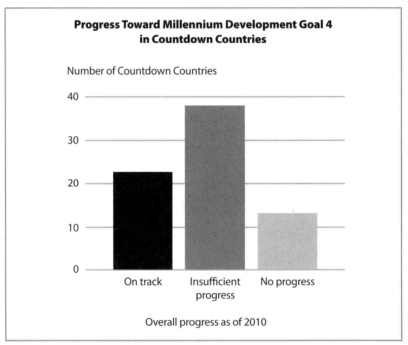

Figure 2-1. Progress toward Millennium Development Goal 4. Source: Countdown to 2015 analysis based on UNICEF, WHO, World Bank and UNDESA 2011.

The Countdown to 2015 project[11] is now focusing attention on the countries that have failed to make progress toward the MDGs with the hope of changing their trajectories. Twenty-three countries are on track, but disappointingly, 40 countries have made insufficient progress and 12 have made no progress (Figure 2-1).

Clearly, work needs to continue with increased and sustained commitment at local, national, and international levels.

Clinical Promotion of the Millennium Development Goals at the Local Level

Within the context of the MDGs, what does it mean for child health professionals at the local level? What are the day-to-day clinical implications of the worldwide pursuit of improved child survival?

Child health covers the medical, social, and educational sectors at home and school and in the community. The professional team involved with promoting child health should be transdisciplinary and inter-sectoral comprising doctors, nurses, midwives, allied health professionals, teachers, social workers, parents, and others. All the professionals need to collaborate toward optimum management of the continuum of care, from parents to newborn, then to babies, children, and adolescents (boys and girls), who then become good parents.

Promotion of Exclusive Breastfeeding as the Bedrock of Improved Young Child Feeding

The promotion of infant and young child feeding is a key strategy for achieving the targets of MDG 4. In addition, MDG 1 (the eradication of poverty and hunger) is advanced by the achievement of optimal breastfeeding and use of appropriate complementary feeding for children younger than 2 years.[12] The Global Strategy for Infants and Young Child Feeding provides a structure for the promotion of breastfeeding worldwide. Its implementation is a critical component in ensuring appropriate growth and cognitive development of children. Breastfeeding plays a key role in the prevention of infectious diseases. Furthermore, the achievement of routine breastfeeding will address emerging noncommunicable disease (NCD) problems such as overweight, obesity, and rapidly increasing numbers of type 2 diabetes mellitus and arterial hypertension.

Early Childhood Development

Increasingly, child experts are emphasizing the importance of early childhood development. Children's development depends on genetics, biology, anatomy, physiology, biochemistry, ecology, and the scaffolding and stimulation provided to them by the adults around them. Many of the disparities in health and function between people in developed and less developed nations (and within the different socioeconomic strata of all countries) can be traced to differences in early childhood opportunities and support. Children who are not exposed to active learning environments may lag behind their peers in receptive and expressive language, concept formation, and executive functioning. Children who are malnourished, suffer recurrent infections, or have a chronic condition learn less well than children who are healthy and well nourished. To achieve a full state of health for children, it is incumbent on child health providers to screen for developmental concerns and support children and families in obtaining quality educational and developmental services. Parents must be empowered to help achieve the universal childhood education outlined in MDG 2.

Global Immunization as Priority for Children's Health

Immunization is a core component of MDG 4 and human rights to health. Each year, more than 1.5 million children die of diseases that can be prevented by vaccines. Approximately 1 in 5 children do not receive vaccines because of inadequate health services, extreme poverty, or armed conflict. Vaccines are one of the most cost-effective public health interventions, costing only a small fraction of the full price to treat the illnesses they prevent and shielding communities from the huge burden of preventable morbidities.

In 2010, the Global Vaccine Action Plan (GVAP) announced the Decade of Vaccines Collaboration and the $10 billion commitment of the Bill & Melinda Gates Foundation. Through a broad consultation with stakeholders, the GVAP includes efforts to strengthen country programs and coordinate activities of all partners. Countries must strengthen and sustain their investment in GVAP goals: a polio-free world; meeting elimination and vaccination targets in every community; development and use of new and improved vaccines; and exceeding the MDG 4 target for reduction in child mortality. The success of the GVAP leading to reducing the frequency of measles and rubella has demonstrated that concerted and coordinated global action can have a major effect on infectious diseases.

Global Action Plan for Prevention and Control of Pneumonia

Pneumonia is the top killer of children younger than 5 years and the second top killer of neonates. As a tool for achieving MDG 4, the Global Action Plan for the Prevention and Control of Pneumonia advises that child health workers emphasize 1) good personal habits (eg, hand washing); 2) immunization for vaccine-preventable illness; 3) healthy nutrition with exclusive breastfeeding for the first 6 months; 4) zinc supplementation; 5) the avoidance of smoke and other indoor environmental hazards; and 6) timely treatment with inexpensive antibiotics.

Integrated Management of Childhood Illness

Integrated Management of Childhood Illness (IMCI) was designed by WHO to enhance children's health and reduce mortality and morbidity due to the most prevalent diseases in developing countries. This strategy includes the early diagnosis, treatment, and timely referral of children younger than 5 years with the most common diseases. It also contributes to improving parental skills and practices associated with the home care of children.

A community-based approach is essential for childhood health because it promotes healthy habits in the family, adequate care of children (eg, feeding, clothing, stimulation), disease prevention, and prompt seeking of medical care when alarming signs and symptoms are noted. The IMCI strategy also helps health care professionals take advantage of opportunities for prevention, promote childhood development, and encourage the rational use of drugs and medications. This strategy is not meant for chronic disease, less frequent disease, or acute emergencies. As a complement to ambulatory care, this strategy includes procedures and practices at different referral levels and types of hospitals.

The IMCI strategy is based on the importance of simple clinical signs and symptoms, the proper classification of the disease, timely treatment, and interventions for prevention and follow-up. It is particularly useful in the first level of care, ie, camps, medical offices, health care centers, or hospital primary care departments. The practical IMCI guidelines are based on the following principles:

- All sick children must be assessed for general danger signs, which indicate the need for immediate referral or admission to a hospital.
- All sick children must be routinely assessed for major symptoms (for children from 2 months to 5 years old: cough or difficult breathing,

diarrhea, fever, ear problems; for newborns aged 1 week to 2 months: bacterial infection and diarrhea). They must also be assessed for nutritional and immunization status, feeding disorders, and other potential problems.

- The combination of individual signs leads to a child's classification rather than a diagnosis. This classification indicates the severity of the condition and calls for specific actions based on whether the child should be urgently referred to a higher level of care, requires specific treatments, or can be safely managed at home.
- The IMCI strategy addresses most but not all of the major reasons why a sick child is brought to a clinic.
- A basic component of the IMCI strategy is the counseling of caregivers about home management issues, such as feeding, fluids, and when to return to a health facility.

Adolescent Health: Prevention of Early Marriages and Young Pregnancies

The health and development of adolescents is crucial to the sustainable achievement of MDG 5 (improve maternal health), MDG 4 (child mortality), MDG 6 (HIV/AIDS, malaria, and other diseases), MDG 2 (universal primary education), and MDG 3 (gender equality and empower women).

The health of the world's 1 billion adolescents is the focus of the 2011 World Health Assembly (WHA) resolution on youth health risks; 2012 WHA paper on early marriages and young pregnancies; UNICEF *The State of the World's Children 2011;* 2012 UNICEF *Progress for Children: A Report Card on Adolescents;* 2012 report of the UN Commission on Population and Development; the 2012 *Lancet* adolescent health series; 2011 UN Summit on NCDs; and the 2011 decision by GAVI Alliance to support human papillomavirus (HPV) vaccination of adolescent girls.[13–20]

Evidence-based interventions in adolescent sexual and reproductive health can prevent early pregnancy and sexually transmitted infections and decrease HIV transmission. Increasingly, there is a need to focus on the behaviors (eg, unhealthy eating habits, lack of sleep and physical exercise, tobacco and alcohol use) that underlie NCDs, mental health, and injuries that cause much of the morbidity and mortality in this age group. These largely preventable disorders have been left unattended until recently.

Addressing the Prevention of Noncommunicable Diseases

Noncommunicable diseases such as hypertension, heart disease, diabetes, and cancer account for 63% of global deaths. Eighty percent of these deaths occur in low- and middle-income countries. Many NCDs have their roots in childhood, often associated with social determinants including stress and poor nutritional practices. In 2011, the UN General Assembly adopted a declaration on the global rise in NCDs. Countries focused on this as a public health issue because it is becoming clear that preventing and treating NCDs is critical to social and economic development and that failing to do so threatens successful achievement of the MDGs. Vaccine-preventable NCD programs (eg, hepatitis B, HPV) build on these successful systems. Noncommunicable disease efforts must collaborate with maternal, newborn, and child health systems to achieve efficiency and effectiveness. It is imperative that country leadership engage with pediatric and other child health clinicians to strengthen national efforts and provide advocacy for achieving global immunization targets as well as addressing the prevention, treatment, and care of NCDs among children and adolescents at all levels of the health care system.

All of these clinical interventions should be carried out using evidence-based practice, with strong professional preparation resource availability, social justice, and government support. Successful management depends on transdisciplinary and inter-sectoral collaboration of professionals within the medical, social, education, and other domains. Advocacy therefore should follow the golden principles of policy, financing, technical program implementation, and effective outcome measures, while efficacious management depends largely on close cooperation among the public, professionals, policy makers, and government in a sustainable, equitable, and qualitative manner. It thus follows that the professional team taking care of child health should be transdisciplinary and inter-sectoral, comprising doctors, nurses, midwives, allied health professionals, teachers, social workers, parents, and others. An effective health care team demands a good coordinator to bring the team into harmonious function and realize the best health effects on the children it serves.

Advocacy by the International Pediatric Association on the Rights of the Child and the Millennium Development Goals

The International Pediatric Association (IPA) is a nongovernmental organization with a membership of 144 national pediatric societies from 139 countries, 10 regional pediatric societies representing all areas of the world, and 13 international pediatric specialty societies. The vision of the IPA is that "Every child will be accorded the right to the highest attainable standard of health, and the opportunity to grow, develop, and fulfill to his or her human potential."[21] Founded in 1910 in Paris, the IPA is the central clearinghouse for global child health for its member societies. The IPA collects epidemiologic data and outcomes of child health programs and drafts strategic plans for intervention. Through member associations, the IPA provides pediatric service and consultation at the national, regional, and international levels.

The IPA has been very active in the promotion and implementation of the MDGs. Examples include IPA participation in the following activities:

- The Nairobi Declaration: Child Watch Africa in 2002 issued at Nairobi.
- The New York call to action in 2002 at the time of the UN General Assembly Special Session on Children.
- The IPA Millennium Declaration in 2005, followed by the formation of the world-renowned Partnership for Maternal, Newborn & Child Health in Delhi, India, in May 2005.
- At a congress in Athens in 2007, the IPA Council of Delegates reaffirmed its commitment to newborn and child survival, health, and development; promotion of breastfeeding; the MDGs; and maternal and family health.

The IPA facilitates country-level action of IPA member societies to address one or more of the MDGs, with special attention to MDGs 4 and 5. This includes getting involved in breastfeeding promotion, early childhood development, immunization campaigns, IMCI, adolescent health, and NCD prevention. The IPA has made a special commitment to promote and support optimal breastfeeding by addressing the economic, social, health, and nutritional needs of mothers and families for exclusive breastfeeding in the first 6 months and continued breastfeeding for up to 2 years and beyond. In addition, the IPA is supporting its member associations in their work with ICMI. The IPA has taken a special interest in adolescent health as an essential key for achieving the MDGs and positively affecting well-being throughout life and across generations.

The IPA collaborates with its member societies at country, regional, and global levels and works to focus and strengthen the response of the international pediatric community to the challenge of the MDGs and newborn and child survival. The IPA coordinates with professional partners in maternal, newborn, and child health at all levels and with the

Partnership for Maternal, Newborn & Child Health. The IPA correlates with the Countdown to 2015,[22] with attention to tracking of newborn and child survival and health at the country level.

One special focus of the IPA as it relates to the MDGs is the ethics of child health. Advocating for child survival, health, and development within the context of the MDGs sometimes can raise controversial and conflicting issues. The leadership of the IPA strongly holds that pediatricians should be well equipped with the most up-to-date information on ethics and be ready to safeguard and strive for the rights and welfare of children. In 2004, the IPA established an ethics committee to review its relationships with industries whose procedures and products might have a negative effect on global child health. Through the report of the committee,[23] the IPA upheld a number of standards including the independence of the IPA and the assurance that all activities of the IPA would be directed at the promotion of child health. The report, "IPA Guidelines for relationships with Industry," states that the IPA will not accept donations from industries that produce, distribute, market, or sponsor tobacco and tobacco products, alcohol, and firearms. It will also not accept donations from groups engaging in negative practices, including violations of the International Code of Marketing of Breast-milk Substitutes or other unethical marketing practices, exploitation of children or child labor, or engaging in discriminatory business practices.[23]

The report has been promulgated to all IPA member societies via mail, e-mail, and the IPA Web site as well as all partners of IPA in the international child health arena including WHO, UNICEF, International Federation of Gynecology and Obstetrics, World Bank, and others. The report has also been circulated to all potential donors to IPA activities, and the principles have been under close surveillance of the IPA ethics committee and passed the review at the IPA congresses at Cancun (2004), Athens (2007), and Johannesburg (2010). The report serves as the gold standard on ethics for accepting donations from industry.

Other IPA guidelines in the pipeline include "Global ethical standards and review procedures of human research conducted in children," "Training of Paediatricians on Ethical Issues related to clinical practice and research with emphasis on developing countries," "How Pediatricians can contribute to prevent gender discrimination in meeting the specific needs of children," "Effect of Religion on Ethical Issues including End of Life Consideration, Gender Counseling, Abortion and Others," "Ethical issues related to advertising and acceptance of money from International Congresses of Pediatrics," "Declaration Form for Multinational Enterprises with involvement of multiplicity of commercial products," and "Definition of Endorsement of Commercial Products." The IPA leadership strongly believes in ethics for professionals and is confident that good ethical practice is the cornerstone of the IPA target for achieving "Healthy Children for a Healthy World."

Conclusion

Global child health advocacy is greatly needed for the achievement of the MDGs, particularly in middle- and low-income countries. Advocacy must be targeted to all levels of government, health and non-health professionals, and the public at large. Interventions can be grouped into 5 tiers: counseling and education; clinical interventions; protective interventions; enabling environment; and socioeconomic interventions. Creating an enabling environment and socioeconomic interventions have the greatest population effect, such as legislation to protect children from exploitation and efforts to reduce poverty and increase employment. Some preventive and clinical interventions also have a population effect, such as vaccination and treatment of communicable diseases and NCDs. The inclusion of adolescents within goals and targets is critically needed to ensure that development assistance includes support for future child and adolescent health interventions.

Many highly effective interventions that have a significant effect on the health of women and children are severely under-resourced. Financing for child health should promote sustainability and enhance fairness to achieve the ultimate targets of not only saving lives but also creating a healthy future for all children. People can be protected from financial hardship through national health financing policies that promote pooling of risks and resources. Extending health protection through insurance and tax-financed systems aims to achieve universal coverage.

Successful implementation of each of the MDGs depends on transdisciplinary and inter-sectoral collaboration of various cadres of workers and professionals of all disciplines and departments, thus making MDG 8 the main strategy for achieving the other 7 MDGs. Most expenditure for the MDGs will continue to come from domestic sources. The poorest and least stable countries will continue to need external aid for the foreseeable future. Aid for health must be predictable, aligned with nationally defined priorities, provided in ways that minimize transaction costs, and designed to enhance sustainability and limit dependency on external funds. Financing for child health should promote sustainability, enhance fairness, and enable our ultimate targets of not only saving lives but also creating healthy futures for all the children we serve.

References

1. World Health Organization. Constitution of the World Health Organization: *Basic Documents*. 45th ed. Supplement, October 2006. http://www.who.int/governance/eb/who_constitution_en.pdf. Accessed April 30, 2013

2. Institute of Medicine Board on Children, Youth, and Families. *Children's Health, the Nation's Wealth: Assessing and Improving Child Health*. Washington, DC: National Academy of Sciences Press; 2004

3. Chan CW. Paediatricians and Global Child Health. Keynote Lecture. Children's Hospital of Debrecen University, Hungary. September 26, 2010

4. Chan CW. Changing Patterns of Global Child Health and New Challenges for Paediatricians of the 21st Century. 25th International Pediatric Association Congress of Pediatrics, 2007, Athens, Greece

5. Office of the United Nations High Commissioner for Human Rights. Convention on the Rights of the Child General Assembly resolution 44/25 of 20 November 1989. http://www.un.org/documents/ga/res/44/a44r025.htm. Accessed May 31, 2013

6. Office of the United Nations High Commissioner for Human Rights Committee on the Rights of the Child. Monitoring children's rights. http://www2.ohchr.org/english/bodies/crc. Accessed April 30, 2013

7. United Nations Development Programme. The Millennium Development Goals: Eight Goals for 2015. http://www.undp.org/content/undp/en/home/mdgoverview.html. Accessed April 30, 2013

8. You D, Wardlaw T, Salama P, Jones G. Levels and trends in under-5 mortality, 1990-2008. *Lancet*. 2010;375(9709):100–103

9. Black RE, Morris SS, Bryce J. Where and why are 10 million children dying every year? *Lancet*. 2003;361(9376):2226–2234

10. UN Inter-agency Group for Child Mortality Estimation. *Levels and Trends in Child Mortality: Report 2012*. New York, NY: United Nation's Children's Fund; 2012. http://www.who.int/maternal_child_adolescent/documents/levels_trends_child_mortality_2012.pdf. Accessed May 18, 2013

11. Countdown to 2015. Country profiles. http://www.countdown2015mnch.org/country-profiles. Accessed April 30, 2013

12. World Health Organization. *Global Strategy for Infant and Young Child Feeding.* Geneva, Switzerland: World Health Organization; 2003. http://www.who.int/nutrition/publications/gs_infant_feeding_text_eng.pdf. Accessed April 30, 2013

13. World Health Organization. WHA64.28: youth and health risks. In: Sixty-Fourth World Health Assembly. Geneva, 16–24 May 2011. Resolutions and Decisions. Annexes. http://apps.who.int/gb/ebwha/pdf_files/WHA64-REC1/A64_REC1-en.pdf. Accessed April 30, 2013

14. World Health Organization. Early marriages, adolescent and young pregnancies: Report by the Secretariat. Sixty-Fifth World Health Assembly. Provisional agenda item 13.4. 16 March 2012. http://apps.who.int/gb/ebwha/pdf_files/WHA65/A65_13-en.pdf. Accessed April 30, 2013

15. United Nations Children's Fund. *The State of the World's Children 2011: Adolescence: An Age of Opportunity.* New York, NY: United Nations Children's Fund; 2011. http://www.unicef.org/sowc2011/pdfs/SOWC-2011-Main-Report_EN_02092011.pdf. Accessed April 30, 2013

16. United Nations Children's Fund. *Progress for Children: A Report Card on Adolescents. Number 10, April 2012.* http://www.unicef.org/publications/files/Progress_for_Children_-_No._10_EN_04272012.pdf. Accessed April 30, 2013

17. The Partnership for Maternal, Newborn & Child Health. 45th UN Commission on Population and Development: New Report stresses reproductive health care for youth. http://www.who.int/pmnch/media/news/2012/20120426_45_cpd/en/index.html. Accessed April 30, 2013

18. Adolescent health. *Lancet.* April 25, 2012. http://www.lancet.com/series/adolescent-health-2012. Accessed April 30, 2013

19. NCD Alliance. A Focus on Children and Non-Communicable Diseases (NCDs). Remembering Our Future at the UN Summit on NCDs, September 2011. http://ncdalliance.org/sites/default/files/resource_files/20110627_A_Focus_on_Children_&_NCDs_FINAL_2.pdf. Accessed April 30, 2013

20. GAVI Alliance. Human papillomavirus vaccine support. http://www.gavialliance.org/support/nvs/human-papillomavirus-vaccine-support. Accessed April 30, 2013

21. International Pediatric Association. Mission & objectives. http://www.ipa-world.org/page.php?id=141. Accessed April 30, 2013

22. Countdown to 2015. http://countdown2015mnch.org. Accessed April 30, 2013

23. International Pediatric Association. IPA Guidelines for relationships with Industry. http://www.ipa-world.org/uploadedbyfck/IPA_Guidelines2005.pdf. Accessed April 30, 2013

Chapter 3

Improving Access to Care in Nigeria

Adenike O. Grange, MBChB, DCH, FMCPAED, FWACP, FAAP(Hon)

Foundation

Access to health care means an individual, a family, a community, or a nation receives appropriate quanta of quality affordable health care when needed. Lack of or reduced access to health care can be caused by problems at the level of the individual household, community, or health facility or at the health policy-making level. Women and children often have limited access to health care. This is not simply a health system problem; it involves all the systems that should promote the quality of life of the individual, family, and community. Household needs include the provision of potable water, sanitary facilities, income-generating opportunities, housing, education, and everything that positively influences the lifestyle of all.

At the individual household level, the major problem is usually lack of awareness of the need to seek care or lack of decision making power, which may be of economic, spiritual, or sociocultural origin. Under these circumstances, the decision to seek appropriate care is not made at all or made too late. The implementation of the 8 Millennium Development Goals (MDGs) is a comprehensive attempt by the global community to address these problems at the grassroots level.

The second major factor that affects access to care is maldistribution of health facilities and inequitable coverage with services, or poor content and quality of services. The underlying factor that is responsible for putting into motion the changes required for improving access to health care is the administrative machinery of the health system.

All nations have health systems, which are described as "all the activities whose primary purpose is to promote, restore or maintain health."[1] Health systems exist to produce some benefit for societies and their citizens. A health system mobilizes and channels resources into institutions for individual or social consumption. This consumption of goods and services should produce a flow of benefits to the population in terms of health care, which should result in improvement in health status and quality of life and increased life expectancy. The resources needed for the delivery of health care include governance/leadership, finance, health workforce, medical products, vaccines and medicines, information, technologies, and physical infrastructures. All these in varying proportions are the components of the health care delivery system, which is organized in 4 systems: health facility, outreach, village-/community-based, and commercial. The organizers of any of the systems could be governmental, nongovernmental, private, or mixed.

For a health system to give rise to positive health outcomes, it must provide effective, qualitative, efficient, and affordable services. It must also be equitably and sustainably accessible to the entire population, responsive to its varying needs and capacities, and with its full participation.

The purpose of developing an advocacy strategy for improved access to health care is to improve the health status, survival, quality of life, and increased life expectancy of different segments of the entire population. The segment of population that is targeted by groups of health professionals depends on the professional focus of that group. For pediatricians the focus is on children 0 to 18 years of age. Children together with women are the most vulnerable segment of society. Advocacy for this dyad is intense and involves many medical and nonmedical professional groups. This chapter covers opportunities and challenges for advocacy by pediatricians for improving access to health care in a developing country as compared with developed countries.

Example: Nigeria

Economic and Cultural Setting

Nigeria is a federation of 36 states plus the Federal Capital Territory of Abuja. With an estimated 148 million people (2009), Nigeria holds approximately one-sixth of Africa's population and is the most populous country on the continent. Its population is expected to rise to 200 million by 2025. Urbanization in Nigeria is occurring rapidly, with the percentage of the population living in urban areas expected to rise from 42% to 55.4% by 2015. The country's population is largely young; the median age is 17.9 years and about 43.9% of the population is younger than 15 years.[2]

The country is very diverse, with more than 250 ethnic groups, 500 indigenous languages, and diverse religions including Islam, Christianity, and traditional African beliefs. The population in the north is predominantly Muslim, while the south is predominately Christian. The major ethnocultural spheres are the Hausa in the north, Yoruba in the southwest, and Ibo in the southeast.

The economy largely relies on the oil and gas sector, which accounts for 99% of export revenues, 85% of the government budget revenue, and 52% of gross domestic product (GDP).

According to the World Bank, Nigeria's annual economic growth rate from 2008 through 2012 averaged 7.4% per annum. Agriculture, mining, light industry, and banking sectors also contribute significantly to the GDP.[3]

In spite of the large revenue generated from oil wealth and natural resources, Nigeria is one of the poorest countries in the world, with a GDP per capita of only about US $1,161. Approximately 54% of the population lives on less than US $1 per day.[3] Moreover, inequalities have widened across income groups and between rural and urban areas in recent years.

Health status statistics in Nigeria leave much to be desired. Of the 2,300 children younger than 5 years who die daily worldwide, Nigeria contributes 10%. This is greatly disproportionate to the relative size of the country, which is approximately 2% of the world's population. More concerning is that nearly a quarter of a million newborns die each year. Information from 50 Demographic and Health Surveys from 1995 to 2002 reveals that within regions, neonatal mortality rates are around 20% to 50% higher for the poorest 20% of households than for the richest quintile. Similar inequities are also prevalent for maternal mortality.[4,5]

According to the United Nations Children's Fund, Africa and Asia account for 95% of the world's maternal deaths, with particularly high burdens in sub-Saharan Africa (50% of the global total) and South Asia (35%). The lifetime risk of maternal death for a woman in a least-developed country is more than 300 times greater than for a woman living in an industrialized country. The gap in risk of maternal death between the industrialized world and many developing countries, particularly in the least developed, is often called the greatest health divide in the world.[3]

The Health System in Nigeria

Nigeria is a federation with 3 tiers of government—federal, state, and local. While the federal government develops policies that are relevant across all 3 levels, responsibility for health service provision in the public sector reflects the 3-tier structure. Thirty-eight percent of all registered facilities in the Federal Ministry of Health facilities database are privately owned, of which about 75% are primary care and 25% are secondary care facilities.[6] Private facilities account for one-third of primary care facilities and are a potentially important partner in expanding coverage of key health services.

Governance

Since Nigeria's independence from colonial rule in 1960, the health system has evolved into a broad-based scheme that is backed by policies and programs, including the development of a new cadre of primary health care (PHC) workers to run the services. The first National Health Policy, which has PHC as its cornerstone, was launched in 1988. The overall policy goal is the provision of "adequate, accessible and affordable health services for Nigerians at all times." The federal government, through the Federal Ministry of Health, has overall responsibility for the health sector in terms of setting policies, providing guidelines for the states, and monitoring their performance.[7] It also has direct operational responsibilities (Box 3-1).

Box 3-1. Operational Responsibilities of the Federal Ministry of Health, Nigeria

Coordination of state efforts toward a nationwide health system

Monitoring and evaluation of the implementation of national health strategies

Training of doctors in tertiary care hospitals and their outreaches

Setting uniform standards for all health workers

Control and operations of institutions and services that provide tertiary health care, such as teaching, psychiatric, and orthopedic hospitals

Control of communicable diseases

Supplies of vaccines and provision of seed money for drug funds

The states have the responsibility of setting up secondary care hospitals, while local governments are required to establish and run the primary care system.

The performance of the health sector under this fragmented leadership setup has often led to a blurring of hierarchy. It has resulted in some tension among the members of staff and several stakeholders, retarding progress in the execution of a holistic plan of action.

An example of such a problem was the delayed passage of a health bill that has the potential of streamlining and empowering the health system, especially at the primary care level. After 7 years of intense advocacy, the bill was finally passed by the legislative councils around 2010. However, the bill is still in the process of being passed into law. It is important that this bill is unanimously seen by all stakeholders as a bill that will reform the system in a way to improve access to care for masses of underprivileged people, especially in rural areas, without posing a threat to the harmonious working relationship among all the segments of the health workforce.

Governance across the health sector is rather weak. For example, institutional arrangements for channeling advocacy and participation are not functioning well. There is significant variation on the level of effectiveness of health programs across zones. Furthermore, there are few organizations that are informed and capable enough to link members of the public with providers and policy makers or engage with public officials in the establishment of policies, plans, and budgets for health services.

There has been a recent effort to assemble an advocacy group, Civil Society on Health, comprising the leaderships of all health professional groups as well as grassroots umbrella stakeholders such as women organizations and faith-based health advocacy groups. It is in its early days yet, but it promises to bridge the information gap between people and policy makers.

Human Resources for Health

Although great disparities exist across zones and the rural-urban divide, Nigeria has a good supply of human resources for health (HRH) compared with other countries in the region. However, functional HRH planning and management units with sufficient personnel and adequate human resource planning skills within the Federal Ministry of Health and state level are generally not adequate. The bill provides for the establishment of health committees at ward and village levels and improved funding of PHC. However, the health system pillar that may not be adequately addressed by the bill is that of human resources. A sustainable solution must be found to tackle the country's maldistribution of clinical personnel and ensure a reversal of the brain drain of specialists abroad.

Delivery of Health Services

The coverage of most key preventive and curative health services is relatively low in Nigeria. This is compounded by geopolitical zone, rural-urban, and socioeconomic disparities in coverage. Overall national hospital bed availability of 9.2 per 10,000 people is above the sub-Saharan average of 5.6 beds per 10,000 people. However, the distribution varies, falling as low as 4.3 beds per 10,000 people in one of the zones.

Many of the solutions for newborn deaths link closely to reducing the country's 33,000 annual maternal deaths. An integrated approach for implementing evidence-based interventions is required. In 2007, the Federal Ministry of Health developed a strategy to address gaps in care, making Nigeria one of the first countries in Africa to plan an integrated continuum of care. The Integrated Maternal, Newborn and Child Health Strategy (IMNCH) was developed by my advocacy team with the support of the World Health Organization (WHO) and ratified during my tenure as the Minister of Health.[8] The strategy encourages stakeholders and health personnel to work together to ensure integration across the continuum of care for maternal, newborn, and child health through collaboration among health care professionals across the spectrum, as well as through alliances with development partners, indigenous nongovernmental organizations, and civil society organizations (CSOs). The implementation plan aims at reducing newborn mortality by 57% by 2015. Rollout of the IMNCH strategy has taken place in 23 states. A subgroup of the implementation team is making a great deal of effort to continue with the advocacy plan to keep the country on course with this program.

Pharmaceuticals in Nigeria

Access to essential medicines is a critical component of achieving the MDGs. The pharmaceutical management system has had mixed performance results. While the government has made tremendous progress in developing national pharmaceutical policies and regulations, implementation and enforcement of these policies lag far behind. Despite these efforts, studies have shown that the Nigerian system continues to be challenged by poor availability, high cost, and irrational use of essential medicines in the pharmaceutical sector. Additionally, these efforts are impaired by a lack of information about and collaboration with the private sector. In its effort to make essential drugs accessible and affordable, the federal government of Nigeria has continued to support an essential drug program. One important area that has required a great deal of advocacy effort is the reduction of the menace of circulation of fake medicines in the system.

Health Information Systems

Health information system (HIS) capacity across the country varies widely. Most states have limited budgets for activities that provide adequate support for HIS. Few states have an adequate, well-trained cadre of HIS personnel and sufficient resources with all positions filled, particularly at state and local levels. There is significant variation among states by level and type of available health information cadres.

Health Financing

Relative to its high burden of disease and large population, health financing levels in Nigeria remain low on a per capita basis and as a share of the state government budget. At the federal level, budgetary allocations highlight systematic underfunding of capital projects. Data show that relatively higher levels of financing are observed in states with significant donor presence, and even in these states, total health expenditure per capita is less than US $4. The WHO Commission on Macroeconomics and Health recommended US $34 per capita to finance a basic package of health services.

Absence of financial protection in health can be regarded as a disease of the health system. The most obvious symptom is that families face economic ruin and poverty as a consequence of financing their health care. The findings of the first National Health Accounts of Nigeria, cited by WHO,[9] provide important insights into sources of health care financing in Nigeria. According to this report, household out-of-pocket expenditures remain the single largest source of health care financing in Nigeria, providing 65.9% of total health expenditures. This is followed by the government at 26.1% (federal 12.4%, state 7.4%, local government 6.4%), firms at 6.1%, and development partners at 1.8%. Per capita expenditures on health were US $50 by 2006.[10]

Addressing Access Issues

In May 1999, the Nigerian government established the National Health Insurance Scheme, which encompasses government employees and the organized private sector that has the capacity to contribute to the scheme. Theoretically, the scheme also covers children younger than 5 years and persons who are permanently disabled; however, in most instances, children are not exempt from hospital admission fees.

Among the recommendations made for achieving improvement in the performance of the health sector, the following illustrates the importance of getting civil societies to be engaged in health advocacy. It has been recommended to strengthen public participation in policy development and implementation through strengthening of voice indicators in the health management information system, supporting independent policy analysis and advocacy groups to "demystify" health expenditures and service delivery so that ordinary citizens can understand them, and working with one or more CSOs to develop local knowledge about health and health services and budgets and thereby become effective intermediaries and advocates for citizens.[11]

Recommendations for Change

My interest in this issue is driven by my experiences in various leadership positions—as head of a pediatrics department, dean of clinical sciences, minister of health, and recently the head of a private maternal and child health hospital in a semirural location. On the civil society front, I have been engaged in advocacy as the president of 3 national professional associations, president of a global health professional association, currently the representative of the International Pediatric Association on the CSO Steering Committee of the GAVI Alliance, and most recently the chair of the newly established Civil Society Initiative on Health in Nigeria. As I pass through all these positions, I have become convinced that the underlying obstacle to ensuring equitable access to health care is the weakness of the national health sector, which is further hampered by weaknesses in other development sectors such as basic infrastructures, education, agriculture, and the economy. Only civil society organizations with combined memberships of health care providers, consumers, and other stakeholders can generate the motivation to explore the fundamental problems underlying poor access to health care.

I would like to see a health sector that is more holistically coordinated with the informed participation of the grassroots leading to measurable outcomes that are in line with planned objectives and interventions at every level of the health sector. Access to health care is a very important issue because it is an effective tool for breaking the cycle of ill health and poverty, especially for the most vulnerable in the community. Availability of services and barriers to access have to be considered in the context of differing perspectives, health needs, and material and cultural settings of diverse groups in society. Therefore, equity of access should be measured not only in terms of the availability of services but also by the utilization and outcomes of services. Providers of health services do not always adopt this holistic approach in the evaluation of their own performance. Thus, a great deal of advocacy by informed stakeholders is required to broaden the perceptions of health care providers in the planning and implementation of health programs. Achieving a high level of access to equitable health care is an eloquent indicator of the nation's state of socioeconomic development.

The problem of inadequate access to health care has been defined and analyzed from the perspective of determining what can be done through advocacy to improve the situation. My understanding of the issue came through personal experience, which included active participation in committees that are engaged in health advocacy.

The team of support was built by first identifying a host organization with the capacity to assist member organizations to come together under one umbrella. This coalition organization now has the potential to influence policies, implement health interventions directly, and be the voice of the people at the grassroots level. The highlight of problems is done through coalition of associations of the media, who are in partnership with us.

Challenges to Improving Access

Challenges to be overcome include the existence of professional rivalry and funding problems. To overcome these challenges, a constitution and strategic plan that are acceptable to all have been designed in which roles and responsibilities are clearly defined and individual CSOs continue to maintain their own identities.

Professional evaluations are to be conducted regularly and outcomes measured against expected level of performance. Indicators of success are determined in terms of achievement of set objectives of the strategic plan.

This advocacy work simply confirms to me that advocacy is an essential and feasible tool for making desired changes. It has helped to consolidate my feeling that being engaged in advocacy for health is a big step in the right direction.

References

1. World Health Organization. *The World Health Report 2000. Health Systems: Improving Performance.* http://www.who.int/whr/2000/en. Accessed April 30, 2013

2. US Central Intelligence Agency. The World Factbook. https://www.cia.gov/library/publications/the-world-factbook. Accessed May 13, 2013

3. World Bank. Data: indicators. http://data.worldbank.org/indicator. Accessed May 13, 2013

4. United Nations Children's Fund. *The State of the World's Children 2009: Maternal and Newborn Health.* New York, NY: United Nations Children's Fund; 2008. http://www.unicef.org/sowc09/docs/SOWC09-FullReport-EN.pdf. Accessed May 13, 2013

5. Borghi J, Ensor T, Somanathan A, Lissner C, Mills A. Mobilising financial resources for maternal health. *Lancet.* 2006;368(9545):1457–1465

6. Ademiluyi IA, Aluko-Arowolo SO. Infrastructural distribution of healthcare services in Nigeria: an overview. *J Geogr Reg Plann.* 2009;2(5):104–110

7. Nigerian Federal Ministry of Health. The National Health Policy and Strategy to Achieve Health for All Nigerians. 1988

8. Federal Ministry of Health, Abuja. *Integrated Maternal, Newborn and Child Health Strategy.* Abuja, Nigeria: Federal Ministry of Health; 2007. http://www.healthresearchweb.org/files/IMNCHSTRATEGICPLAN.pdf. Accessed April 30, 2013

9. World Health Organization. National health accounts: Nigeria. http://www.who.int/nha/country/nga/en. Accessed May 13, 2013

10. World Health Organization. Global Health Observatory. http://www.who.int/gho/en. Accessed May 13, 2013

11. Kombe G, Fleisher L, Kariisa E, et al. *Nigeria Health System Assessment 2008.* Abt Associates Inc. http://www.healthsystems2020.org/files/2326_file_Nigeria_HSA_FINAL_June2009.pdf. Accessed April 30, 2013

Chapter 4

Creating a Public Child Medical Insurance System in China

Zonghan Zhu, MD

In China we have large regional disparities in child health and well-being, particularly between poor rural areas and wealthier urban centers. Our strategy to narrow these disparities included developing a public child medical insurance system to make health care affordable for all families. Pediatricians must be strong advocates for ensuring that all children have equal access to appropriate pediatric medical services.

To reach this goal in China it was necessary to establish a nationwide medical insurance system for children and to make a commitment to construct more children's hospitals across the country. To accomplish this goal, we implemented a comprehensive health strategy called "Da Wei Sheng," which mobilized the community's involvement, developed multi-sector collaboration, and focused the agenda of the pediatric society on influencing governmental child health policy. Chinese pediatricians played an important role in implementing this strategy and achieving success. They spoke out strongly for the protection of children's rights and benefits and fought hard for local and central governments to make the social interests of children a high priority.

Chinese traditional culture considers children to be owned by their parents. This traditional social consciousness implies that parents should and will take full responsibility for paying for children's medical care without help from the government. Therefore, it has been traditional that families pay for pediatric medical services themselves. Because many families could not afford to pay for medical care, their children did not receive care when needed. This was especially true for the unfortunate families whose child had a severe or chronic illness. Many of these families became impoverished by paying for their child's medical care and still could not afford to pay for ongoing needed care. For example, it was estimated that more than 1 million children with leukemia in the country did not get adequate treatment because of the inability of families to pay for care.

Chinese pediatricians and other child advocates disagreed with the approach that government plays no part in funding child health and believed that our government has a responsibility to help families pay for their child's health care expenses. We proposed the creation of a Children's Medical Security System (CMSS) to address this problem with funding from governmental tax revenue. Because of China's economic growth, tax revenue had increased significantly. The national revenue in 2004 was 2.41419 trillion yuan, an increase of 500 billion yuan over the previous year, with 92% of the revenue being generated from tax revenue. Therefore, we wanted and needed to make a compelling case that the public would support using tax money to establish the CMSS.

To assess the level of public support, we first solicited taxpayers' views on their willingness to spend their taxes to help families pay for their children to see a doctor and get needed medical care. We surveyed thousands of people who were almost unanimously in support of this approach. During the same period, we collaborated with the media to tell the stories of families who were having difficulties accessing care for their children. Because of this media attention, the annual National People's Congress and the National Committee of the Chinese People's Political Consultative Conference (CPPCC) took note. There was a heated discussion on this issue that was covered by television and newspaper media. Our message was that families had great unmet needs related to accessing health care for their children, particularly for the children that needed care the most. It was time for government policy makers to address these needs.

Fortunately, the elevated public awareness of this problem and our advocacy efforts had an effect on local governments. Several local governments started to pilot different forms of medical insurance for children. Beijing and Shanghai introduced the Mutual Aid Benefit System for children with special needs. Suzhou City, Jiangsu Province, in 2005 introduced the government-run CMSS through local legislation, funded by multiple stakeholders including government, organizations, and families. These pilot programs improved our understanding of important issues and provided a solid foundation for the establishment of a more national CMSS.

In 2004 several CPPCC National Committee members joined me in putting forward a proposal to establish a children's medical insurance system at the CPPCC meeting. While it was not accepted in 2004, we continued to introduce this proposal every subsequent year. We also proposed the same motion to the Women and Children Working Committee of the State Council. Although policy makers realized the severity of the problem, they only approved studies rather than action to address it. However, we were persistent and kept up our media campaign and yearly proposals.

In 2007, the proposal was ultimately accepted by the government, as it had won the support of premier Wen Jiabao. That year, the CMSS was implemented in 70 cities, and in 2010 it was expanded throughout the entire country. However, due to funding limitations, families can only get 60% to 70% of children's medical expenses reimbursed. Although it is a significant improvement, many families with children who have special needs and conditions such as congenital heart disease, leukemia, and renal failure still cannot afford care. Through our advocacy efforts, a medical aid fund of catastrophic medical expense was added to the CMSS in 2010 to provide additional subsidies for children and their families suffering from these serious diseases. The establishment of the CMSS and the medical aid fund for catastrophic medical expenses has significantly improved access to needed care, especially for children living in poor families.

In recent years, there has also been progress in improving preventive care and health promotion for children. For example, the Expanded Program on Immunization is now fully funded by the government and provides 13 vaccines that can prevent 15 diseases. Also, free health checks for all children 0 to 3 years old and free newborn disease screening have been implemented nationwide.

Capacity Building of Pediatric Services

A program to help families pay for medical care must be combined with adequate capacity in the delivery system in terms of health care professionals and facilities. Without quantitative and qualitative improvement of pediatric services, improving access through payment subsidies will not have a sufficient positive effect in reducing childhood morbidity and mortality. The first step in addressing adequacy of the delivery system was carrying out a comprehensive survey on the capacity of pediatric services by the Chinese Pediatrician Association in 2010. The survey assessed the numbers of pediatricians and children's hospitals and the needs of pediatric services. It revealed a serious shortage in the number of pediatricians and pediatric facilities and hospitals. Moreover, compensation of pediatricians was significantly lower than doctors in other specialties. According to health statistics, in 2008 only 1.6% of physicians were pediatricians and 6.4% of hospital beds were pediatric, and there were only 68 children's hospitals, of which 48 were government owned. Nationally there were only 0.26 pediatricians per 1,000 children. There was a huge mismatch between supply (pediatrician and pediatric beds) and demand for pediatric services. In comparison with developed countries, the shortage of pediatricians was estimated as 200,000. This pediatrician shortage did not consider likely future retirements, so needs were considerably underestimated. In addition, geographic misdistribution is a problem, as most pediatricians practice in relatively few professional pediatric medical institutions. As a result, these hospital settings are overstaffed while many areas are underserved. For example, the total number of outpatient visits in Children's Hospitals of Beijing, Shanghai, and other places are more than 5,000 daily.

In early 2011, we reported survey findings to the media and government policy makers. Our findings were brought to the attention of the Chinese vice premier and health minister. As a result of their support, development of pediatric medical institutions was included in the national health development plan and the central government developed a special budget to support the construction of children's hospitals at various levels in the coming years. There will be a significant increase in the number of children's hospitals. In addition, programs to train primary care and subspecialty pediatricians have been initiated. In 2011, the Chinese Pediatrician Association invited the American Academy of Pediatrics to hold a pediatric career development forum in Shanghai addressing the acceleration of pediatrician training and development of pediatrics. The same forum was held in Shanghai again in 2012. However, because medical education is under the management of the ministry of education, additional advocacy must occur to ensure that more pediatricians are trained in medical schools.

While much work still needs to be done, our "Da Wei Sheng" strategy has been successful. The combined efforts of China's pediatricians and a mobilized community have influenced governmental child health policy. However, we cannot relax our efforts to improve access to high-quality pediatric primary and secondary care. We must find creative solutions to providing care to our underserved and vulnerable pediatric populations.

Section 2

Immunizations

Chapter 5

Nurturing Partnerships: Implementing a National Immunization Program in the United States

Walter Orenstein, MD, FAAP
Louis Z. Cooper, MD, FAAP
Katherine Seib, MSPH

"Making systems work is the great task of my generation of physicians and scientists. But I would go further and say that making systems work— whether in health care, education, climate change, making a pathway out of poverty—is the great task of our generation as a whole. In every field, knowledge has exploded, but it has brought complexity, it has brought specialization. And we've come to a place where we have no choice but to recognize, as individualistic as we want to be, complexity requires group success."

— From April 2012 TED Talk "How do we heal medicine?"
  by Atul Gawande

Vaccines and Global Health

Right now we are in an important and exciting era for global immunization efforts. Because vaccines are such effective instruments of disease prevention, charitable organizations see focusing money and attention on immunization as a big bang for their buck. Many countries around the world are working hard to develop or enhance their nationally scaled immunization programs. Driven by efforts to eliminate and eradicate diseases like polio and measles, as well as efforts to better control endemic diseases and build sustainable public health infrastructures, developing countries are experiencing an unprecedented influx of attention, pressure, and money.[1] These efforts are unquestionably the right thing to be doing—no other public health intervention except clean water is more effective at preventing morbidity and mortality than vaccines.[2] The best way to achieve a successful immunization program requires not just having the right goals but also having effective approaches to reaching goals and successfully unifying all the moving parts that must come together to drive objectives forward.

Lessons From Building the US Immunization Program

The building of the US immunization program offers important insights into how coalitions of key organizations were able to engage critical agencies and institutions and develop an infrastructure that has led to record high levels of immunization coverage in children and record low levels of disease. Though the US immunization system is very different than the systems in most countries, there are universal lessons that should apply to any immunization program.[3] The US immunization program was based on reducing disease rather than achieving some "artificial level" of immunization coverage. Polio spread fear and panic in the United States, particularly in the early 1950s when annual epidemics caused more than 15,000 persons, most of whom were children, to be paralyzed.[4] President Franklin Delano Roosevelt, perhaps the most famous polio victim, used his political clout to form the March of Dimes (originally known as the National Foundation for Infantile Paralysis), whose major focus at the time was development of a polio vaccine. The licensure of the Salk inactivated poliovirus vaccine proved to be a milestone not only in providing a tool to prevent polio but in galvanizing the US Congress to specifically appropriate funds for vaccination for the first time in its history.[5] Congress provided funds for 2 years, 1955 and 1956, for the federal government to provide support to states and local communities to buy and administer polio vaccines. Aside from a one-time appropriation of $1 million in 1960, this funding was time limited. But a precedent had been set.

317 Program

In 1962, President John F. Kennedy signed into law the Vaccination Assistance Act, which supported the Communicable Disease Center, now the Centers for Disease Control and Prevention (CDC), in supporting mass immunization programs and initiating maintenance programs. The act, which is more widely known as the 317 Program because it authorized grants to state and local health departments under Section 317 of the

Public Health Service Act, has been the basis for federal immunization infrastructure since that time. Specifically, the first grants made in 1963 included the provision to supply vaccines to grantees in lieu of cash, eventually setting up development of federal contracts with vaccine manufacturers to purchase vaccines at reduced prices. Further, the 317 grants allowed grantees to return funds to the government and receive for those funds, experienced public health advisors to help direct immunization activities in the state or locality and build state or local capacity to eventually take on these activities.

Long-term Success

But what really led to the long-term success of the US immunization program was its focus on elimination of measles. When measles vaccines were licensed in 1963, they became the first new vaccines available since passage of the Vaccination Assistance Act.[3] The CDC chose to focus the program on measles elimination, acting vertically to do what was needed to stop transmission of the virus in the United States, but at the same time thinking horizontally as to how the work on measles could help build the overall vaccination system. The success of that program was the result of a massive public/private partnership that included academic and other researchers; vaccine manufacturers; policy makers; public and private vaccine deliverers; third-party payers; federal, state, and local agencies; political leaders; parents; and many others. And it was years of success followed by failure, with management of the failures to make needed changes in the system, success, and then more failures in cycles, which led to present successes. In 1966, David Sencer, then director of the CDC, announced the goal to eradicate measles in the United States. Measles met criteria for eradication in that there was no known animal reservoir (ie, human-to-human transmission was essential for maintaining the virus; there were no chronic shedders of infectious virus; when immunity levels were high enough, as on some island populations, transmission ceased). There was an infusion of federal funding to support a strategy consisting of 4 components: 1) enhancing routine immunization of children; 2) vaccination of the unvaccinated at school entry; 3) surveillance to determine where disease was occurring, who was getting disease, and reasons for development of disease; and 4) outbreak control.

Failure and Refocus

Major efforts during the initial US measles eradication effort included mass catch-up campaigns for school-aged children. Reported measles incidence dropped from more than 500,000 cases per year in the pre-vaccine era to a low of approximately 22,000 cases in 1968. This led to redirection of federal funding to newly licensed rubella vaccines in 1969 and a major resurgence of measles, peaking at more than 70,000 cases in 1970. Reasons for the resurgence included low immunization coverage in preschool- and school-aged children. Enactment and enforcement of school immunization laws were not common at the time. Another reason was the misguided thinking that the low level of measles disease in 1968 of 22,000 cases would remain constant despite the elimination of federal funding for measles vaccine. Each year, one birth cohort arrives and becomes susceptible. If not vaccinated, this cohort will fuel the next epidemic. Measles is episodic. If vaccination is stopped today, outbreaks do not start tomorrow. Instead it takes times for susceptible cohorts to accumulate before the next epidemic is seen, something that politicians and other lay individuals often fail to understand.

Success in smallpox eradication using a strategy of outbreak containment led to efforts to try to focus measles elimination activities on outbreak control. However, measles was much more contagious than smallpox, spread in unpredictable manners, and was hard to contain. But the frustrations and failures in measles outbreak control played a major role in galvanizing political support to prevent outbreaks rather than try to contain them. In addition, data began accumulating that school mandates for measles vaccination were remarkably effective in reducing disease incidence. Perhaps the seminal event was a measles outbreak in Los Angeles, CA, in 1977. Despite efforts to provide vaccines for free and make them easily accessible, the outbreak persisted. The health officer issued an emergency decree requiring children to be vaccinated to remain in school. After extensive clinics were conducted to provide vaccines to children in school, approximately 50,000 of the 1.4 million children in the school system remained unvaccinated and were excluded. Most returned with proof of immunity within days. But a precedent had been set: "No shots—no school." Soon it was realized that it was better to prevent outbreaks than control them, so "no shots—no school" became the standard everywhere to enroll in school.

In 1977, the United States again saw a resurgence of measles with more than 57,000 cases, many of them occurring in unvaccinated school-aged children not covered by existing school laws. And in 1977, a new administration came into office. Mrs Betty Bumpers, wife of former Governor and now Senator Dale Bumpers of Arkansas, was already a major immunization advocate. She had led an effort in the early 1970s in her state to improve immunization coverage. Mrs Bumpers was a governor's spouse at the same time as Mrs Rosalynn Carter and when Mrs Carter became the first lady in 1977, Mrs Bumpers approached her to try and do something about the sorry state of immunization in the country. This led to a presidential initiative entitled "The Childhood Immunization Initiative" (CII) in 1977 with a major infusion of federal funding and a focus on the enactment and enforcement of comprehensive school immunization laws covering children in all grades.

Partners and Politics

In the mid-1980s, the Children's Defense Fund (CDF) had on its Board of Directors future First Lady Hilary Clinton and Donna Shalala, who would later become the secretary of the Department of Health and Human Services. The CDF was interested in developing a measure of access to health care for poor children. It settled on immunization coverage as that measure because vaccination was the one medical intervention (ie, injections) recommended repeatedly for all children. They noted immunization coverage was low in preschool-aged children, especially among poor and minority children. The CDF was invited by the CDC to address the National Immunization Conference about its concerns and an alliance was formed to further immunization coverage in the United States.

Between 1989 and 1991, a major resurgence of measles occurred that was quite different from earlier outbreaks. This time, the focus was on unvaccinated preschool-aged children, many of whom were minorities living in large inner cities. This resurgence showed that ensuring vaccination at school age was not enough. Vaccination was needed when recommended during the first 2 years of life. At the same time, an already vigorous relationship with the CDC and American Academy of Pediatrics (AAP) was reinvigorated because many of the under-vaccinated children were receiving some but not all of their care at private physicians' offices. Because of the costs of vaccines and lack of insurance coverage, many private providers were referring children out of those offices to public health clinics, where vaccines were free. However, the parents of the children, for whatever reasons, were not making the extra visits. Thus, there was a natural alliance between public health and practicing physicians to seek ways to provide free vaccines for these children to private providers so the children could be vaccinated in their medical home without having to make separate visits for vaccines.

In 1993, the Clinton administration came to power and fixing the vaccination problem received top priority, with a second presidential initiative (again entitled CII) established with the goal of achieving at least 90% immunization coverage in preschool-aged children.

The federal government, working with the AAP and CDF, sought to establish universal federal purchase of all vaccines for children. This was opposed by a number of groups because of fears that universal purchase would lead to low vaccine prices and stifle innovation, critical to development of new and better vaccines. What emerged was a compromise entitled the Vaccines for Children (VFC) program, which provided free vaccines to private or public providers for children on Medicaid, those without insurance, and Alaska Natives/American Indians. In addition, those children whose insurance did not cover immunization (underinsured) were covered but only if immunizations were received at Federally Qualified Health Centers. There were fears by some that even this purchase program would be a stepping stone to universal government purchase and attempts to eliminate VFC. But groups like the AAP and CDF were staunch defenders and overcame the opposition. In 2010, approximately 82 million VFC vaccine doses were administered to an estimated 40 million children at a cost of $3.6 billion.

The resurgence of measles between 1989 and 1991 also helped build other critical components of the National Immunization Program. For example, in the mid-1980s, because of budget limitations, the system to measure immunization coverage of preschool-aged children was eliminated in the United States. Through the second CII, the National Immunization Survey was started, a random-digit–dialing survey covering all 50 states and a number of major localities. This allowed tracking of program performance and focusing efforts on areas with lower immunization coverage.

Lessons From Building Japan's Measles Immunization Program

Prior to and during 2001, Japan's immunization rates for measles were low (83.2% in 2001). Measles remained uncontrolled in Japan, resulting in an outbreak of 265,000 cases during 2001 alone.[6] Sixty-seven cases of measles were imported to the United States from Japan from 1993 to 2001, more than from any other country.[7]

How could this happen? Why, in fact, did so many Japanese parents and even physicians fear measles vaccine more than they feared the disease itself? During the 1980s, the United States demonstrated the value of using a combined measles, mumps, and rubella (MMR) vaccine. The Japanese government embraced the US success and attempted to replicate the program in Japan. However, Japanese manufacturers chose a different strain (Urabe) for the mumps component of their locally produced MMR vaccine instead of the mumps strain used in the US MMR vaccine (Jeryl Lynn). The Japanese mumps vaccine strain caused a significant number of cases of mumps meningitis. When deployed in a campaign started in 1989 many children experienced this frightening complication, and the vaccine was removed from use in 1993.[8] The understandable public furor that led to the cancellation of the MMR vaccine program along with enduring fear left Japan with relatively poor control of measles throughout the remaining decade.

Public health authorities and private pediatricians recognized that uncontrolled measles was costly in terms of morbidity and mortality. However, for more than a decade, no entity felt empowered to change the policies and practices that allowed persistently low utilization of measles vaccine. Recognition that Japan's situation was unfortunate not only for Japanese children but also for US (and other) children infected with disease exported from Japan sparked an opportunity to build on the existing high level of respect between the AAP and the Japan Pediatric Society (JPS) along with the US and Japanese public health ministries. The key was translating the successful public and private partnership structure and lessons of the US immunization programs to their Japanese counterparts.

Support from the Aprica Childcare Institute (ACI) allowed the AAP to initiate a series of meetings involving leading Japanese and US pediatricians and public health officials. After discussions clarified the dynamics behind low immunization rates, and with the help of a Japanese child advocacy group, a meeting was held with the Japanese Ministry of Health, Labour and Welfare. Attendees also included the president of the JPS, the president-elect of the AAP, a leader of Japan's Senate, and the ACI. The president of the JPS presented data from the United States on Japanese importations of measles. The minister, a pediatrician, understood the magnitude and implications of the problem and made a commitment for Japan to match US immunization levels. After the meeting, the minister's counterpart, the US Secretary of Health and Human Services, sent a follow-up letter of support to the Minister of Health, Labor and Welfare. Throughout, the

ACI ensured good coverage of the events from Japan's major print and television media.

Although it took several years to put all the pieces together, in 2006 Japan adopted a 2-dose measles and rubella policy similar to that used in the United States (and now many other countries). In December 2007, Japan adopted a National Measles Elimination Plan and is now well on the way to eliminating measles. A contributing factor leading to this triumph was outreach by the AAP and sharing information and strategies on multilateral advocacy by US pediatric and public health leadership. That approach links governmental public health, organized private pediatrics (the AAP and JPS), reputable citizen child advocates, and the media. These voices from outside Japan likely would not have been heard absent long-standing, respectful relationships. The AAP continues to build its relationships with other national pediatric societies, working through bilateral programs and the International Pediatric Association, the organizational home of more than 160 national and regional pediatric societies.[9]

Lessons From the US and Japanese Experiences

Disease Motivates

A focus on disease rather than coverage can be much more motivating. Low immunization coverage is a theoretical problem. Disease outbreaks covered in the media with pictures of families grieving for lost children on television is far more captivating than the theoretical possibility of an outbreak, given low coverage. However, the real goal is to avoid outbreaks and drive home the message that low coverage will eventually mean a major outbreak unless the problem is addressed.

Build Relationships Outside Your Program

Government officials within immunization programs need help in reaching the highest levels of government to secure resources and support. Private and nongovernmental organizations have proven that they can advocate for programs and motivate people at the grassroots level, including politicians, often in ways that cannot be accomplished from within a government. Nongovernmental organizations can focus media attention on a governmental issue at critical times to bring attention, money, and support from outside as well as higher up in the government. Bureaucratic constraints usually prevent technical programs within government from reaching out directly to key decision-makers. In the United States, outside groups such as the CDF, AAP, and many others have the ability to reach out more directly to high government levels, including senior people in the highest levels of government, to get the message across that under-immunization is a problem and something needs to be done about it. It is critical for government officials within an immunization program to find common ground with outside groups. For example, with the CDF, common ground was ensuring poor children get needed access to lifesaving interventions such as vaccines. For the AAP in the United States, common ground was improving immunization status of preschool-aged children and at the same time improving their overall health by providing immunizations in the medical home instead of fragmenting care. For the AAP and others in Japan, common ground was protecting citizens in and outside of Japan from measles outbreaks and exportations.

In addition, active involvement of high-level officials can play critical roles. Betty Bumpers had developed a relationship with Rosalynn Carter when they were both governors' spouses and visited Mrs Carter when she initially became first lady, bringing renewed emphasis to a vaccine program that had failed to prevent a major resurgence of measles in 1976–1977. Mrs Bumpers had become interested in immunization because of low coverage in her home state of Arkansas. She was informed by and worked closely with her state immunization program. Similarly, in Japan, a presentation of data showing that Japan was the major exporter of measles to the United States captured the attention of Japan's Minister of Health, Labour and Welfare and led to an *immediate* commitment.

Manage and Exploit Failures
Frustration and failure can lead to success, if managed appropriately. For example, in the United States, repeated redirection of federal funding away from measles each time measles appeared under control led to outbreaks. This showed that there must be sustained funding to keep vaccine-preventable diseases at low levels so each new birth cohort is highly vaccinated, avoiding the accumulation of susceptible cohorts. With progressive CIIs, funding for immunization has been increased and sustained. Difficulties in conducting outbreak control for measles led to stronger efforts to prevent outbreaks, including the enactment and enforcement of comprehensive school immunization laws preventing entry to school of unvaccinated children unless they have specifically permitted exemptions to vaccination. In Japan, implementing a case-based surveillance system and expanding measles and rubella immunization to

middle school children in response to large-scale outbreaks in 2007 and disruption of an international Little League baseball tournament led to more accurate disease detection and control. New actions are easier to take when people are frustrated with the current situation than when they are satisfied.

Manage and Exploit Successes

A vertical focus on measles in the United States led to development of a horizontal immunization program including removal of vaccine cost as a barrier, vaccination in medical homes, and systems to measure and track immunization coverage for all vaccines.

Build in Accountability and Metrics

Accountability is critical, and having systems to measure coverage not only at the national level but also at the lowest local level possible help in galvanizing action in poor performers. Sometimes embarrassment, such as being the state with the lowest immunization coverage, can garner political support to make changes necessary to improve that coverage.

Sustained Political Will Is Essential

It can be difficult to establish and sustain political momentum for a program, and often outside forces are essential. Programs may have the enthusiasm and support of internal staff and resources but sometimes are unable to advocate for vital support and resources from external sources due to political constraints or hierarchic limitations. Building relationships with outside partners and coalitions is critical to achieving and sustaining these elements and bridging this gap. Moreover, obtaining political support is easier when you have an intervention that is proven to be highly cost-effective, as with immunizations.[10]

In the United States, being part of a presidential initiative allowed our technical immunization program people in low levels of government to have access to people in decision-making roles at high levels and in diverse programs, working together for a common goal. Presidential initiatives were critical in enhancing support for immunization from programs like Women, Infants, and Children of the Department of Agriculture to ensure the children they served were protected from vaccine-preventable diseases and for the Centers for Medicare & Medicaid Services to enhance its efforts to ensure populations they serve are vaccinated.

Let Science Prevail

Immunization programs must be grounded in vaccine and health systems science that is relevant to the country setting. For example, the measles resurgence in the United States of 1989–1991 was initially thought to be due to parents not bringing their children in for immunization. But careful analysis showed that many of the unvaccinated children had interacted with the health care system and that the system had missed many opportunities to vaccinate.[11] This research led to focusing interventions more on providers of vaccines than on parents, with marked success.

Let Your Program Grow Over Time

The US and Japanese programs took decades to become successful in disease reduction and sustained population coverage, and each took different paths. At any given time programs should have a limited number of measureable goals with crosscutting impact. This facilitates communication and focus. Goals should be "ultimate outcome" such as "measles elimination" or "90% routine immunization coverage" so they are readily understandable by not only technical program managers and employees but also lay government officials, private and public health care practitioners, collaborating groups, the media, and the lay public.

Conclusion

Immunization programs operate as a large system that must be coordinated to be agile and effective. Strong partnerships and focused plans are routinely the key to this coordination. While new and developing immunization programs won't take the exact same path as the United States or Japan, they needn't reinvent the wheel. Advocacy and political will are not a science but a craft honed by many players. Being willing to ask for help from partners and allowing partners to do the work of advocacy for an immunization program can go a long way toward building a foundation for success.

References

1. Cochi SL. *The Future of Global Immunization: Will the Promise of Vaccines Be Fulfilled?* Washington, DC: Center for Strategic and International Studies; 2011. http://csis.org/files/publication/111205_Cochi_FutureGlobalImmun_Web.pdf. Accessed April 30, 2013

2. Plotkin SA, Orenstein WA, Offit PA, eds. *Vaccines.* 6th ed. Edinburgh: Elsevier/Saunders; 2013

3.   Orenstein WA. The role of measles elimination in development of a national immunization program. *Pediatr Infect Dis J.* 2006;25(12):1093–1101

4.   Oshinsky DM. *Polio: An American Story.* New York, NY: Oxford University Press; 2005:342

5.   Orenstein WA, Rodewald LE, Hinman AR, Schuchat A. Immunization in the United States. In: Plotkin SA, Orenstein WA, Offit PA, eds. *Vaccines.* 6th ed. Edinburgh: Elsevier/Saunders; 2013:1479–1510

6.   Centers for Disease Control and Prevention. Progress toward measles elimination— Japan, 1999-2008. *MMWR Morb Mortal Wkly Rep.* 2008;57(38):1049–1052

7.   Vukshich Oster N, Harpaz R, Redd SB, Papania MJ. International importation of measles virus—United States, 1993-2001. *J Infect Dis.* 2004;189(Suppl 1):S48–S53

8.   Ueda K, Miyazaki C, Hidaka Y, Okada K, Kusuhara K, Kadoya R. Aseptic meningitis caused by measles-mumps-rubella vaccine in Japan. *Lancet.* 1995;346(8976):701–702

9.   American Academy of Pediatrics. AAP Global. Pediatric societies. http://www2.aap.org/international/pediatric-societies.html. Accessed April 30, 2013

10. Zhou F, Santoli J, Messonnier ML, et al. Economic evaluation of the 7-vaccine routine childhood immunization schedule in the United States, 2001. *Arch Pediatr Adolesc Med.* 2005;159(12):1136–1144

11. Grabowsky M, Orenstein WA, Marcuse EK. The critical role of provider practices in undervaccination. *Pediatrics.* 1996;97(5):735–737

Chapter 6

Preventing Neonatal Tetanus in Haiti

Warren L. Berggren, MD, MPH, DrPH

Foundation

Neonatal tetanus and its prevention are well understood by health officials and workers throughout the world. Practical applications of this knowledge during the past 40 years have greatly diminished the frequency of neonatal tetanus worldwide.[1-3]

Neonatal tetanus remains frequent where prenatal care and clean birthing facilities are not available to all women and systematic, timely anti-tetanus immunization is not provided to all fertile women. The World Health Organization (WHO) reports that neonatal tetanus accounts for at least 3.4% of all neonatal deaths,[4] and this is probably underestimated. Ministries of health may be slow to recognize the problem. As Carl Taylor[5] observed in India, parents of newborns with tetanus usually do not bring their babies to health facilities, and their deaths are not reported, so health officials may not be alerted to the frequency of deaths from tetanus of the newborn.

Example: Rural Haiti

A Partnership to Control Tetanus of the Newborn

We describe how one rural Haitian population (115,000 persons), in partnership with a private hospital, achieved long-term control of neonatal tetanus among its newborns. It especially focuses on how these partners advocated for maternal immunization, informally and formally, by communicating their successes and how those successes may have encouraged policy makers in the Ministry of Health, United Nations Children's Fund (UNICEF), and Pan American Health Organization (PAHO)/WHO to consider controlling tetanus of the newborn on a nationwide basis. One formal, peer-reviewed report of the partnership's success seemed to have played a role in modifying an important WHO technical guideline essential to eliminating tetanus of the newborn through use of tetanus vaccine.[6]

Choice of Target and Interventions

Hospital Albert Schweitzer (HAS) of Deschapelles, Haiti, has implemented 3 important tetanus-preventive strategies since it opened in 1956.

1. *Training and supervision of traditional birth attendants (TBAs):* Beginning in 1957, HAS staff educated 175 TBAs and supplied them regularly with sterile cord-cutting materials. This activity had been initiated in Haiti by UNICEF in 1947, 9 years before the hospital was built.

2. *Hospital and outpatient newborn care:* Since 1957, HAS provided an outpatient service that included examination of the newborn, aseptic cutting of the umbilical cord, and injections of antibiotics and antitetanus serum to babies who had very recently been born at home. Local families realized that if tetanus developed, their baby would require skilled nursing care and expensive medications. Furthermore, it became known that advanced care of patients with neonatal tetanus at HAS saved the lives of many babies every year. Haitian families brought their babies to the hospital because they realized that tetanus of the newborn causes intense suffering—most families had seen newborns with tetanus locked motionless and voiceless in painful muscular spasms or else desperately panting for breath to replace the oxygen used up during spasms. Their attempts to comfort these babies with the mother's breast, lullabies, or caresses provoked more spasms. However, once hospitalized, parents observed that care and medications diminished spasms even though these might push the patient dangerously close to respiratory arrest. They knew that without hospital care, most such babies would die. Even with excellent care at HAS, 51% of hospitalized newborns with tetanus were lost, nearly all deaths occurring early in the first week of hospitalization.

3. *Immunization of pregnant women willing to come to HAS for prenatal care:* When Schofield, Tucker, and Westbrook reported in 1961 their successful anti-tetanus program in Papua New Guinea,[7] HAS nurses immunized pregnant women against tetanus as an essential part of prenatal care. Decline in numbers of new tetanus cases from women living in the defined "hospital district" followed slowly as many women still lacked the necessary 3 doses recommended. They consulted late in pregnancy if at all and attended no more than 1 or 2 prenatal care sessions during their pregnancy.[8]

In 1967, HAS organized its preventive services as a community health department (CHD) with professional leadership, a dedicated budget, and a mandate to provide village-based preventive services to Haitians living in its rural district. Hospital records showed that since HAS opened in 1956, numbers of admissions for patients with tetanus of the newborn, malnutrition, tuberculosis, and diarrheal diseases had steadily increased. There was no evidence that these increased numbers of admissions resulted from increased incidence of these diseases in the community. Rather, much of it was later shown to have resulted from increased use of the hospital, especially by patients who lived outside the hospital district.[1]

Hospital policies at first required that all care be given in the hospital, its outpatient services, or outlying schools where doctors and nurses maintained service quality. These policies supported high service standards but impeded community access to high-volume preventive services such as vaccinations. Accordingly, the CHD searched for venues and work methods that accommodated more persons in less time while maintaining high standards of care and accountability.

Haitian and ex-patriot hospital staff members agreed that there should first be an implementation plan, local residents should be recruited and trained as health workers, and prevention of tetanus of the newborn should have highest priority.

Despite disciplined implementation of the first 3 strategies in the hospital's assigned district, by 1967 tetanus remained the most frequent final diagnosis among hospitalized patients. The preventive strategies worked mainly among women living close to the hospital. But many patients arrived from outside the hospital district where the 3 strategic services were not easily available for preventive care.

At that time, Ministry of Health (now known as the Ministry of Public Health and Population [MSPP]) officials and their multilateral and bilateral counselors saw no need for special attention to tetanus prevention. The disease was rarely reported from Haitian health facilities other than HAS. An extensive chart review by the ministry's epidemiologist confirmed the HAS reports about frequency of tetanus, but this did not immediately stimulate any new national policies.

In the meantime, HAS success in treating babies with "jaw sickness" encouraged parents of newborns with tetanus to bring more and more of them to HAS.

Advocating With Local Hospital Policy Makers for New Methods

Hospital staff members knew that tetanus of the newborn was reliably prevented by vaccination. They had read the Schofield, Tucker, and Westbrook report of preventing tetanus of the newborn by vaccinating pregnant women[7]; they had quickly added tetanus vaccination to HAS prenatal care services. Hospital professionals agreed that the CHD should vaccinate all in-district women of childbearing age, whether pregnant or not, with 3 doses of tetanus toxoid, given at 1-month intervals, and follow with booster injections every 5 years.[9]

Hospital professionals questioned whether the CHD could vaccinate and maintain vaccination records in venues outside the hospital or schools and do it to HAS quality standards. A written action plan, detailed budget, printed immunization cards protected with plastic envelopes, ledgers for keeping a central registry of all vaccinations, and promise to post all vaccinations to the vaccinated person's hospital chart, if she had one, finally won their approval.

Advocacy in the Community

Since 1947, Haitian and multinational programs had educated rural Haitians about cause and prevention of tetanus, but most were not impressed. They had their own explanations concerning tetanus of the newborn and were comfortable with them. Hospital educators' different explanations seemed to blame the mother, grandmother, or traditional birth attendant. No one, of course, appreciated feeling blamed for the death of a newborn.

The hospital produced a film concerning prevention of tetanus in Creole using local actors. The film successfully dramatized the conduct of a clean home delivery as well as consequences of not keeping the umbilical cord clean. A team showed the film in many villages and urged their audiences to go to the local government maternity for their next delivery. The team's work resulted mainly in increased attendance at the HAS outpatient clinic for umbilical cord prophylaxis.

Engagement of Community Residents

The CHD created a plan to engage its community in a high-profile tetanus immunization program that would not challenge any beliefs and would give highly visible, verifiable outcomes. The plan was developed in 3 phases.

1. A closely monitored pilot study and showcase of methods in a 23-village census tract

2. Extension of vaccination services to HAS district marketplaces

3. Integration of vaccination services with other village-level health services in the other 300 villages in the hospital district

The Pilot Study

To monitor preventive service uptake, service-related effect, and newborn birth and death rates, the CHD took a census of 23 contiguous villages and established a local information system. Locally recruited, HAS-trained enumerators mapped and numbered all dwellings. They then registered each resident in her biologic family by address, name, gender, birth month/year, pregnancy status, hospital ID number, and other variables. This population registry stored each family's demographic, health, and family relationship information on one census sheet. Census sheets were bound by village in folders and filed for reference on shelves in the CHD office.

To monitor vital events prospectively, the CHD also created registries to record new pregnancies, pregnancy outcome, births, deaths, and migrations for the registered families and established a system for community health workers to report births and deaths to a central register. To identify and offer vaccinations to every female resident in the census tract, the CHD created rosters of female residents aged 10 to 49 years for each village.

The CHD recruited literate volunteers from each census tract village. The 2 largest villages (populations 1,200 and 1,000, respectively) were allowed 2 volunteers. Each volunteer used a copy of his village's roster to invite women of childbearing age to be vaccinated on highly visible premises of the hospital, where it could be witnessed outside HAS inner clinics. The volunteers visited homes, not only to invite women to be vaccinated but also to monitor the immunization cards and ensure that all women aged 10 to 49 years actually received 3 doses of tetanus toxoid at appropriate intervals.

Volunteers received a reward when all women in their village rosters received at least 3 doses of tetanus toxoid with an interval of 1 month between doses and the last dose received fewer than 5 years previously. This process was completed in 3 months and no further cases of tetanus of the newborn occurred among residents of the census tract.

Volunteers and census-tract residents took pride in their accomplishments. They maintained the census tract tetanus-free for 2 decades, by which time vital event reporting had been discontinued as an economy measure. The feat is remarkable in that tetanus immunizations provide no herd immunity and an immunized woman must receive booster doses at 5-year intervals to maintain her immunity. Health workers knew and acted on the fact that each girl who eventually entered the population's fertile age group had to be vaccinated to protect her and future newborns from tetanus.

The complete coverage rate is also remarkable because no newspapers, radio announcements, or other media were available to the CHD or its many new local partners. Rural Haitians called their medium of communication telejowel-la, the Creole expression meaning the gossip they communicated face-to-face with remarkable speed, high fidelity, and a generous amount of humor. Later on, this communication system was key to the enthusiastic welcome of vaccination by thousands more rural Haitians.

Expansion to Marketplaces

The CHD next took its immunization services to marketplaces. Every rural Haitian woman visited and traded in a marketplace at least once per week during that village's market day. Meeting them there saved much effort that might otherwise have been spent assembling women at a convenient meeting place or visiting women who wished to be vaccinated and convincing them to keep 2 more appointments at 1-month intervals.

At first, immunizations seemed an unwelcome interruption of market activities; however, when CHD staff offered women photographs of themselves for successfully inviting their neighbors, the numbers of women vaccinated increased to more than 300 per market day. The project also swelled attendance at the market, much to the joy of truckers and businesspeople in the town.

After 6 months in the first marketplace, many vaccinated women had given birth and realized that none of their newborns had contracted tetanus. Immunization services were moved to another market. Attendance for vaccination in the second market exceeded 1,000 women per weekly market day and appointments for first, second, and third doses of vaccine to be accomplished. Photographs or other promotional activities were no longer needed to stimulate attendance. Women had heard from those who attended the first marketplace immunizations that the vaccinations were free, did not make them ill, and were preventing tetanus of the newborn.

Quickening the Pace

The CHD had to work faster in each marketplace to accommodate women who were understandably impatient to get their immunization card, get vaccinated, and get back to their marketing as soon as possible. Community health department teams arrived at dawn and arranged the marketplace vaccination venues to shorten waiting times. The flow of women through the stations of education, vaccination card emission, registration, and vaccination was made laminar and rapid. Soon jet injectors (widely used at that time) replaced needles and syringes. The CHD recruited more day workers to fill in vaccination cards. Attendance rose on a few occasions to 8,000 per 7-hour market day.

Workers Become Advocates

More important than the numbers recorded, the day workers realized that they were implementing a successful program, saving lives, and being admired by their community for their services. Several village volunteers acquired all the skills needed to make vaccination sessions work smoothly while maintaining impeccable relations with the community. They and some of the day workers transformed quickly from being barely literate farmers and grossly underpaid schoolteachers to confident and respected advocates for the health of women and children. They became salaried resident home visitors, able to mentor families in the practice of habits that protect health.

The large markets attracted great numbers of women who lived outside the hospital district. This was appropriate, given that more tetanus patients were coming from outside than inside the partly vaccinated district. During the CHD's second year, Haitian men demanded tetanus vaccinations also. This demand was quickly granted and the change greatly increased attendance, not only of men but also of women.

As marketplace vaccination clinics finished their work, the CHD concentrated more on children's and adult's village-level health services to prevent, in addition to tetanus, tuberculosis, malnutrition, and diarrheal diseases.

Impact at the Hospital Level

Annual hospital admissions for tetanus of the newborn declined from 461 in 1967 to 72 in 1972.[8] Staff members found satisfaction at having fewer neonatal tetanus patients and were happy to have more beds available for patients more likely to survive.

Advocating at the National Level

Before 1967, the HAS mission, goals, and policies rarely included scientific research or publication of its strategies, activities, or results. The hospital submitted its required monthly statistical reports to the MSPP. Hospital policies kept its health, hospital, and development activities focused on the 115,000 persons residing in the hospital district as it was defined geographically.

There were several opportunities for advocacy among Haitian and ex-patriot health professionals, academic institutions, and colleagues from many countries during rare visits to the capitol city and to the CHD leader's academic home. A club formed by Haitian physicians and professors of medicine practicing in the capitol city invited CHD leaders to present findings from the tetanus control program at HAS. This club, the Mercredi Medicale, met weekly to exchange news, experiences, and a discussion of at least one original scientific article, preferably authored by one of their number. Community health department leaders were also privileged to converse informally with the leaders of multinational and bilateral agencies that were major supporters of Haiti's health-related programs.

By 1972, the MSPP, in presenting plans and strategy for funding by PAHO, mentioned tetanus of the newborn as a major health problem.

In 1975, 2 years after CHD leaders completed their first 5-year term at HAS, the Haiti Division of Family Hygiene (DHF) of the MSPP invited them to help create a 4-year project with objectives similar to those of the CHD. The project repeated the HAS village-level disease prevention program in 3 rural sections, each with a registered population of approximately 10,000 residents. The new project was staffed entirely by MSPP employees and coordinated nationally by a senior physician-director in the DHF and technically by the 2 former leaders of the CHD.

The project closed as promised in 4 years, having demonstrated that MSPP professionals could implement successfully the activities that delivered preventive care to rural families (total population of 30,000) and lower infant and child mortality rates. The DHF published a description of the project and its results in 4 paperbound volumes that were distributed by the DHF to MSPP physicians.

The DHF adopted several of the project's techniques for bringing services, including prevention of tetanus of the newborn, to the village level. The

MSPP later developed its Expanded Program on Immunization (EPI), supported by UNICEF, PAHO/WHO, and the US Agency for International Development. The local EPI, among its many impressive benefits, provided tetanus toxoid for all Haitian women, including those living in rural areas.

Advocating Beyond National Borders

Community health department leaders published a scientific paper describing the HAS tetanus control program in a peer-reviewed journal. The article stressed the importance of immunizing all fertile women rather than just those women who attend prenatal care 2 times or more before their delivery and was among the documents that informed the WHO Global advisory Group Meeting of 1983[7] (Figure 6-1). At that meeting, the WHO tetanus immunization target was changed from "pregnant women" to "fertile women."[6]

Call to Action

Many countries still report tetanus vaccination activities by the number and percent of women who received 2 doses of tetanus toxoid before they delivered and a third dose 6 months after the second dose. That indicator focuses monthly reports on pregnant women, prenatal care, and deliveries conducted and reported in organized, official birthing facilities.

Because in some countries vaccinations of nonpregnant women are not recorded in monthly activity reports, vaccinators may conclude that nonpregnant women are not within their target after all. Thus, unvaccinated, fertile women may become pregnant and fail to consult for prenatal care early enough in pregnancy to complete their immunizations. If vaccinations are not completed 6 weeks before delivery, maternal anti-tetanus antibodies may not have had time to cross the placenta and adequately immunize the mother's newborn.

Reports should include the number and percent of fertile, nonpregnant women who have completed 3 tetanus toxoid injections and those who have received their 5-year boosters on schedule. If fertile, nonpregnant women are not included in vaccination reports, their vaccinations cannot be measured, so they will not be vaccinated until they become pregnant. If they are not fully vaccinated against tetanus in a timely manner, their newborns will be at risk for neonatal tetanus.

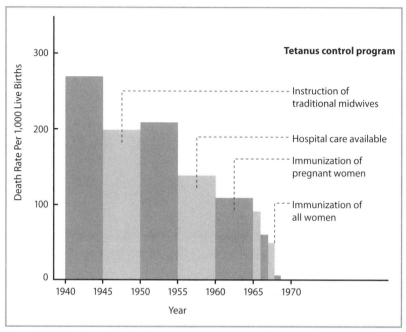

Figure 6-1. The changing rate of death due to tetanus of the newborn among children born within the Albert Schweitzer census tract, Deschapelles, Haiti, between 1940 and 1972. The rates are expressed as deaths due to tetanus of the newborn per 1,000 live births. The data are based on the results of interviews of 1,629 mothers aged 15 to 59 years who were living within the Deschapelles census tract in 1968. The broken arrows denote the period of operation of each of the tetanus control programs specified in the column at right. From Berggren WL. Administration and evaluation of rural health services. I. A tetanus control program in Haiti. *Am J Trop Med Hyg.* 1974;23(5):936–949, with permission.

References

1. Marshall FN. Tetanus of the newborn. With special reference to experiences in Haiti, W.I. *Adv Pediatr.* 1968;16:65–110

2. Weinstein L. Tetanus. In: Feigin, Cherry, Demmler-Harrison, Kaplan, eds. *Feigin & Cherry's Textbook of Pediatric Infectious Diseases.* 13th ed. Philadelphia, PA: Saunders Elsevier; 1992

3. World Health Organization. *WHO Vaccine-Preventable Diseases: Monitoring System. 2010 Global Summary.* Geneva, Switzerland: World Health Organization; 2010. http://www.who.int/immunization/documents/who_ivb_2010/en. Accessed May 1, 2013

4. World Health Organization. *The Global Burden of Disease: 2004 Update.* Geneva, Switzerland: World Health Organization; 2008. http://www.who.int/healthinfo/global_burden_disease/2004_report_update/en/index.html. Accessed May 1, 2013

5. Taylor-Ide D, Taylor CE. *Just and Lasting Change: When Communities Own Their Futures.* Baltimore, MD: Johns Hopkins University Press; 2002

6. Foster SO. Immunization and respiratory diseases and child mortality. In: Mosely WH, Chen L, eds. Child survival: strategies for research. *Population and Development Review.* 1984;10(suppl):119–140

7. Schofield FD, Tucker VM, Westbrook GR. Neonatal tetanus in New Guinea. Effect of active immunization in pregnancy. *Br Med J.* 1961;2(5255):785–789

8. Berggren WL. Administration and evaluation of rural health services. I. A tetanus control program in Haiti. *Am J Trop Med Hyg.* 1974;23(5):936–949

9. Newell KW, Dueñas Lehmann A, LeBlanc DR, Garces Osorio N. The use of toxoid for the prevention of tetanus neonatorum. Final report of a double-blind controlled field trial. *Bull World Health Organ.* 1966;35(6):863–871

Chapter 7

Haemophilus influenzae Vaccine Advocacy in Guatemala

Edwin J. Asturias, MD

"Never be afraid to raise your voice for honesty and truth and compassion against injustice….If people all over the world...would do this, it would change the earth."

— William Faulkner

Understanding the Problem of Meningitis and Pneumonia in Guatemala

In 1906, a baby was born in a remote area in southwest Guatemala to a young woman. This was her fourth child with her physician husband. The baby was growing well, healthy and rosy, until one day close to his second month of life, he became ill with high fevers and was lethargic and less eager to breastfeed. After 2 days of fever and persistent crying, the father noted a rigidity throughout his young son's body. It was then he knew his child had meningitis, a bacterial infection that invades the bloodstream and attacks the brain. Before antibiotics became available in the mid-20th century, meningitis was a death sentence. Against the odds, this young infant survived meningitis and became a prosperous coffee farmer. He was a miracle among millions of children dying and suffering from bacterial infections in the era before penicillin was discovered. Later in the 1960s, antibiotics and other supportive treatments made the outcome of bacterial meningitis a bit better, with 60% to 90% surviving the disease if treated on time, but more than half of these survivors were left with severe sequelae including deafness, mental retardation, and seizures.

Before the 1990s, *Haemophilus influenzae* type b (Hib) was a leading cause of childhood meningitis, pneumonia, and inflammation of the epiglottis in the United States, causing an estimated 20,000 cases a year, mostly in children younger than 5 years. Since routine vaccination began in 1991, the incidence of Hib disease has declined by greater than 99%, effectively eliminating Hib as a public health problem. Similar reductions in disease occurred after introduction of the vaccine in Western Europe.

In low- and middle-income countries around the world, meningitis was a recognizable severe and feared disease, killing 1 of every 3 to 5 children that got the infection and leaving at least half of its survivors with disabilities. However, in many of these countries, Hib was not recognized as an important cause of meningitis or pneumonia, mainly because of the lack of appropriate techniques and resources to isolate the organism from infected children. Children presenting with meningitis were treated as if they were infected with Hib, pneumococcus, or meningococcus, usually spending numerous days in intensive care units with prolonged hospitalizations and incurring a tremendous cost to the already limited health care system.

The first task at hand was to find out if Hib and pneumococcus were as important causes of meningitis as they were reported in the United States and European countries. Some data were available from Chile and Uruguay demonstrating the importance of Hib as pathogen in meningitis, sepsis, and pneumonia. Neal Halsey, MD, and I decided to evaluate how many cultures from the spinal fluid of children suspected of having meningitis at the San Juan de Dios General Hospital in Guatemala were positive for Hib and pneumococcus. To our surprise, for a full year in 1994, from 365 samples of spinal fluid taken from children with meningitis, only one case of Hib was detected, yet many of these children had clear signs of bacterial meningitis and were being treated as such. What was preventing the pediatricians at the hospital from correctly identifying Hib infections? We decided to test some of the new fresh samples from patients with meningitis using a simple technology available in the United States, latex agglutination. This method identified Hib antigen present in the fluid of children with meningitis even when the culture result was negative. Soon the first cases of Hib meningitis became evident. The problem was in the laboratory. We uncovered that the specimens from spinal taps had transport delays and were mishandled in ways that made it more difficult to culture Hib bacteria. Also, the blood and chocolate agar in the petri dishes needed to grow Hib were prepared from discarded human blood from the blood bank rather than the recommended sheep blood. This prevented Hib from growing properly and being isolated. We sought the help of Ralf Clemens, a German physician and scientist leading the efforts to provide lifesaving vaccines for the world's poorest children, to provide funds for a surveillance study that could allow us to demonstrate that Hib was indeed a serious public health problem.

Within 3 years, with the help of several physicians and microbiologists at the 3 major hospitals in Guatemala City, we were able to show that Hib was responsible for 46% of the cases of acute bacterial meningitis in children younger than 5 years. While Hib was clearly the most important cause of bacterial meningitis, it also caused pneumonia, sepsis, arthritis, cellulitis, and epiglottitis. Most Hib infections were in infants 6 to 11 months of age, and the mortality associated with these infections was 5%. We also identified pneumococcus as the second leading cause of bacterial meningitis and primary cause of pneumonia. Pneumococcus was more common in infants younger than 6 months, and only 2 of 3 children survived the brain infection, meningitis. So Hib was an important infection, causing thousands of hospitalizations and hundreds of deaths in Guatemala despite the best efforts of our physicians and hospitals.[1]

Having shown the burden of Hib disease, the next step was to prevent these infections with the vaccine that had been introduced in the United States and Europe with great success. The solution was obvious. The challenge was how to get children in Guatemala immunized with Hib vaccine.

Engaging a Solution

The Hib vaccine was a very effective vaccine in high-income countries. Within a few years of its introduction, Hib meningitis, sepsis, and pneumonia became diseases of the past, saving thousands of children's lives and millions in health care cost. *Haemophilus influenzae* type b vaccine, a highly effective technology produced by at least 3 manufacturers, cost $10 to $15 per dose. At a time when most low- and middle-income countries were spending no more than $3 to $5 to completely immunize children during their first year of life against diphtheria, tetanus, pertussis, poliomyelitis, tuberculosis, and measles, increasing the cost of immunization programs 10-fold to prevent an infection that only pediatricians and infectious disease specialists recognized as a problem was a challenge.

Establishing the burden of illness in Guatemala City highlighted for everyone that Hib infections were an important public health problem. Now if Hib vaccine should be introduced into the national vaccine program, public health and policy officials had to decide which formulation, the population to be immunized, and whether the costs would be acceptable. To determine if the costs were acceptable, it would also be critical to understand the offsets related to decreased costs within the health system due to reduced Hib disease burden. As in many countries in Latin America, the Guatemalan health care system has 3 major players: the small private sector that takes care of people with means to pay out of pocket; the social security system that is a public retirement program and also provides care for permanent workers by law; and finally the Ministry of Health, which cares for the poor and underemployed. *Haemophilus influenzae* type b vaccine had been introduced into the private sector within 3 years of being available in the United States, protecting less than 1 in 20 children, and these protected children lived mainly in the capital city. Preventing severe Hib infections throughout the country would require coverage of the public sector and strong support of the Ministry of Health. That support from the ministry could only be obtained if the effectiveness of Hib vaccine could be demonstrated from studies carried out in Guatemala. Guatemala needed to have its own data to make an evidenced-based decision. Although the Hib vaccine had been introduced and proven to be effective in 2 middle-income countries, Uruguay and Chile, it was unclear whether the vaccine would be as effective in a low-income country like Guatemala. Evidence from studies led by Joel Ward in Alaska and Mathuram Santosham in the Navajo reservation showed that Native Americans suffered an increased burden of Hib disease and did not appear to respond to at least one of the Hib vaccines as well as others. Therefore, it was important to learn how the large indigenous population of Guatemala would respond to Hib vaccine. Dr Halsey and I were able to convince Ralf Clemens again to fund a study to evaluate how young indigenous children, ladino, and malnourished infants responded to a new combination vaccine, the pentavalent diphtheria, tetanus, whole-cell pertussis, hepatits B, Hib (DTwP-HepB/Hib) vaccine. Anticipating that the study would demonstrate substantial benefits, we proposed that a vaccine manufacturer provide free vaccine for the full cohort of children in Guatemala City for 1 year, half in the second year, and one quarter in the third year. This commitment would create an incentive for the Ministry of Health and national government to add Hib to its vaccine program by helping to reduce the costs of introduc-ing the vaccine. The national cost would be more manageable as it would gradually increase over the 3 years. With that in hand, we held a meeting with the Vice-Minister of Health, consultants, and epidemiologists to discuss this proposal. However, our plan was not accepted because the Ministry of Health had decided to expand the national immunization by replacing the measles vaccine with measles-mumps-rubella vaccine. *Haemophilus influenzae* type b was considered less of a priority than protecting children from rubella and mumps. Yet Hib was killing many more children than measles, rubella, and mumps together. The challenge was to have these officials stop thinking about vaccines as a zero-sum game between these 2 options. Fortunately, at a conference of the Technical Advisory Group on Immunizations from the Pan American Health Organization (PAHO) convened in Guatemala, I sat by Carlos Mayorga, MD, a pediatrician who headed the Maternal Infant Division at the Guatemalan Institute of Social Security (IGSS). When I mentioned to him that the Ministry of Health turned down the project, he recognized the importance of Hib vaccine for Guatemalan children and proposed to do the study and the project within the IGSS system. A few months later, we began our study in Guatemala City and San Juan Sacatepéquez, a town of Kaqchikel native Indians. By the end of 1998 we documented that the Hib vaccine was protective for children from different ethnic backgrounds, and even malnourished children responded well.[2] In March 1999, IGSS was the first public health institution in Mesoamerica to begin universal immunization against Hib using the pentavalent vaccine. The introduction of Hib vaccine for children receiving care at IGSS was a success; within 2 years the number of cases of Hib meningitis and pneumonia had been reduced by 83%. Dr Mayorga and the pediatricians working at IGSS clinics were proud to demonstrate that Hib prevented so much childhood disease and death. This created a strong advocacy force to extend this benefit to the poorest children who were cared for by the Ministry of Health.

The Challenges of *Haemophilus influenzae* Vaccine Introduction for All Children in Guatemala

Our surveillance study of Hib infections and vaccine trial within IGSS provided strong evidence to convince the Ministry of Health to incorporate this effective vaccine into the national immunization schedule. The PAHO was also recommending that countries try to include Hib vaccine as part of vaccine programs for young children, and many other nations in Latin America had done so. However, the political atmosphere had changed in Guatemala. A populist corrupt government had won the elections in 2000, and despite the possibility of securing funding from the Japanese Agency for International Development in 2002, the government failed to submit the project and the funding was lost, delaying introduction once again.

In 2004 a new government was elected and I was able to secure a meeting with the Minister of Health of Guatemala. An engineer by career, Marco A. Sosa was returning as the only Minister of Health who had ever served twice in that position in the cabinet. We had a positive meeting; he was convinced that if we could implement policies that would reduce infant mortality rapidly, the country would move forward in its efforts to tackle the high poverty and health disparity we suffered. He asked me to take charge of the Hib introduction, and for the first time I became an official of the Ministry of Health.

Within 8 months, the National Immunization Program, PAHO, and Pediatric Association of Guatemala agreed to collaborate and after several productive meetings in partnership with the United Nations Children's Fund and other agencies, a plan was designed to introduce Hib vaccine. Financing purchase of the vaccine was a key issue. Sosa had set aside half of the $5 million needed to purchase enough to cover a birth cohort of 350,000 newborns. We contacted GlaxoSmithKline, who agreed to pay for an additional quarter of the needed funds. The remaining money was provided by the Peace Fund, an entity that had been created after the signing of the peace accords in 1999 to help Guatemalans rebuild their infrastructure after a 36-year civil war. This was the first time the Peace Fund funded a vaccine project. One of the former vice presidents of the country was directing the institution, and he became convinced that introducing Hib vaccine would do as much for the population as any infrastructure project. It now has been shown that the return on investment of vaccines in developing countries for the creation of wealth is around 15% to 20%—as good as education.

In March 2005, the Ministry of Health of Guatemala introduced Hib vaccine for all children. Since then, the number of infections and deaths from meningitis and pneumonia from this bacterium has been reduced by 86%, and the country has enjoyed a steady reduction in child mortality.

Lessons for Vaccine Advocacy for Low- and Middle-Income Countries

Introducing new lifesaving vaccines in low- and middle-income countries is not an easy process, not because decision-makers are not concerned about the well-being of children or their potential public health effect but mainly due to competing strategies, reduced budgets, and the lack of political will.

The 5 key elements in advocating for the introduction of a new, needed vaccine in a country that should be taken into consideration are the following:

Element 1: Make the problem visible. Before one can enlist public health officials, community physicians, and even parents in the process of advocating for the introduction of a new vaccine, it is critical that the burden of disease is recognized. You need to embark on a search for the evidence that will document the burden of disease and demonstrate that the prevention of disease will affect children's health. As an example, it is harder to convince public health authorities to introduce a vaccine against rotavirus infection in a country with very low mortality from diarrhea compared with a country where rotavirus infection causes two-thirds of all hospitalizations and diarrhea is the second leading cause of death in children.

Element 2: Show and tell. Obtaining data and recognizing the burden are not enough. One needs to become a public advocate of the problem. Physicians, nurses, health care workers, public officials, and the population respond well when one is able to convey a compelling message. That message is more effective when it is based on good data and communicates feasible solutions and technologies that can change the situation.

Element 3: Engage decision-makers and influencers. One must recognize that spreading the message is not enough. Partnering with key decision-makers and people with influence, especially when they come together to promote change, is crucial. There are many examples of advocacy in developing countries in which failure to work with public officials has resulted in blockage or delays in adapting transformative solutions because those decision-makers resent that they have not been an active partner. Working to ensure that responsible agencies are invested in the program is usually more effective than trying to change the agency with outside pressure. This approach strengthens those who will carry the workload ahead.

Element 4: Moving to action as a champion. Advocacy means hard work and taking advantage of all possible partners to produce transformation or introduce the solution. This work may take years, but at the end the solution may improve with time.

Element 5: Help measure the impact. No advocacy work is complete, particularly related to controlling vaccine-preventable diseases, if we do not measure the effect of the change or solution. This monitoring will give partners the pride of having transformed the problem and provide additional information to strengthen the change and make it sustainable.

References

1. Asturias EJ, Soto M, Menendez R, et al. Meningitis and pneumonia in Guatemalan children: the importance of *Haemophilus influenzae* type b and *Streptococcus pneumoniae*. *Rev Panam Salud Publica*. 2003;14(6):377–384

2. Asturias EJ, Mayorga C, Caffaro C, et al. Differences in the immune response to hepatitis B and *Haemophilus influenzae* type b vaccines in Guatemalan infants by ethnic group and nutritional status. *Vaccine*. 2009;27(27):3650–3654

Chapter 8

Advocating for Equity Through Immunization

Jon Kim Andrus, MD

Introduction

Communicating the truth about how vaccines prevent fatal diseases in children should be simple, but clearly it is not. Why is it so difficult to translate truth into action? Is it a lack of understanding, commitment, finances, trained professionals, or systems to supervise and monitor impact? Are these challenges perceived too often as insurmountable? Advocacy and perseverance can overcome these challenges.

The last week of April 2012 marked the 10th anniversary of the Pan American Health Organization (PAHO) Vaccination Week in the Americas (VWA). With support from PAHO, VWA began when the Ministers of Health of the Andean countries decided to conduct a vaccination campaign to stop the spread of a measles outbreak that threatened the rest of the hemisphere. It was an act of solidarity, putting the health and security of the hemisphere above that of any one country. At the community level families responded extraordinarily well. I have been fortunate to have participated in 9 of those 10 annual events, always occurring the last week of April. It is an honor for those of us working in global health to see how every family puts their full faith in their public health authorities to do the right thing, to protect their children from unnecessary harm, and to do so in a way that contributes to the whole of society. Indeed, that act of faith is an act of love, a motto we adopted for VWA use. In April 2012 VWA expanded globally for the first time with the involvement of more than 180 countries.[1] Families around the world should be acknowledged for their part in the chain of vaccination—hearing and understanding the truth, placing trust and faith in their public servants, and translating that truth into action.

Using polio eradication as a case study, this chapter provides a unique opportunity to examine the challenges of child advocacy and the pursuit of equity on the front lines.

Understanding the Problem of Polio Eradication in India

Drawing on my experience in the World Health Organization (WHO) region of South-East Asia, I focus here on 1) how a specific public health problem may be defined and analyzed; 2) how interventions are assessed and implemented to address the problem; 3) how outcomes are defined and assessed; and 4) how flexibility should be injected into the initiative to allow for adjustments in the interventions whenever appropriate.

In 1993, I arrived in New Delhi to lead the polio eradication efforts for the WHO South-East Asia Regional Office (SEARO). I had been assigned by the Centers for Disease Control and Prevention (CDC) to WHO for this role. That year India reported more than 4,000 polio cases, half of cases worldwide.[2] The polio epidemic was apparent for all to see. Almost every street corner of New Delhi had a "crawler," or polio victim. The reported cases were perhaps only one-tenth of the actual disease burden because surveillance was passive and variable across the hundreds of districts of India. Active case detection with stool specimen collection for documentation, so important to eradication efforts, had not been implemented everywhere in India. Many Indian health policy makers doubted it ever could be. Obtaining laboratory results would be critical because of the numerous other causes of acute flaccid paralysis (AFP) in children, including Guillain-Barré syndrome, transverse myelitis, coxsackievirus, and other enteric enteroviruses.[3]

In 1993, the administrative system for the Indian vaccination programs was centralized in the office of the national immunization manager. This national manager was in charge of all the nation's vaccine purchases. In addition to the manager there were one secretary and one data-entry specialist. The only data on coverage were maintained on one desktop computer. These 3 people sat in a single, non–air-conditioned office, smaller than the smallest airport restroom. In contrast, at that time the United States, with roughly a quarter of the population of India, had the National Immunization Program at the CDC supported by more than 50 epidemiologists, countless computer programmers, analysts, and other support staff.

The challenge of eradicating polio in India was complicated by multiple factors. First, the estimated disease burden was overwhelming. Second, surveillance was poor so that this disease burden was markedly underestimated. Third, government leadership and administrative support for achieving the polio eradication target by 2000 was nonexistent. There was no consistent Indian leadership committed to accelerating efforts to establish active surveillance systems for AFP needed to accelerate polio eradication strategies. The high-level Ministry of Health & Family Welfare (MHFW) staff responsible for immunization programs did not consider polio eradication a feasible or worthwhile priority. While WHO had adopted a resolution in 1988 to eradicate polio globally by 2000, it had only begun to establish the beginnings of a regional polio laboratory network in South-East Asia by 1992. When I arrived in India, 5 years of the 12-year clock had passed. Despite having only 7 years remaining to achieve the WHO goal of polio eradication, there was little sense of urgency or commitment from the regional WHO and United Nations Children's Fund leadership to recognize the crisis and rapidly accelerate polio eradication activities. The Chinese language has 2 symbols for crisis, one indicating "danger" and the second indicating "opportunity." Advocacy for polio eradication in India was essential. Opportunities soon emerged. A critical component of the advocacy involved creating new partnerships that would deliver one united message—that polio eradication was feasible in India, and with assistance from partners, Indians themselves could achieve this goal.

Analyzing and Selecting Appropriate Interventions

Strategically, the first step was to address the need for political support of key Indian child health policy makers in the MHFW. Two events helped to build this support. The first involved the very successful Bangladeshi nationwide mass polio vaccination campaign in March 1995 that reached 83% of the 18.9 million children younger than 5 years with 2 doses of oral polio vaccine.[2] Given this was the first such campaign in Bangladesh, it was a remarkable achievement. Bangladesh had a much better capacity than India to gear up rapidly for polio eradication. The Ministry of Health of Bangladesh had a 3-story building staffed with offices fully dedicated to their childhood immunization program. Bangladesh had successfully built on their smallpox eradication efforts to create a strengthened capacity for their national immunization program. Leaders of Bangladesh embraced proven polio eradication strategies. Bangladesh authorities remained committed to their routine immunization program by conducting mass campaigns that ultimately led to the interruption of wild poliovirus transmission.

When Bangladesh received global and regional press coverage for its successful polio eradication program, parliamentarians in India were astounded. How could Bangladesh eradicate polio before India? If Bangladesh could do it, why cannot India? These questions where taken up by the Indian press and began to flood the hallways of the Indian Parliament. The World Health Organization and Rotary International took advantage of what was happening to hold countless meetings with members of the president's staff and friends in parliament to advocate for a commitment to polio eradication from the MHFW. The Minister of Family Welfare finally embraced the polio eradication initiative and authorized the first polio vaccination campaign during the winter of 1995–1996, reversing prior policy that failed to support polio eradication.[2]

The second event that lent political support to polio eradication efforts involved the Danish International Development Agency (DANIDA), which had a long-standing track record of providing India with support for infrastructure and capacity development. We had several discussions, official and unofficial, about ways DANIDA might support polio eradication efforts in India. The discussions progressed to considering the need of enhancing infectious disease surveillance capacity and developing the necessary public health laboratory support.

Fortunately, DANIDA recognized that infectious disease surveillance in India was sorely needed; a suspected plague outbreak of 1994 clearly demonstrated this fact to Indian policy makers. One year after my arrival, the plague scare proved to provide enormous opportunities to advocate for improved infectious disease surveillance in India. In September 1994, Indian health officials in Maharashtra became extremely alarmed by reports from Surat city of a cluster of deaths and large numbers of people who were seriously ill.[4] Largely because of an increased occurrence of respiratory presentations, concomitant with a recent history of the rodent die-off, officials feared the worst, the pneumonic plague. Misinformation about the exact number of deaths, perhaps falsely exaggerated, caused nationwide panic and eventually global fear. Several foreign embassies in New Delhi closed and sent their staff back home to their countries of origin. Several international jet airlines refused to fly to India. To this day, the cause of the outbreak remains unclear. Some reputable scientists still doubt that plague was the cause. At the time, though, the crisis and resulting chaos directly resulted in India losing millions of dollars in tourist and other revenue. The Danish International Development Agency agreed to provide SEARO with a $12 million AFP surveillance grant. The first core group of 59 surveillance medical officers (SMOs) was trained in 1997 at the Maulana Azad Medical College, a Muslim school located in

New Delhi. A substantial burden of polio occurred among Muslim minority communities of the northern Ganges River valley. The choice of the Muslim school as the first training site was a subtle but certainly strategic advocacy message. Immediately after their 2-week crash course, the newly trained SMOs fanned out across the country to their local assignments, supported by the centrally located National Polio Surveillance Project (NPSP) to begin their assignments to rapidly implement active AFP surveillance. Simultaneously, more than 10,000 official AFP reporting sites were established across the country for SMOs to manage and supervise.[5]

The Danish International Development Agency support was absolutely critical in those initial phases of establishing and implementing what many have called state-of-the-art polio surveillance. Later, when funding streams were more difficult to sustain, other partners like the CDC, UK Department for International Development, US Agency for International Development, and Canadian International Development Agency stepped forward to support this critical public health function. Linked to this was support for the laboratory network, particularly the capacity provided by the CDC to Indian scientists to develop the necessary understanding of molecular epidemiology to monitor the program's progress in reaching zero polio cases.

During the plague scare, the Minister of Health, Harsh Vardhan, of the Federal District of New Delhi, became committed to the global polio eradication effort and was an amazing champion of the cause. He and his dedicated team, with support from SEARO and Rotary International, organized the first state-based polio mass vaccination campaign on Mahatma Gandhi's birthday, October 2, 1994.[6] The team used advanced micro-planning techniques and highly sophisticated social mobilization and communication strategies. Of the approximately 1 million children younger than 3 years targeted, approximately 89% received the oral polio vaccine.[7] Despite the background chaos created by the plague scare, the campaign proved to be a huge success. Many of the vaccinators wore surgical masks over their faces while vaccinating to diminish the risk of contracting the much-feared plague. The minister exerted an extraordinary amount of courage to conduct the campaign, despite many leaders calling for its cancellation because of the plague scare. I know personally that the minister worked all night prior to the campaign to ensure all vaccination teams and vaccines were in place (Figure 8-1). One year later, the nation targeted more than 93 million children younger than 4 years in the first nationwide mass polio vaccination campaign in India.[8] The last isolate of wild poliovirus type 2 reported in the world was from India in 1999, largely a result of these and other efforts described as follows.

Implementing Acute Flaccid Paralysis Surveillance and Immunization Activities

Implementation of surveillance was launched with the first training of SMOs. Each SMO, after receiving the initial training, had use of a 4-wheel-drive land cruiser, a laptop computer and printer, and a cell phone. They also had authority to rent office space, pay support staff, and operate on an expense account. The centralized office set up in New Delhi, dubbed the NPSP, supported their work.

The NPSP would rely on Indian nationals as the SMOs to do the brunt of the work, not foreigners as occurred with smallpox eradication. This ensured Indian "ownership" of the program, which inspired the initial

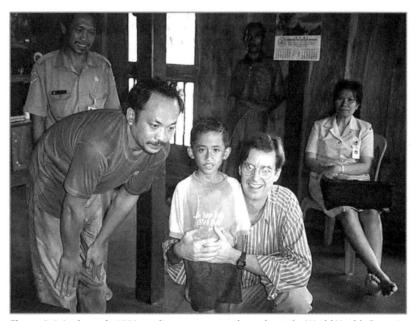

Figure 8-1. In the early 1990s, polio was rampant throughout the World Health Organization region of South-East Asia. The advocacy and technical strategies implemented in India were the same implemented in Bangladesh, Nepal, Myanmar, Indonesia, Thailand, and other countries of the region. This young Burmese boy on physical examination had mild asymmetry of the gluteal folds and mild weakness on the same side of the large muscles groups of the leg. The case, although mild, was used as an advocacy tool with the Ministry of Health to help accelerate the development of surveillance of acute flaccid paralysis in Myanmar and assure authorities that no reservoirs of wild poliovirus transmission would be missed.

group of SMOs trained at the Muslim college because they were to be the ones to eradicate polio in their own country. The SMOs consistently worked from dawn to the wee hours of the night. In a matter of months, AFP reporting and stool specimen collection rates skyrocketed to more acceptable standards.[5]

Good public health practice is good program management. That was a key guiding principle of enhanced polio surveillance. Attention to capacity development includes the human resource as well as system capacity. Human and system development are inextricably linked. People get the job done, but they need to be supported by the system. Surveillance medical officers were constantly supervised within a management structure that was decentralized but supported by the centralized NPSP. The SMOs were instructed to fill their office walls with charts of key surveillance performance indicators so local government administrators and others walking into their offices for the very first time could determine the level of surveillance and gaps by district. These visits helped to insure local government buy-in. The SMOs attended decentralized quarterly meetings and an annual meeting to sustain the spirit corps of the SMOs and provide technical updates on local, regional, and global progress.

It was important for the sustainability of the polio eradication program to have the NPSP housed in the central offices of the MHFW of Nirman Bhawan. After advocating for this decision for almost a year, we were finally successful in obtaining the ministry's approval to be located in their confines. However, when the NPSP outgrew the small space made available, there was no choice but to move operations outside to the Nehru Stadium.

Monitoring and Evaluation of Interventions

As stated in various WHO global resolutions, the outcome of polio eradication is defined as the interruption of wild poliovirus transmission. Fortunately, the PAHO had developed and used indicators that evaluated the quality of surveillance with this target in mind.[9] For disease eradication, the surveillance system has to be sensitive enough to capture all reservoirs of transmission of the agent targeted for eradication, while specific enough that only disease caused by the agent can be accurately identified. Indicators for surveillance assessment were streamlined to be simple, practical, and easy to understand while maintaining the scientific rigor necessary to interrupt wild virus transmission.

Initially, the stool collection rate indicator required 2 stool specimens to be collected within 2 weeks of paralysis onset for laboratory testing. We targeted that 80% of AFP cases reported should have at least 2 stool specimens collected within 2 weeks after paralysis onset; the bar was set relatively high. Later, data indicated that one stool would be sufficient, so the indicator was changed from 2 stools to 1 stool, but the 80% criterion remained unchanged. There were 2 very key indicators: the AFP reporting rate per 100,000 population younger than 15 years, and the percentage of AFP cases with stool specimens collected within 2 weeks of paralysis onset.[9] The AFP reporting rate indicator was a proxy for the sensitivity of surveillance. The AFP reporting rate should be at least 1 per 100,000 largely because several studies indicated that would be the expected background rate for Guillain-Barré syndrome.[10] Achieving that reporting rate assures us that the surveillance system was sensitive enough to capture cases of paralysis caused by wild poliovirus. The stool collection rate was the proxy for surveillance specificity. The experience of the Americas demonstrated that a stool collection rate of 80% was sufficient to ensure specificity in determining that wild poliovirus was the cause of a child's paralysis. Evidence was used not only to improve the indicator definitions but also the case definitions.[11] The AFP reporting rate and stool collection rate indicators were sufficient to determine that once zero case status was achieved, wild poliovirus transmission was unlikely to have been missed.

Call to Action

Vaccination of a child is the culmination of countless hours, if not decades, of hard work linked to the second the needle pricks the skin. That act saves lives. Hard work must be done by scientists who develop the vaccine, volunteers who mobilize the community, the janitor who maintains the cold boxes for vaccine delivery and storage, the nurse who gives the shot, and child advocates who influence government policy makers. Families around the world should also be acknowledged for their part in this chain—hearing and understanding the truth, placing trust and faith in their public servants, and translating that truth into action.

While our interventions led to an incredibly motivated team and state-of-the-art surveillance for polio in India, we failed to strengthen substantially the system for other routine immunizations. We also hoped to use the polio platform to improve infectious disease surveillance in general. Unfortunately, we never fully realized this vision. With global polio eradication now feasible, we must take full advantage of new vaccines that have been developed by improving primary care and infectious disease prevention and control. Advocacy should embrace the successful immunization lessons related to the elimination of polio, measles, rubella, and congenital rubella syndrome in many less-developed parts of the world. Science and technology have introduced new life-saving vaccines against *Haemophilus influenzae* type b, pneumococcal, rotavirus, and human papillomavirus infections.[12] Building on the capacity resulting from successful polio and other immunization interventions should be the cornerstone of our work to bring these immunization opportunities to scale.[13] This will take sustained advocacy for these immunization programs. Advocates must position themselves to take advantage of whatever fortuitous events become available to promote the cause of reducing vaccine-preventable disease. We owe it to our children.

Acknowledgments

I want to acknowledge the amazing faith and commitment the children and families of India gave in support of the program, as well as my own children, Claire and Elizabeth, who participated in many polio eradication activities during their 7-year stay in India.

References

1. World Health Organization. Special report on the first World Immunization Week. *Global Immunization News.* April 30, 2012. http://www.who.int/immunization/GIN_April_2012.pdf. Accessed May 2, 2013
2. Andrus JK, Banerjee K, Hull BP, Smith JC, Mochny I. Polio eradication in the World Health Organization South-East Asia Region by the year 2000: midway assessment of progress and future challenges. *J Infect Dis.* 1997;175(Suppl 1):S89–S96
3. Dietz V, Andrus J, Olivé JM, Cochi S, de Quadros C. Epidemiology and clinical characteristics of acute flaccid paralysis associated with non-polio enterovirus isolation: the experience in the Americas. *Bull World Health Organ.* 1995;73(5):597–603
4. Ramalingaswami V. Psychosocial effects of the 1994 plague outbreak in Surat, India. *Mil Med.* 2001;166(12 Suppl):29–30
5. Andrus JK, Thapa AB, Withana N, Fitzsimmons JW, Abeykoon P, Aylward B. A new paradigm for international disease control: lessons learned from polio eradication in Southeast Asia. *Am J Public Health.* 2001;91(1):146–150
6. Vardhan H. *A Tale of Two Drops.* New Delhi, India: Ocean Books Ltd; 2005
7. Bandyopadhyay S, Banerjee K, Datta KK, Atwood SJ, Langmire CM, Andrus JK. Evaluation of mass pulse immunization with oral polio vaccine in Delhi: is pre-registration of children necessary? *Indian J Pediatr.* 1996;63(2):133–137
8. Banerjee K, Andrus J, Hlady G. Conquering poliomyelitis in India. *Lancet.* 1997;349(9065):1630

9. Andrus JK, de Quadros CA, Olive JM. The surveillance challenge: final stages of eradication of poliomielitis in the Americas. *MMWR CDC Surveill Summ.* 1992;41(1):21–26

10. Olivé JM, Castillo C, Castro RG, de Quadros CA. Epidemiologic study of Guillain-Barré syndrome in children <15 years of age in Latin America. *J Infect Dis.* 1997;175(Suppl 1):S160–S164

11. Andrus J, de Quadros CA, Olive JM, Silveira CM, Eikhof RM. Classification and characteristics of confirmed polio cases, The Americas 1989. VIII Meeting of the Technical Advisory Group on EPI on the Eradication of Poliomyelitis in the Amercias (Oral Presentation), Mexico City, Pan American Health Organization

12. Andrus JK, de Quadros C, Matus CR, Luciani S, Hotez P. New vaccines for developing countries: will it be feast or famine? *Am J Law Med.* 2009;35(2-3):311–322

13. Andrus JK, Solorzano CC, de Oliveira L, Danovaro-Holliday MC, de Quadros CA. Strengthening surveillance: confronting infectious diseases in developing countries. *Vaccine.* 2011;29(Suppl 4):D126–D130

Chapter 9

Community Partnerships for Polio Eradication in India

T. Jacob John, MD

"Your dream is not big enough if it doesn't scare you."
— Matthias Schmelz

Introduction

Public health projects begin simply with an idea. If that idea catches on with others, some projects may progress to the point of imagining solutions. Occasionally a champion arises behind whom many may rally around and the project grows. Successful public health programs involve several people, each pushing forward the concept, idea, intervention tools, expansion, logistics, political agenda, financial support, and global networking. When a certain threshold of activity is reached, the public health program becomes a reality. Among the many propelling forces of the progression of ideas to programs is advocacy. Advocacy acts as a selector of a specific problem and catalyst in its solution.

The process of prioritization and program development should be systematic and analytic. But that is not what often happens. An individual may be seized with one problem, chosen for some reason, perhaps in the emotional realm of mind. That reason may appear to be trivial to others, but it may be the seed for the birth of an idea, a dream. In the early days of recognizing a problem and exploring its solutions, there may be loneliness on the path of the mental journey—for it is not possible to infect others with one's inner perceptions or drive. Everyone sees the same problem from a different angle. When one has to venture forth alone, one must muster inner strength.

Understanding the Problem

Christian Medical College in Vellore is India's first private not-for-profit teaching and tertiary care hospital. The head of the department was John Webb, OBE, MBBCh, from England, a great clinician. Dr Webb sent me for training in infectious disease—2 years in the United Kingdom for Membership of Royal College of Physicians (Pediatrics) of Edinburgh and 2 years in the United States in Denver, CO, working with C. Henry Kempe, MD, and Vincent Fulginiti, MD. While living in Denver, my son was due for vaccination against polio; in 1964, inactivated poliovirus vaccine (IPV) of Salk and live oral poliovirus vaccine (OPV) of Sabin were available in the United States. Jules Amer, MD, an astute pediatrician, chose to give 1 dose of IPV and 3 doses of OPV. In 1962, OPV had been introduced, and soon vaccine-associated paralytic polio (VAPP) was recognized. There were some 20 cases of VAPP in just one year, 1962, and many more since. According to Dr Amer, no child had gotten VAPP if at least 1 dose of IPV preceded OPV. When a solution was available, why should he take even the slightest risk of VAPP? Today, 48 years later, I recall his rationale because the very same question, or rather its ramification, is hotly discussed today. Will IPV help contain circulating vaccine-derived poliovirus (cVDPV)? I learned there was VAPP in vaccinated children and contacts of vaccinated children, and also "community-acquired VAPP" in children far removed from those vaccinated. Sabin's attenuated vaccine viruses did have the potential to circulate in the community, but thankfully it was rare. Rare, yes, but not to be neglected when OPV is used to eradicate wild polioviruses (WPVs) and not to be tolerated when WPVs are eradicated.

Efficacy Problems With Oral Poliovirus Vaccine in Vellore

In Vellore in 1962, polio was a common problem—we saw at least one case per month. In 1965, Dr Webb introduced OPV in the immunization clinic. In 1967, Lakshmi, a little girl, presented to our clinic with typical polio. But why did she get polio in spite of taking 3 doses of OPV, the last dose some 3 months earlier? It could not have been VAPP because VAPP has an incubation period of fewer than 30 days. It was unlikely to have been contact VAPP for 2 reasons: one, the vaccine was given to too few children to secondarily infect that many children and cause a case; second, Lakshmi had taken 3 doses of OPV already. I discussed the case with my senior, who said it could not be polio at all, as everyone knew OPV protected 100%. I thought to myself, I have got to prove Lakshmi had polio, for if she had vaccine-failure polio, that was a bad omen. We had to understand and overcome that problem. The definition of *vaccine failure* is the development of the vaccine-targeted disease in spite of giving the standard recommended 3 OPV doses.

I collected and tested Lakshmi's stool sample and grew poliovirus in primary monkey kidney cell culture. A sample of vaccine from the pharmacy showed excellent potency. A literature search through Index Medicus showed no precedent for 3-dose OPV failure. Was this just a one-off, or could there be more such cases? I requested colleagues to refer all polio cases and offered free virology. Sure enough, more cases were slowly detected. I had no clue why OPV protection was incomplete. Oral poliovirus vaccine was flown on dry ice, brought in wet ice containers from the airport, and straightaway put in pharmacy refrigerators. So the vaccine's quality was not the problem. Why were vaccinated children acquiring polio?

Gathering Support

In 1967 Dr Webb was flying out of England, and the gentleman sitting next to him happened to be W. Chas Cockburn, MD, the World Health Organization (WHO) chief of virology. He wondered if Dr Webb knew where to investigate OPV efficacy in a tropical center—Dr Cockburn had data from Kenya suggesting lower than expected antibody response, but he was sure the vaccine had lost potency in the tropical heat. He wanted a study in which the potency of OPV was ensured and to measure immune response. Dr Webb said he had the right site, person, and infrastructure. On return he introduced me to Dr Cockburn by mail.

Dr Cockburn organized a meeting in Helsinki in 1968, with Albert Sabin, MD; Joseph Melnick, PhD; John Fox, MD; Isamu Tagaya, MD; Nils Oker Blom, MD; and David Montefiore, MD, plus Dr Cockburn and myself. The experts suggested 3 possible reasons for the OPV problem in Kenya and Vellore: 1) heat affecting vaccine potency; 2) interference by concurrent enterovirus infections; or 3) inhibition by maternal antibody in the young infant.

A WHO grant allowed me to investigate vaccine efficacy (VE) of OPV in Indian children. The results were disturbing: very low efficacy for types 1 and 3 but reasonably good efficacy for type 2. This was reported to WHO and published in *Indian Pediatrics* and the *American Journal of Epidemiology*. Careful study proved absence of interference by other enteroviruses on response to OPV. Today we know that polioviruses use a unique cell receptor quite different from receptors used by all other enteroviruses, so lack of interference has biological reasons.

We found additional OPV doses improved the efficacy—the response to each dose was proportional to first-dose efficacy. Each dose resulted in a "hit" or "miss," "take" or "no take." So one simple solution to improve VE was to give multiple doses. When WHO launched the Expanded Programme on Immunization (EPI) in 1974 with 3 doses of OPV, I was disappointed. India adopted EPI in 1978 with the 3-dose schedule. When I pleaded for an increase to 5 doses (EPI has 5 contacts in infancy), I was asked first to convince WHO. When I requested WHO consider this, I was asked first to convince the Indian government.

I thought national policy makers would read and understand, so we wrote 18 papers until 1980 on the problem of polio and how to control it to change national policy to control polio. By 1980, more than 15% of children with polio in our region had received 3 doses of OPV. National statistics (based on sentinel reporting) on polio cases showed no decline in the 9 years after introduction of OPV in EPI. The government ignored this disturbing information.

Implementing Solutions

1981 was declared the International Year of Disabled Persons. We felt we had a moral duty to keep our town, Vellore, free of disability caused by polio. *If we know how to prevent a disease but do not, we become a cause of that disease.*

So a system was established to count all cases through a daily search in all local hospitals. We did this from January 1980 onward. In Vellore, population approximately 200,000, there were new cases reported each month during the next 21 months; the monthly average was 4.2 cases. After a massive public education campaign and with full support of the Rotary Club of Vellore, we conducted a pulse vaccination campaign through 16 clinics, one day each in October, November, and December 1981, offering OPV to all children younger than 5 years, regardless of the number of doses taken previously. The VE of OPV given in this pulse campaign appeared to be higher than in routine, age-based vaccination. The vaccine for the campaign was donated by Save the Children UK, courtesy of Peter Poore, MBBS.

Then, as if a tap was turned off, there were no cases for 9 months. This was great news, and the town administration and rotary members were thrilled and excited. During October to December 1982, as polio was just beginning to reappear, it was time for the next annual pulse vaccination. In those 3 months there were only 5 cases, one-third of the expected number in the pre-intervention era. In 1983 again, there were no cases for 9 months. A similar effect was observed when we pulsed a community with measles vaccine. Because measles vaccine does not have vaccine-associated disease, what likely happens is that the sudden shrinking of the pool of susceptible children by the pulse vaccination limits transmission dynamics of the agent, whether WPVs or measles virus. In other words, pulse vaccination resulted in higher herd effect for a limited period. In Vellore it lasted 9 months after one pulse with 3 doses. *Herd effect* is defined as the reduction of incidence of disease in the unvaccinated segment of a well-vaccinated community.

Despite our success we were instructed by the national government to stop giving vaccine by campaign as it was against EPI policy. National policy was age-based vaccination. The municipal health officer, Rajasekhara Pandian, who cooperated with our pulse vaccination campaign, was transferred to a distant town. I felt very sad for him, but he kept telling me he was proud to have eliminated polio is his own town.

In India we have a behavior pattern of implementing interventions as rituals or duty rather than as efforts for achieving results. Results are of less concern than following the rules. Furthermore, results were of no concern, for health is in *God's hands*. This realization explained a lot of India's many less-than-successful public health activities.

I did not give up. The EPI was a program of the national government. Under our constitution, health care is the responsibility of the state government. We had made use of this as an opportunity. From 1979, the rotary movement had been working closely with the state health ministry to eliminate measles mortality by massive measles vaccination campaigns— measles vaccine was not then included in India EPI because measles was believed to be caused by the visitation of a spirit or goddess. There was a fear that including measles in the EPI would create a backlash against the EPI. I had personally discussed with village elders and grandmothers who assured me that anything we do before the goddess's visitation would be acceptable, but nothing should be done once a child develops measles. They asked: did we not accept smallpox vaccination? Is not the smallpox goddess more powerful than the measles goddess?

The state government had seen the disappearance of measles-related deaths and blinding keratomalacia with immunization. So the state government was very supportive of vaccination by campaigns that were outside the purview of the EPI. The message of measles vaccination success was presented to the union government planning commission in Delhi, and it forced the health ministry to license measles vaccine in 1984 and to include it in the India EPI in 1985.

The success of measles vaccination in Tamil Nadu led the rotary movement to partner with the state government to increase the per capita number of OPV doses. The EPI gave 3 doses and rotary gave an additional 5 doses. Polio was quickly brought under control during the late 1980s/early 1990s. By then we had nearly eliminated polio in our district by achieving very high OPV coverage (97%), thus creating herd immunity.

Global Program Expansion

Our efforts on polio control did not go unnoticed globally. Our method and success caught the attention of Clem Renouf of Australia, president of Rotary International (RI), who was impressed. Renouf was instrumental in RI taking on polio as a global challenge. He saw the simplicity and success of pulse vaccination and the role of rotarian volunteers. The Vellore model was modular and could be replicated.

Until then, health issues were not on the rotary service agenda, with a few local exceptions, particularly in surgical interventions and providing calipers for children paralyzed by polio in African countries. Polio paralysis evoked immense compassion and empathy. Everyone in RI knew the tragic aftermath of paralytic polio.

Renouf asked John Sever, MD, of the National Institutes of Health, a pediatric infectious diseases expert and an RI leader, what should be the next disease that could be eradicated globally, after smallpox. Dr Sever said polio. Three reasons encouraged Renouf to accept the challenge: sympathy-evoking disease, worthy of global confrontation, and a plan to go forward. He dreamed that RI could create a world without polio—a gift to the children of the 21st century from RI to celebrate its birth centennial in 2005. Renouf didn't say eradicate polio, but he made Dr Sever the chairman of the Polio 2005 Committee established by RI, and I was invited to become a committee member in 1984 (Figure 9-1). During the 1970s and 1980s, childhood immunization had been nicknamed "John's gospel" in India's pediatric circles. I began preaching it at every available occasion from 1966 onward; my reason was simple—measles and pertussis, both vaccine preventable, were frequent proximate triggers to push marginally nourished

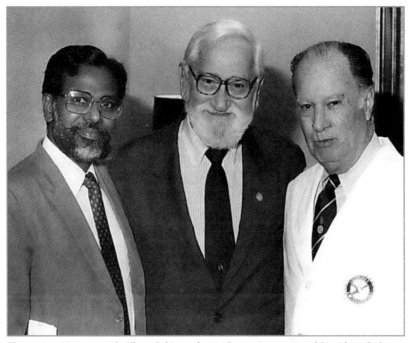

Figure 9-1. Meeting with Albert Sabin and 1984 Rotary International President Carlos Canseco.

children into kwashiorkor. Kwashiorkor, gross calorie deficiency resulting in whole body swelling and slow death, and keratomalacia (blinding eye disease, a common complication of measles in vitamin A-deficient children) were rampant in Vellore and surrounding villages. It made sense to use the opportunity to push for more immunizations given the need for multiple doses of OPV to predictably protect children from polio. Should we allow a child protected from polio to die of diphtheria or measles? Should RI go alone? Why not work with WHO and the United Nations Children's Fund (UNICEF), which were promoting EPI?

Albert Sabin argued that RI should go all out against polio and not dilute its goal of preventing polio globally by involving itself with broader childhood immunizations. According to him, the EPI was not doing well in many countries. By its second meeting the Polio 2005 Committee had been renamed PolioPlus, signaling our full support for EPI but with special thrust on polio. Four people were instrumental in this change of course: Carlos Canseco, then the RI president and a dermatologist from Mexico; Hector Acuna, former head of the Pan American Health Organization (PAHO); John Sever, MD (all of them physicians); and Herbert Pigman, the RI general secretary. They were convinced that RI should support all immunizations while keeping polio elimination as our focus. Soon PolioPlus became partners with WHO and UNICEF. Indeed, after the polio eradication resolution was passed in 1988, the very first staff unit for polio eradication in WHO was funded by a grant from PolioPlus.

In 1985, PAHO declared an all-out war on polio with an initial grant from PolioPlus to purchase OPV. Brazil had already faced the problem of 3-dose OPV failure and shown the success of annual 2-dose national immunization days—equivalent to our pulse vaccination. There was great progress in polio control in all South American nations under the leadership of Ciro de Quadros, MD, MPH.

In 1988, the World Health Assembly unanimously passed a resolution committing WHO and member nations to polio eradication by 2000. Rotary International was right at the head table with the Global Polio Eradication Initiative, joining WHO, UNICEF, and the Centers for Disease Control and Prevention. On behalf of PolioPlus, I became the rotary volunteer to promote polio control in Zimbabwe, Lesotho, Swaziland, Somalia, Ethiopia, and Sri Lanka.

Jonas Salk's Visit to Vellore in 1983

To obtain the best efficacy from vaccination against polio in the 1970s, we had tried extra doses of OPV and pulse vaccination. Both were successes, but this was not enough for the Indian government to change its policy. Then we tried higher potency OPV and monovalent OPV (mOPV). The former was not practical, but mOPV-1 and mOPV-3 showed 2 to 3 times higher VE than that of trivalent OPV (tOPV). The eye-opener was the effect of type 2 virus in tOPV on infection frequency of types 1 and 3 vaccine viruses. Type 2 vaccine virus was already highly infectious—increasing its potency would not help. Wild poliovirus type 2 had been eradicated by 1999, attesting to the satisfactory VE of tOPV for type 2 polio. Obviously, tOPV coverage was sufficient. Had the VE of tOPV been equally high for types 1 and 3, they would also have been eradicated. But that was not the case.

Types 1 and 3 vaccine viruses, when given as a single agent in oral vaccine (mOPV), elicited a better immune protective response. So type 2 was interfering with the take rate of types 1 and 3. I had no clout to get mOPV licensed, but I also knew that mOPVs would make the vaccination schedule quite complex for the health worker. These studies were done in the late 1970s. In 2005, when polio eradication was floundering over the problem of very low VE of tOPV against WPV types 1 and 3 in Northern India, Roland Sutter, MD, MPHTM, and Bruce Aylward, MD, MPH, wise colleagues in WHO, used our data and convinced India's National Regulatory Authority to license mOPV types 1 and 3 in India. The National Regulatory Authority stipulated that the superior VE of mOPV had to be confirmed within 1 year. Studies confirmed it, and since then mOPVs and later bivalent OPV with types 1 and 3 are sharper tools in current use, promising success in those regions where vaccine failure had been an insurmountable obstacle. The Tamil Nadu state health ministry accepted the 5-dose OPV schedule and drastically reduced the burden of polio. By 2000, WPV transmission had been eliminated in Tamil Nadu, including types 1 and 3.

Epilogue

India was removed from the list of WPV-endemic countries by WHO on February 25, 2012. The day of onset of paralysis of the very last child with WPV polio in India was January 13, 2011. This is proof that all obstacles for polio eradication, sociocultural and biomedical, can be overcome if they are identified, defined, and solved. During the stormy years when WPVs continued to arise in major parts of northern India, I had the privilege of chairing the India Expert Advisory Group that guided eradication activities through the National Polio Surveillance Project. Monovalent and bivalent OPVs are used in India and elsewhere where WPVs are still endemic—Pakistan, Afghanistan, and Nigeria. Wild polioviruses were eliminated in Chad, but WPV-1 importation caused a polio outbreak continuing into 2012.

India had on average 500 to 1,000 children developing polio paralysis daily in the 1970s and 1980s. The humanitarian and economic burdens were disturbingly huge. Today these are things of the past. Soon India will enter the second phase of polio eradication, introduction of IPV in the EPI and under the umbrella of its immunity withdrawal of OPVs. We have to preempt the emergence of cVDPVs and if some escape, intercept them, using IPV.

Call to Action

The rotary movement is an underappreciated global force for public service and public health. There are thousands of other polio stories that joined in spiral after spiral to form a rope. We see the rope and its member fibers and wonder about the rope, made up of individual single fibers, each vulnerable and not strong enough alone to pull weight. But together the rope is strong enough to create global change.

The partnership between state health ministry, RI, and Christian Medical College worked wonders. Today we are planning to recreate history with the same partnership to control tuberculosis (TB) in our district. Tuberculosis is not controlled in India. Experts tell us TB *cannot* be controlled in India. I say, I have heard that one before, more than once.

Tamil Nadu state health ministry and professional medical and pediatric associations intend to join forces to control TB. Tuberculosis is a major health problem that impoverishes families. While polio had just one intervention tool, the polio vaccines, TB control will require the convergence of multiple interventions. Together we promise to get TB under control in Vellore district in 10 years and thus build a model that every district in India can adopt.

Section 3

Undernutrition

Chapter 10

Malnutrition Crisis Intervention in Niger

Susan Shepherd, MD, FAAP
Stéphane Doyon, BA
Jonathan M. Spector, MD, FAAP

"It is no longer possible to regard protein-energy malnutrition simply as the result of poverty, so that its solution must wait on improvement in economic conditions. It must, on the contrary, be regarded as an evil in its own right, causing millions of unnecessary deaths, which we must and can prevent."

— Professor John C. Waterlow

Introduction: Niger 2005, the Year Everything Changed

Hot, dusty winds were blowing down from the Sahara Desert across the Sahelian city of Maradi, Niger, in late March 2005, and along with the winds came droves of thin, malnourished young children. They were streaming into the therapeutic feeding program run by the international, independent medical humanitarian organization we work for, Médecins Sans Frontières (MSF) (Doctors Without Borders). Although the weather was typical for the season, the numbers of malnourished children were exceptional—3- to 4-fold more than March the previous year. At the time, no one had a clear understanding of why this was. There had been no obvious trigger, no epidemic disease, no war. The 2004 harvest had been less productive than expected, but there was food in the markets. Yet there they were, thousands of emaciated children.

Médecins Sans Frontières field teams scrambled to set up more than 20 outpatient feeding centers and field hospitals across the region. By June, journalists and television cameras arrived and the stage was set for a tense and public debate—was this an emergency or just the usual state of affairs in this Western African country where child malnutrition and mortality rates were among the highest in the world? By insisting on medical treatment with therapeutic food for these acutely malnourished children, was MSF, a veteran emergency humanitarian actor, in some way derailing the progress of development?

The Niger crisis in 2005 is as fitting a lens as any through which to critically examine affairs relating to advocacy for children affected by malnutrition. The crisis prompted what was by far the largest nutrition emergency response in the history of MSF. It was also the most effective. By the end of the year, MSF alone had treated more than 60,000 children for severe acute malnutrition (SAM) with recovery rates that surpassed 80%, much higher than those achieved in previous emergencies.[1] Lessons we learned in the process, in particular those yielded by the successful scale-up of an outpatient treatment strategy that had been recently developed by colleagues in Sudan and Ethiopia, continue to inform the way we approach the programmatic management of nutrition emergencies and our advocacy activities.[2]

Understanding Malnutrition

Childhood acute malnutrition, defined as muscle wasting (marasmus) or nutritional edema (characteristic of kwashiorkor), is as old as humankind—yet precisely assessing disease burden remains challenging even in the 21st century. The accurate assessment of a child's nutritional status is a complex undertaking with practitioners usually limited to body measurements and clinical examinations. A child's weight and arm circumference can fluctuate rapidly, and the onset or resolution of nutritional edema can take place in a matter of days. With these limitations in mind, it is estimated that between 16 to 20 million children younger than 5 years suffer from SAM, as defined by a mid-upper arm circumference (MUAC) less than 115 mm, weight-for-height z score (WHZ) less than -3, or nutritional edema.[3,4] Children with SAM are anorexic and have markedly increased susceptibility to infections. They have a high risk of death from common childhood illnesses such as respiratory infections, diarrhea, malaria, and measles. Three-quarters of SAM-affected children live in South Asia (8.3 million) or sub-Saharan Africa (3.1 million).

Despite its high prevalence, SAM represents only a fraction of the global burden of nutritional deficiency. Moderate wasting (ie, WHZ between -3 and -2) affects tens of millions more. Stunting (ie, height-for-age <-2) is the most common manifestation of growth failure, affecting 200 million children younger than 5 years.[5] Isolated micronutrient deficiencies such as vitamin A deficiency are even more widespread. In all its myriad manifestations, childhood malnutrition underpins at least one-third of the

7 million deaths recorded annually in children younger than 5 years, the vast majority occurring before age 2.[6]

Treatment strategies for acute malnutrition have evolved in important ways over the past decade. Core principles underlying treatment of SAM-affected children have essentially remained the same: for those who are sick or cannot eat, we must manage and prevent life-threatening complications of malnutrition (eg, hypothermia, hypoglycemia, infection) and slowly refeed to gradually rebuild tissue mass and promote growth. But the vast majority of children with SAM can be detected and treated prior to developing these signs of severe disease, thanks to a new treatment strategy that emerged in the early 2000s, one driven by frustration with aspects of traditional models of care and made possible by advanced technologies in foodstuff production.

Traditional models of malnutrition treatment were based on the belief that children with SAM required inpatient therapy; children were therefore treated for the most part in "nutrition hospitals" that provided therapeutic milk and required admissions ranging for periods of weeks to more than a month. Drawbacks to this approach were many: limited hospital space, heavy human resource requirements, grouping together of highly vulnerable children in close proximity (increasing the risk of infectious complications), and the need for mothers (or other caregivers) to stay in the center with their children, thereby leaving household duties unattended.[7] Clinicians were often forced into untenable decisions of which children would be admitted, and mothers were faced with impossible choices between caring for their malnourished child at the inpatient center and the others at home.

The new way forward was developed originally by Steve Collins, at Valid International and called *community-based therapeutic care;* we now refer to this strategy as Community-based Management of Acute Malnutrition (CMAM). Trailblazers have been able to demonstrate what was previously heresy: if children with SAM are detected early, they can largely be treated as outpatients. Community-based Management of Acute Malnutrition works by providing high-quality nutritional care in or near families' own communities.

Community-based Management of Acute Malnutrition only became possible because of innovations in food technology; specifically, the development of a semisolid, ready-to-use therapeutic food (RUTF) that provides an energy-dense, complete, balanced nutrition specially formulated to support lean-tissue growth in young children. Ready-to-use therapeutic food combines fortified milk powder with peanut butter and delivers the same nutritional value as therapeutic milk in a therapeutic feeding center but in a form that is safe for mothers to feed at home. Because it contains no water and is eaten directly from the sachet, it does not expose children to potential food-borne illness.

In CMAM programs, a weekly or biweekly RUTF ration is distributed to the child's caregiver. Growth progress and assessment for complications (for which hospital referral may be indicated) can be carried out at the time of RUTF distribution. At last there was an effective treatment for SAM that was safe for home-based care. Clinicians redirected their efforts toward screening large numbers of children for SAM and identifying and referring those few who required hospitalization; children who still had appetite and no serious infections could now be cared for by their mothers at home. Instead of programs being limited to treating children by the hundreds in inpatient care, it was now possible to treat them by the thousands.

Progress in Niger

In the heat of the 2005 crisis in Niger, major disagreement ensued on the part of United Nations agencies, the Nigerian government, donor governments, and nongovernmental organizations over the true nature and severity of the emergency. To its credit, however, the Nigerian Ministry of Health worked to quickly enact evidence-based health policy that endorsed the treatment of SAM with RUTF for children 6 months and older. This paved the way for the opening of hundreds of outpatient feeding centers and treatment on an unprecedented scale. As a result, many lives were saved.

In the years since, the Ministry of Health in Niger, supported by groups including the United Nations Children's Fund (UNICEF), Save the Children, Action Against Hunger, Helen Keller International, Concern Worldwide, and MSF, has acted on a common understanding of how best to tackle malnutrition at scale and in so doing has facilitated the treatment of more than 1 million children with SAM. This focus on SAM-affected children has played a role in a virtuous cycle of child health in Niger. Despite its ranking near the bottom of the UN Human Development Index, child mortality rates in Niger are decreasing twice as fast compared with its larger, richer neighbor to the south, Nigeria.[8]

Measures of malnutrition are also improving, vaccination coverage rates are better, use of mosquito nets has dramatically increased, and the number of children receiving appropriate treatment for malaria has quadrupled. All of these improvements have occurred without any detectable improvement in economic circumstances.

Advocacy for Nutrition: "Starved for Attention"

The major advances that have taken place for treating SAM and other nutritional deficiencies have been translated to crucial gains in well-being for children globally. Still, an enormous gap exists between need and necessary action, and food-based nutrition programming has received uneven recognition in influential channels. In 2007, the main UN agencies concerned with child health and nutrition formed a common policy establishing CMAM as standard care for children with SAM,[9] but this policy recommendation was absent from the 2008 Lancet Maternal and Child Undernutrition Series. *Science in Action: Saving the Lives of Africa's Mothers, Newborns, and Children,* a 2009 report from the African Science Academy Development Initiative, identified malnutrition as 1 of 5 major challenges to survival, yet failed to recommend treatment of SAM. In the World Bank analysis *Scaling Up Nutrition: What Will it Cost?*[10] CMAM programming and complementary feeding account for half of the estimated US $12 billion required annually to adequately address childhood malnutrition. Food-based nutrition programming, therapeutic or preventive, is often pushed down the list of priorities due to cost considerations.

"Starved for Attention" is a multimedia campaign launched to further expose the crisis in childhood malnutrition.[11] It was born largely from MSF experiences in Niger and has sought to challenge humanitarian actors, governments, and donors to identify economic models that will provide access to nutritionally appropriate foods for severely malnourished children and prevent SAM. Instead of rejecting out of hand the idea of enhanced nutritious food for young children as too costly, the campaign steadfastly seeks to find ways to make it possible.

The capacity of the MSF to undertake and sustain its nutrition-related advocacy initiatives is grounded in 4 key principles.

1. *Speak from experience and make patients count.*
   Médecins Sans Frontières is a large organization and brings its size to bear to make severely malnourished children more visible. By working to harmonize program monitoring and reporting across all operations,

we have been able to count programs and children more reliably, track our program results, identify programs that are falling short, and work to make them better. Through the "Starved for Attention" campaign we worked with the VII photojournalist group to put real-life stories of affected children and families front and center. These accounts are vivid and compelling and have been successful at engaging new, important audiences. This work earned an Emmy nomination in 2012.

2. *Willingness to innovate.*
   Confronted with large CMAM programs in Niger, some within MSF saw the need to develop new ways to reach children before they developed SAM. In collaboration with the main manufacturer of RUTF, MSF piloted a ready-to-use supplementary food (RUSF) that provides the same micronutrient value as RUTF but is concentrated in a smaller caloric amount.[12] Another form of innovation is experimentation with different MUAC thresholds for identifying severely malnourished children; MUAC is easier to use than weight and height tables, requires fewer personnel and less training, and is easier for mothers to understand.

3. *Commitment to building evidence.*
   As MSF has become more deeply involved in nutrition programming, the organization has committed itself to help build evidence necessary to inform sound policy making. Médecins Sans Frontières and Epicentre (the epidemiologic branch of MSF) have conducted randomized trials within CMAM projects in Niger. Epicentre has shown that RUTF reduces the incidence of SAM when administered to children before they begin to lose weight[13] and demonstrated RUTF to be superior to corn-soy blend porridge for children with moderate acute malnutrition.[14] During a subsequent nutritional emergency in Niger in 2010, Epicentre documented the effects of a large-scale RUSF distribution to more than 70,000 children younger than 2 years and showed a 50% reduction in all-cause mortality.[15] Ongoing studies are examining the effects of various food supplements on the incidence of malnutrition and mortality; to the extent possible MSF is trying to pinpoint the optimal balance between food quality, food cost, and outcomes.

4. *Willingness to engage professionally, publicly, and politically.*
   Médecins Sans Frontières not only has large medical programs and Epicentre but also its own think tank, Centre de Réflexion sur l'Action et les Savoirs Humanitaires (CRASH), and a unit of policy and advocacy

professionals known as the Access Campaign. We have found that the mix of direct field experience, robust data, and respect for the often complex political dimensions of public health frequently sparks controversy and can establish a framework for powerful advocacy. For example, the CRASH book, *A Not-So Natural Disaster* (based on the 2005 Niger emergency), brought to the forefront the inconsistencies inherent in holding mothers to blame for young children's poor diets. It reinforces a general but essential point that improvements in public health require not only intellectual arguments but also political action to widen perspective on certain visions of the world—in this case, the view that health systems must take responsibility for the quality of young children's diets, in much the same way they are held accountable for other fundamental public health programming such as vaccine delivery.

Taking Stock

What happened in Niger in 2005 was called a "hunger crisis," presumably an extreme and unusual circumstance. Severe malnutrition is often recognized to be the product of war or extreme weather conditions. But looking back through several years of program activity, it is evident that *every year* in Niger has been a crisis to a greater or lesser extent. It took CMAM programs combined with staunch advocacy to make severely malnourished children visible and reveal the massive scale of the public health problem posed by severe malnutrition. What was exceedingly controversial in 2005—the treatment of severely malnourished children and distribution of additional food to families with a malnourished child in the absence of war, epidemic, or extreme drought—has since become common practice. With effective treatment, SAM is becoming one of multiple common childhood pathologies treated according to proven practice, similar to respiratory infections and malaria.

Five years into the "Starved for Attention" campaign, where do things stand? The clearest gains are in the treatment of severe malnutrition in CMAM programs, which has become standard of care due largely to the willingness of UNICEF to provide RUTF free of charge to ministries of health that devise treatment protocols. There are now more than 70 countries where children can receive treatment with RUTF. Annual deliveries of RUTF provide enough of this food to treat approximately 2 million children, and there are more than 20 producers of RUTF in 2012 compared with just one in 2005.

As child health advocates in the current era, we have the benefit of leveraging an increasingly rich base of knowledge and experience to help prevent and treat malnutrition. We know that childhood malnutrition remains a major public health issue in fewer than a quarter of the 195 countries in the world and then only within certain regions and certain population segments in those countries. Moreover, some of those with the heaviest burdens of malnutrition actually have considerable resources of their own (eg, India, Nigeria). Secondly, as public health professionals we have seen similar stories play out before; for example, with vaccines and antiretrovirals, with which costs were initially prohibitive. If effective medicines (or in this case, fortified infant foods) are available and the public health benefit is great enough, eventually an economic model will develop that renders them more accessible. No major innovations in health care occur at initial market conditions. Finally, this is not about handouts. People of all economic strata buy food every day. The success of CMAM has shown us very clearly that mothers understand the benefits of healthy foods for their children and many are likely to be willing customers if offered these foods at a cost they can afford.

Regarding specific practices that many of us can put into action immediately, our support can take many forms. These include 1) focused attention to mothers' diets and multivitamin supplementation during pregnancy; 2) promotion of breastfeeding with recognition that this is not at odds with access to quality weaning foods, even if produced by the food industry; 3) work with governments and the food industry to ensure access to high-quality nutritious weaning foods ranging from coupons for meat, fish, dairy, fruits, and vegetables to multivitamin supplementation to fortified weaning foods; and 4) advocating for treatment for children with SAM with RUTF, wherever they may live.

To call malnutrition a complex issue is clearly an understatement. But because a problem is complex does not imply it is insurmountable. If we are to give children a hand up, to help them climb out of poverty, as child health advocates it is our obligation to make full advantage of these practical solutions that can effectively deliver on Professor Waterlow's call to action.

References

1. Tectonidis M. Crisis in Niger—outpatient care for severe acute malnutrition. *N Engl J Med.* 2006;354(3):224–227

2. Collins S, Sadler K. Outpatient care for severely malnourished children in emergency relief programmes: a retrospective cohort study. *Lancet.* 2002;360(9348):1824–1830

3. United Nations Children's Fund. *The State of the World's Children 2012: Children in an Urban World.* New York, NY: United Nations Children's Fund; 2012. http://www.unicef. org/sowc/files/SOWC_2012-Main_Report_EN_21Dec2011.pdf. Accessed May 2, 2013

4. Black RE, Allen LH, Bhutta ZA, et al. Maternal and child undernutrition: global and regional exposures and health consequences. *Lancet.* 2008;371(9608):243–260

5. Stevens GA, Finucane MM, Paciorek CJ, et al. Trends in mild, moderate, and severe stunting and underweight, and progress towards MDG 1 in 141 developing countries: a systematic analysis of population representative data. *Lancet.* 2012;380(9844):824–834

6. You D, New JR, Wardlaw T; United Nations Inter-agency Group for Child Mortality Estimation. *Levels and Trends in Child Mortality: Report 2012.* New York NY: United Nations Children's Fund; 2012. http://reliefweb.int/sites/reliefweb.int/files/resources/ Levels%2520and%2520Trends%2520in%2520Child%2520Mortality%2520Report %25202012.pdf. Accessed May 2, 2013

7. Collins S. *Community-based Therapeutic Care: A New Paradigm for Selective Feeding in Nutritional Crises.* London, United Kingdom: Humanitarian Practice Network; 2004. http://www.odihpn.org/documents/networkpaper048.pdf. Accessed May 2, 2013

8. Amouzou A, Habi O, Bensaïd K; Niger Countdown Case Study Working Group. Reduction in child mortality in Niger: a Countdown to 2015 country case study. *Lancet.* 2012;380(9848):1169–1178

9. World Health Organization, United Nations Children's Fund, World Food Programme, United Nations Standing Committee on Nutrition. *Community-Based Management of Severe Acute Nutrition.* Geneva, Switzerland: World Health Organization; 2007. http://www.who.int/maternal_child_adolescent/documents/a91065/en/index.html. Accessed May 2, 2013

10. Horton S, Shekar M, McDonald C, Mahal A, Brooks JK. *Scaling Up Nutrition: What Will It Cost?* Washington, DC: The World Bank; 2010. http://siteresources.worldbank.org/ HEALTHNUTRITIONANDPOPULATION/Resources/Peer-Reviewed-Publications/ ScalingUpNutrition.pdf. Accessed May 2, 2013

11. Starved for Attention. About the campaign. http://www.starvedforattention.org/about. php. Accessed May 2, 2013

12. Defourny I, Minetti A, Harczi G, et al. A large-scale distribution of milk-based fortified spreads: evidence for a new approach in regions with high burden of acute malnutrition. *PLoS One.* 2009;4(5):e5455

13. Isanaka S, Nombela N, Djibo A, et al. Effect of preventive supplementation with ready-to-use therapeutic food on the nutritional status, mortality, and morbidity of children aged 6 to 60 months in Niger: a cluster randomized trial. *JAMA.* 2009;301(3):277–285

14. Nackers F, Broillet F, Oumarou D, et al. Effectiveness of ready-to-use therapeutic food compared to a corn/soy-blend-based pre-mix for the treatment of childhood moderate acute malnutrition in Niger. *J Trop Pediatr.* 2010;56(6):407–413

15. Grellety E, Shepherd S, Roederer T, et al. Effect of mass supplementation with ready-to-use supplementary food during an anticipated nutritional emergency. *PLoS One.* 2012;7(9):e44549

Chapter 11

Improving Nutrition and Health in Adolescent Mothers and Children in Colombia

Julio Cesar Reina, MD

Introduction

The health and well-being of children and their families in Colombia are far from ideal. Government and civil society-driven improvements in socioeconomic, cultural, and political systems are necessary to meet the 2015 United Nations Millennium Development Goals (MDGs) of eradicating extreme poverty and hunger, achieving universal primary education, reducing childhood disease and maternal mortality, reducing discrimination against women, promoting gender equality and the empowerment of women, and reducing environment degradation.[1]

Colombia is situated just above the equatorial line in South America and enjoys a tropical climate with dry and rainy seasons. In 2009 the estimated population was 45 million, third most populous in Latin America after Brazil and Mexico. Those younger than 15 years make up about 30% of the population. Approximately 75% of all Colombians live in urban areas, and approximately 50% live in poverty. In terms of food security, 9% of the population is below the minimum level of dietary energy consumption and 16% below $1 per day.[2] Figure 11-1 shows the slow but continuous decline of chronic malnutrition in Colombian children younger than 5 years using World Health Organization (WHO) and National Center for Health Statistics standards to 13.2% in 2010, 5 points above the 2015 MDG.[3]

Life expectancy at birth in Colombia is 76 years, similar to Ecuador, Mexico, Venezuela, and the Dominican Republic and slightly inferior to that registered in Brazil, Chile, Argentina, Uruguay, and Costa Rica. As of 2005 life expectancy in Colombia was 7 years less than the United States.[2]

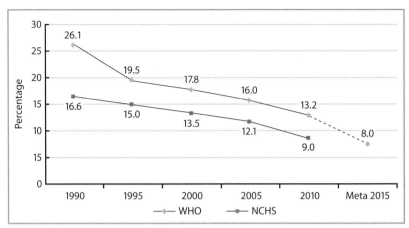

Figure 11-1. Chronic malnutrition rates in Colombia. Decline of chronic malnutrition in Colombian children younger than 5 years. Abbreviations: WHO, World Health Organization; NCHS, National Center for Health Statistics.[3]

In 2009 the birth rate was 19.9 per 1,000 population compared with 17.7 in Argentina, 15.7 in Chile, 14 in the United States, and 11.3 in Cuba, with the worldwide average of 23.2. Overall mortality rate per 1,000 population was 5.8. The rate of low birth weight (<2,500 g per 1,000 live births) was 7, and neonatal mortality (per 1,000 live births) was 11. The infant mortality rate (infants younger than 1 year per 1,000 live births) was 21, and the under-5 mortality rate (per 1,000 live births) decreased from 23 in 2000 to 16. The maternal mortality rate (per 100,000 live births) was 92. There was a low physician and nurse and midwife health workforce (1.5 and 6.2, respectively, per 10,000 population); however, 93.5% of pregnant women received prenatal care and 96.5% of births were attended by skilled health staff. According to WHO and the United Nations Children's Fund (UNICEF), the estimates of national immunizations coverage have shown a decline in the last 5 years, from 96% to 84%. There are, however, some regional differences. For example, in Cali the coverage is close to 98%.[2,3]

Adolescent pregnancy is one of the main public health problems in Colombia. The rate has been increasing in the last 20 years. In 2010, 20% of all pregnancies occurred in adolescents compared with 18% in Latin America, and the adolescent fertility rate (per 1,000 girls aged 15–19 years) was 96, one of the highest in Latin America.[2]

Colombia has important challenges to overcome to improve rates of poverty, unemployment, illiteracy, and inequality. Violence caused by the ongoing armed conflict and drug trafficking must be limited. To progress in these areas, Colombia needs to transform the scattered and fragmented efforts of multiple governmental agencies into a more unified and effective approach that does not tolerate fraud and corruption.

During the last 2 decades the Colombian government has tried to improve the health care and welfare of the population, especially children and women. The Ley 100 (Law 100) was launched in 1993 to promote and improve health care systems, upgrade health care facilities, and improve access to care coverage. One important pediatric initiative has been the WHO-UNICEF strategy of Integrated Management of Childhood Illness (Atención Integrada a las Enfermedades Prevalentes de la Infancia).[4] This program focuses on health promotion and prevention as well as diagnosis and treatment of common childhood illness. The government has also expanded coverage in a public health program to include 96% of the population with an investment equivalent to 7.6% of the gross national product. The national Congress has approved several reforms in addition to Law 100 targeting the MDGs with emphasis on equality for women, ethnic populations, and internally displaced persons. It has also strengthened the child welfare and social protection system. Despite these advances, many difficulties remain with ensuring that services are available and of acceptable quality. The widespread effects of fraud and corruption compromise the availability and quality of care, leading to a great deal of dissatisfaction and disillusionment within affected communities.

Successful advocacy for mothers, children, and families who live in deprived communities requires that an advocate become involved in the community in ways that document problems and improve the lives of people living in the community. My personal experiences illustrate that pediatricians in private practice and academic settings can work in underserved communities, network and create partnerships, and implement sustainable programs. These pediatricians become influential advocates within their communities. I choose to work in Aguablanca, a large socioeconomically and culturally deprived community that makes up 60% of the Cali population. Cali is the third largest city in Colombia with a population of 2.4 million, 60% of which is ethnically Afro-Colombian.

Understanding the Problems of Aguablanca

I first started working in Aguablanca in the late 1970s as the local member of a collaborative working group of investigators who carried out many studies on growth, nutrition, and health in children and adults living in socioeconomically and culturally deprived communities in and around Cali. These studies demonstrated the consequences of inadequate food intake, infectious diseases, malnutrition (Figure 11-2), poor living conditions, and social and cultural marginalization. We demonstrated that the capacity for physical work, as measured by VO_2 max, depends on nutritional status. Undernourished subjects have a depressed work capacity largely because of decreased muscle mass. As productivity is directly

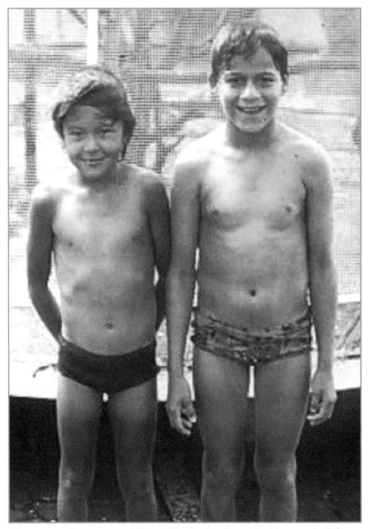

Figure 11-2. Two 11-year-old boys. Marginal malnourished boy on the left.

related to physical work capacity, the productivity of undernourished individuals is depressed.[5] During the growth of schoolchildren, even marginal malnutrition results in growth retardation, slowing of sexual maturation, delay in the adolescent growth spurt, and reductions in physical work capacity because of the smaller body size. In adulthood these smaller boys will be unable to produce physical work as well as their nutritionally normal counterparts.[6,7] Young girls and adult women living in poor communities were also included in similar studies, including energy expenditure.[8,9] These and many other studies document the effects of maternal undernutrition and its consequent effect on fetal and infant nutrition in lesser-developed countries. A high proportion of births in these countries fall in the category of low birth weight, which is a major risk factor for infant morbidity and mortality and subsequent childhood malnutrition.

The problem of maternal undernutrition can be successfully addressed. Antenatal interventions with balanced protein-energy supplements can significantly improve fetal growth and reduce the risk of fetal and neonatal deaths. One such intervention in Colombia in the 1970s significantly increased maternal weight gain and birth weight (+95 g) but had no effect in low birth weight rates.[10] We chose to target adolescent mothers living in Aguablanca to improve maternal nutrition and birth outcomes.

Interventions to Improve Adolescent Birth Outcomes

The adverse effects of malnutrition on adolescent mothers and their babies was highlighted by our research. As a result I have been involved in projects to improve health care and nutrition for adolescent mothers and their children in Aguablanca for the past 18 years. Over this time we have enrolled more than 1,800 pregnant adolescents, 12 to 17 years of age, in a project that promotes prenatal health and nutrition, breastfeeding, care for the newborn, and prevention of repeat pregnancies. We monitored outcomes of our interventions for 335 pregnant adolescents studied between 1996 and 2002.[11] The mean age of these adolescents was 15 years, and weight and height at entry into the program were 50.2 kg and 154.1 cm, respectively. Mean birth weight was 3,115 g. This was similar to our adult controls from the same community. The frequency of low birth weight was 7.7% and was significantly associated with the low body mass index of adolescent mothers. The study used a rigorous prenatal protocol that included screening for intrauterine infections and standard prenatal blood tests and follow-up, as well as health and nutrition education and counseling. The results (Table 11-1) document that adequate prenatal care and frequent follow-up can insure the health and well-being of adolescents and their infants who live in deprived communities like Aguablanca.

This project is currently active in Aguablanca and encourages adolescents who are pregnant or already mothers to attend weekly interactive meetings on educational topics related to healthy pregnancy, optimum nutrition, prevention of pregnancy infections and diseases, normal delivery and care of the newborn, breastfeeding, and vaccines. The project also includes follow-up visits for their babies at 2 and 6 months. When a problem is detected in these meetings or during a follow-up visit, I make arrangements to personally see the baby. During the project I have volunteered at the local Aquablanca public community hospital to work with the hospital director to upgrade pediatric services. This has often involved advocating on the director's behalf for more government staff and resources. Having someone outside the system advocate is often more effective than the administrator requesting funds within the system.

Table 11-1. Outcomes of Interventions for 335 Pregnant Adolescents Between 1996 and 2002

Measures	Averaged Results
Mother's weight 1[a]	50.2±7.2 kg
Mother's weight 2[a]	50.4±7.8 kg
Mother's weight 3[a]	59.2±7.9 kg
Preconception weight	50.0±7 kg
Weight gain	9.2 kg
Mother's height	154.1±5.4 cm
BMI 1[a]	21.1±2.6
BMI 2[a]	22.6±2.3
BMI 3[a]	24.8±2.7
Newborn weight	3,115±445 g
Newborn weight of adult mothers (control)	3,176±537 g
Prematurity (<37 weeks)	9.7%
Low birth weight	7.7%

Abbreviation: BMI, body mass index.
[a] 1: 13.5 weeks; 2: 23.9 weeks; 3: 36 weeks - mean ± standard deviation.

Advocacy Strategies

Implementing advocacy strategies requires creating partnerships that have common aims and goals. In 2005 I helped create Fundaciòn Manos Unidas por Colombia, a nonprofit foundation with the mission of helping people in deprived communities. Sponsoring partners included government agencies and national and local private enterprises and foundations. As a founding member and the current president, I see the power of networking and creating private/public partnerships. Since its inception the foundation has supported Mission Colombia, a project to improve the quality of care provided in community hospitals to low-income patients. The project has provided medical consultations, laboratory tests, x-ray studies, medicines, and surgical procedures. Doctors, nurses, and technical personnel from many disciplines, most of whom live and practice medicine in the United States, come to Cali at their own expense and attend patients during 6 full days. I am in charge of organizing pediatric services. The equipment and medicines that remain after the mission has been completed are donated to community hospitals. Another main goal of the foundation is to build and staff a rehabilitation facility that will care for wounded young soldiers. At the end of 2011 I created another nonprofit foundation with the goal of supporting activities to improve the health and well-being of Cali's under-served and vulnerable children. This foundation is supporting the medical care of children and pregnant adolescents as well as other programs in Aguablanca. I hope that this foundation will be able to obtain financial support from the business community and create an effective voice for the needs of these children and adolescents.

Call to Action

In Colombia, improvements are needed in all programs related to the health and well-being of children, adolescents, and their families. Colombian pediatricians and other physicians need to develop partnerships with government agencies, nongovernmental organizations, and civil society for Colombia to achieve the 2015 United Nations MDGs. These partnerships should
- Focus on disadvantaged children and families.
- Provide government-supported health programs to enable children to learn, so when they become adults they can earn.
- Prevent loss of developmental potential and the cost of this loss for individual children and poverty alleviation.

- Integrate health care, nutrition, education, social and economic development, and collaboration between governmental agencies and civil society.
- Promote sufficient intensity and duration of direct contact with children beginning early in life.
- Promote the idea that parents and families should interact as partners with teachers or caregivers to support children's development.
- Provide quality early child development staff with systematic in-service training, supportive and continuous supervision, observational methods to monitor children's development, and good theoretical and learning-material support.
- Increase schooling for girls because it has a long-term effect on their children's survival, growth, and development.

References

1. United Nations Development Programme. The Millennium Development Goals: Eight Goals for 2015. http://www.undp.org/content/undp/en/home/mdgoverview.html. Accessed May 3, 2013
2. World Health Organization. *World Health Statistics 2011.* Geneva, Switzerland: World Health Organization; 2011. http://www.who.int/whosis/whostat/2011/en/index.html. Accessed May 3, 2013
3. Instituto Colombiano de Bienestar Familiar. *Encuesta Nacional de la Situación Nutricional en Colombia 2010.* http://www.icbf.gov.co/portal/page/portal/PortalICBF/NormatividadGestion/ENSIN1/ENSIN2010/LibroENSIN2010.pdf. Accessed May 3, 2013
4. Organización Panamericana de la Salud. Atención Integrada a las Enfermedades Prevalentes de la Infancia (AIEPI). http://www.paho.org/Spanish/AD/DPC/CD/imci-aiepi.htm. Accessed May 3, 2013
5. Spurr GB. Body size, physical work capacity and productivity in hard work: is bigger better? In: Waterlow JC, ed. *Linear Growth Retardation in Less Developed Countries. Nestle Nutrition Workshops Series.* Vol 14. New York, NY: Raven Press; 1988:215–243
6. Spurr GB, Reina JC, Barac-Nieto M. Marginal malnutrition in school-aged Colombian boys: anthropometry and maturation. *Am J Clin Nutr.* 1983;37(1):119–132
7. Spurr GB, Reina JC. Maximum oxygen consumption in marginally malnourished Colombian boys and girls 6-16 years of age. *Am J Hum Biol.* 1989;1:11–19
8. Dufour DL, Staten LK, Reina JC, Spurr GB. Anthropometry and secular changes in stature of Colombian women of different socioeconomic status. *Am J Hum Biol.* 1994;6:749–769
9. Spurr GB, Dufour DL, Reina JC. Energy expenditure of urban Colombian women: a comparison of patterns and total daily expenditure by the heart rate and factorial methods. *Am J Clin Nutr.* 1996;63(6):870–878
10. McKay H, Sinisterra L, McKay A, Gomez H, Lloreda P. Improving cognitive ability in chronically deprived children. *Science.* 1978;200(4339):270–278
11. Reina JC. El recién nacido hijo de madre adolescente. In: Restrepo C, et al, eds. *Pediatria Catorse.* 2005:30–40

Chapter 12

Improving Nutrition in Rural China

Zonghan Zhu, MD

Introduction

Early childhood nutrition builds the foundation for a healthy adulthood. Improving child nutrition and promoting a nurturing home environment that will support optimal growth and development protects a child's brain development and improves future social abilities that are critical components of human development.

Chinese nutritional studies showed the following[1]:

1. Although there was a significant improvement in the nutritional status of children in China, there were still disparities related to poverty, urban and rural areas, and ages.
2. Underweight, stunting, and anemia were still outstanding problems in rural areas, especially in poor rural areas.
3. The age period of 6 to 36 months was the peak time for undernutrition and this was often not appreciated or ignored.
4. Interventions to address feeding problems during the first 36 months are key to improving early childhood nutrition in rural areas.

A number of nutritional studies on infants and young children in rural China have indicated that early weaning and inadequate complementary feeding in terms of quantity and quality were key problems.[2] For example, Dai Yaohua, MD, and her colleagues from the Capital Institute of Pediatrics surveyed 3 poverty-stricken counties. From the survey, the daily diet for infants in those rural areas did not provide sufficient nutrition. The main reasons for the feeding problems during early childhood in rural areas were

1. Limited knowledge of feeding and understanding of the importance of child nutrition by parents in rural areas.

2. Rural families usually fed their children with rice soup or noodle soup and rarely gave their children meat and eggs. Therefore, the nutritional composition and density of these foods were not sufficient to meet the child's daily requirement.

3. Food supply and cooking methods for complementary feeding were suboptimal. The more remote the area, the more scarce was the food supply. Remote villagers had great difficulty getting the nutritious food needed for their children. The problem was compounded by the lack of refrigeration needed for food storage. Refrigerator penetration was very low in rural families.

4. Economic conditions of poor rural households limited their capability to purchase nutritionally enriched food.

5. The local government and community had not yet recognized the importance of early childhood nutrition and had no plans for improving child nutrition.

To solve the problem of infant nutrition and feeding, our fundamental strategy was to educate parents about infant and young child feeding, change their behavior related to selection and preparation of complementary foods, and improve the food supply in rural areas. Despite its complexity, implementing strategies for nutrition could not wait for economic conditions to change. The nutritional status of millions of rural children had to be improved.

Development of Ying Yang Bao

In 2001, the Chinese Center for Disease Control and Prevention Institute of Nutrition and Food Safety, under the leadership of Chen Chunming, MD, proposed the concept of a nutrient supplement package to meet the needs of rural 6- to 36-month-old children. Therefore, an infant complementary food supplement, also known as Ying Yang Bao (YYB), was developed and implemented. Ying Yang Bao includes protein powder and a variety of vitamins and micronutrients (eg, iron, zinc, calcium). Daily consumption of a package of YYB is able to meet 50% to 60% of the daily nutrient requirements of infant and young children.

Ying Yang Bao provided a way to fortify inadequate homemade complementary food to better meet the needs of infant and young children. In 2001, a pilot test of YYB was conducted in the Gansu rural areas for infants aged 6 to 24 months. From 2004 to 2009, a follow-up study of the effectiveness of YYB was conducted. The results showed that the YYB significantly improved the nutritional status of infants.[3] The program decreased the incidence of anemia, increasing height- and weight-for-age z scores, and improved children's cognitive and development quotient.[4] In addition, the incidence of diarrhea and fever during the prior 2 weeks was reduced.

At the same time, research by Dai Yaohua, MD, and Zhu Zonghan, MD, in Shaanxi Province showed that the incidence of anemia after 3 months of YYB intervention decreased from 34.9% to 29.1% and the incidence of low weight rates was reduced by 50%. These studies provided strong evidence that the use and promotion of YYB was an effective measure to improve the nutrition of infants and young children in rural areas.

In view of these results, in 2008 the National Standards Administration Committee and Ministry of Health developed the general standard for complementary nutritional supplements (GB/T 22570-2008) so that production and promotion of YYB would have national regulation.

Promotion of Ying Yang Bao

On the basis of pilot work that achieved these remarkable results, we designed the following 3 models to scale up implementation of YYB in more areas:

1. A donation model
2. A government's support model
3. A social business model

Donation Model

We first tried to seek donations from nonprofit foundations and international organizations to underwrite the distribution of YYB to infants and young children in poor rural areas. In the past decade, we have gained support and donations from many domestic and international foundations and organizations, including the Global Alliance for Improved Nutrition, United Nations Children's Fund (UNICEF), World Health Organization, Plan International, China Development Research Foundation, Children of China Pediatrics Foundation, and China Foundation for Poverty Alleviation. With support from these organizations and foundations, more than 10 projects on nutrition improvement with YYB were carried out in rural areas and more than half a million infants and young children received YYB. Supported by the Ministry of Health and UNICEF, an assessment of those projects was carried out. The results indicated that the nutritional status of children in the project areas was significantly improved. Disseminating the findings from these projects helped mobilize community support, which led to the government paying more attention to infant and child nutrition.

The donation model is simple to implement and has a rapid impact. However, sustainability is of concern because a project often only lasts for 2 to 3 years. Given the huge number of children in expansion areas, the donation model alone is not enough to achieve the necessary scale.

Government's Support Model

The government should take more responsibility for improving early childhood nutrition through the use of YYB. We reported pilot results and experience to the local and central government to gain support. The first local government to respond was Qinghai provincial government, a poor province in western China. When we reported the pilot results of YYB from Ledu County to the Qinghai provincial government, the local government understood the importance of our work and decided to allocate RMB10 million annually to YYB. The project was piloted in 6 counties and then scaled up for the whole province. Support from the local government raised awareness within central government. Chinese Prime Minister Wen Jiabao adopted the YYB approach, and it was considered at the 2012 National Conference on Women and Children. In July 2012 the Ministry of Health and Ministry of Finance decided to allocate RMB100 million yuan in the current year to purchase YYB for distribution to poor rural areas free of charge and conduct health education on child nutrition, growth, and development. This project will be implemented in 100 counties in 10 underdeveloped areas across the country. This is the first nutritional improvement project with YYB to be included in the national financial budget. If this project is implemented successfully, it will be taken to scale throughout the country.

Social Business Model

In more affluent areas in China, parents can afford YYB. Therefore, we wish to encourage a social business model to promote YYB. Social business involves a "non-loss, non-dividend" company providing a market-based solution to a social problem. The social business model, unlike the traditional business model, is not trying to make a profit. The purpose of this new type of business is to provide public service through a marketing mechanism. We mobilize entrepreneurs and investors, shift the promotion model from donation to investment, and establish a social company to improve infant malnutrition and eliminate anemia in infants and young children. Since 2010, 2 social enterprises that produce and promote YYB have been established: NutriGo and TaitaiAi. These enterprises produce and distribute YYB at a price that is affordable for rural families. The 2 companies have already produced a tremendous amount of YYB and successfully distributed YYB to rural areas (Figure 12-1). However, they will need more support from the government and society to overcome financial challenges.

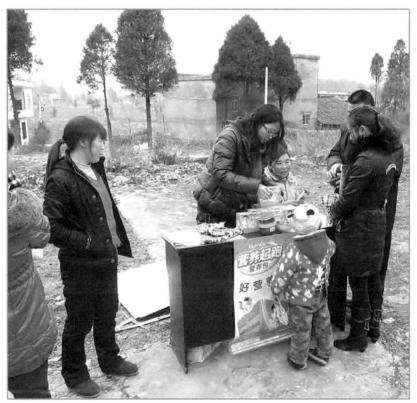

Figure 12-1. Community mobilization. Village health workers were describing the benefits and use of Ying Yang Bao to young parents in Anshi rural area, Henan Province. The photo was provided by Jacky Deng, NutriGo.

Call to Action

In China we face challenges associated with balancing economic development with social human capital development. We have large regional disparities in child health and well-being. Differences in nutrition, growth, and development are related to poverty in rural areas. While we are making progress in improving nutrition in our poor rural areas, we must also develop strategies to educate families about how to provide the stimulation at home that will promote language acquisition and overall development. We know the importance of the quality and quantity of a child's interactions with parents as well as receiving adequate nutrition in promoting brain growth. We need to implement a comprehensive program to promote physical, behavioral, and intellectual development so children will function well in school and have more economic opportunities than their low-income parents.

References

1. People's Republic of China Ministry of Health. *National Report on Nutritional Status of Children Aged 0-6 year (2012)*. http://www.camcn-cns.org/4-report-e.pdf. Accessed May 3, 2013

2. People's Republic of China Ministry of Health. *Report on Women and Children's Health Development in China (2011)*. http://unpan1.un.org/intradoc/groups/public/documents/apcity/unpan051019.pdf. Accessed May 3, 2013

3. Wang YY, Chen CM, Wang FZ, Jia M, Wang KA. Effects of nutrient fortified complementary food supplements on anemia of infants and young children in poor rural of Gansu. *Biomed Environ Sci*. 2009;22(3):194–200

4. Chen CM, Wang YY, Chang SY. Effect of in-home fortification of complementary feeding on intellectual development of Chinese children. *Biomed Environ Sci*. 2010;23(2):83–91

Section 4

Acute and Chronic Health Care

Chapter 13

Diarrhea and Pneumonia: Genesis of a Global Action Plan

Zulfiqar Bhutta, MBBS, FRCP, FRCPCH, FAAP(Hon), PhD
Jai K. Das, MBBS, MD, MBA
Kerri Wazny, MA

Children are a future of any nation, thus accentuating the national and global stakeholder's obligation to safeguard their health and ensure universal access equitably. Achieving this goal can have far-reaching effects on society as a whole, not just limited to health. This can build up to greater gains and serve as a major catalyst for the prosperity, growth, and development of any nation. With this determination, the UN Millennium Summit in September 2000, agreed on by 190 countries, proposed Millennium Development Goal (MDG) 4 to a specific target of reducing mortality of children younger than 5 years by two-thirds from the 1990 baseline by 2015.

In 2011, almost 6.9 million children younger than 5 died, a decrease of 5.1 million from 1990. Despite considerable progress over the last decade, the rate of reduction is less than satisfactory for many countries to achieve MDG 4. The highest burden of child mortality continues to be concentrated in sub-Saharan Africa and South Asia (83%) and with variable coverage of interventions and high birth rates, this gap may continue to widen; in addition, only 5 countries (India, Nigeria, Democratic Republic of Congo, Pakistan, Ethiopia) are responsible for approximately half of these deaths. An estimated 4.4 million (58%) of these under-5 deaths in 2011 were due to infectious causes, of which pneumonia (1.4 million) and diarrhea (800,000) serve as the 2 leading causes of postneonatal deaths (Table 13-1); 15 countries are responsible for two-thirds of total deaths caused by diarrhea and pneumonia (Table 13-2).

Table 13-1. Causes of Mortality in Children Younger Than 5 Years, 2010

Cause of Death	CHERG (%)	GBD (%)
Neonatal	**40.4%**	**41.5%**
Pneumonia	4.3	2.8
Diarrhea	0.7	1.1
Tetanus	0.8	0.6
Preterm birth complications	14.1	11.9
Intrapartum-related events	9.4	7.1
Sepsis/meningitis	5.2	7.7
Congenital anomalies	3.5	2.7
Injuries	0.0	0.4
Others	2.4	7.2
Pneumonia	14.1	9.6
Diarrhea	9.9	8.6
Injuries	4.6	5.4
HIV/AIDS	2.1	1.9
Meningitis	2.4	2.3
Measles	1.5	1.6
Malaria	7.4	9.5
Others	17.8	19.7

Abbreviations: CHERG, Child Health Epidemiology Reference Group; GBD, Global Burden of Disease.
Source for CHERG estimates: Child Health Epidemiology Reference Group. Child causes of death annual estimates by country, 2000-2010. http://cherg.org/projects/underlying_causes.html. Accessed May 3, 2013
Source for GBD estimates: Global Health Data Exchange. GHDx. http://ghdx.healthmetricsandevaluation.org. Accessed May 3, 2013

The total number of deaths in children younger than 5 years has decreased from more than 2 million over the past decade. Four-fifths of this reduction is attributable to the collective reduction in infectious causes, specifically with reductions in deaths caused by pneumonia and diarrhea contributing to 40% of the overall reduction (0.451 million [0.339–0.547] and 0.359 million [0.215–0.476], respectively) (Figure 13-1). Despite this success, pneumonia and diarrheal diseases still account for 2.2 million deaths and remain the major causes of postneonatal child deaths, and pneumonia remains the single largest cause of child deaths globally. Thus, sustained and focused efforts are required to tackle the persistent burden of childhood diarrhea and pneumonia mortality. Trends show that the burden is

Table 13-2. Fifteen High-Burden Countries for Childhood Diarrhea and Pneumonia Mortality

Rank	Country	Deaths Among Children Younger Than 5 Years Due to Pneumonia and Diarrhea, 2010
1	India	609,000
2	Nigeria	241,000
3	Democratic Republic of the Congo	147,000
4	Pakistan	126,000
5	Ethiopia	96,000
6	Afghanistan	79,000
7	China	64,000
8	Sudan	44,000
9	Mali	42,000
10	Angola	39,000
11	Uganda	38,000
12	Burkina Faso	36,000
13	Niger	36,000
14	Kenya	32,000
15	United Republic of Tanzania	31,000
	Rest of the world	537,000
	Total	2,197,000

Source: United Nations Children's Fund. *Pneumonia and Diarrhoea: Tackling the Deadliest Diseases for the World's Poorest Children.* New York, NY: United Nations Children's Fund; 2012. http://www.unicef.org/media/files/UNICEF_P_D_complete_0604.pdf. Accessed May 3, 2013

declining amidst the increasing number of live births, but still the progress is slower and far from achieving MDG 4. The elimination of the remaining deaths would not be easy, will require more concerted efforts, and would not be possible unless major interventions are rapidly scaled up, especially in high-burden regions and countries, in the next few years. Levels of coverage for proven and effective interventions for the 75 countdown countries, where more than 95% of all child deaths occur, must be ensured, and health of populations everywhere must be protected and promoted, not only as a developmental commitment to equity but also an imperative for economic growth and security.

Focused and sustained efforts against pneumonia and diarrhea, while augmenting nutrition, could save the lives of thousands of children globally.

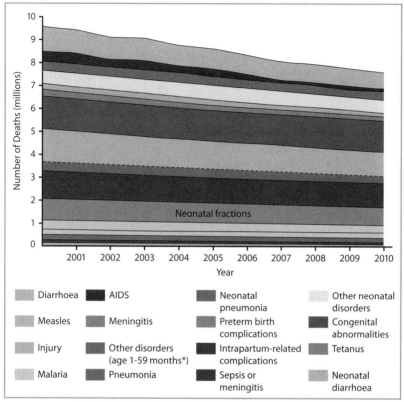

Figure 13-1. Trends in global burden of childhood deaths, 2000–2010. Source: Liu L, Johnson HL, Cousens S, et al. Global, regional, and national causes of childhood mortality: an updated systematic analysis for 2010 with time trends since 2000. *Lancet.* 2012;379(9832):2151–2161.

There is evidence for a range of existing interventions which, if scaled up, can have far-reaching consequences. Of these include exclusive breastfeeding up to 6 months of age, promotion of complementary feeding, vaccinations, use of oral rehydration solution (ORS) and zinc in diarrhea, improved case management of diarrhea and pneumonia, and vitamin A and zinc supplementation. More recently, Fischer-Walker et al estimated that scaling up a combination of 10 interventions for diarrhea in 68 countdown countries could reduce diarrhea-specific mortality by 78% by 2015. They further estimated a mere cost of US $0.49 per capita and an additional US $1.78 per capita if water, sanitation, and hygiene interventions were also included. It is also recognized that many of these direct interventions may have indirect benefits on child survival beyond the specific targeted pathways for reducing deaths and thus can contribute to even greater gains.

Although a global action plan for pneumonia has been in existence for some years, its actual implementation across countries varies considerably. Of the number of countries with high burden of childhood pneumonia, only a few have introduced pneumococcal vaccine and almost none have addressed issues of environmental health and air pollution. Recent findings indicate that only a median of 43% of children in low-income countries with pneumonia are seen by an appropriate care provider and fewer than one-third (29%) receive antibiotics.

The Division of Women and Child Health at the Aga Khan University Hospital took up the challenge of addressing issues related to childhood diarrhea and pneumonia burden and excess mortality. These 2 disorders alone account for half of all postneonatal child deaths in Pakistan, and more than two-thirds of all deaths take place at home. The Department of Paediatrics and Child Health has had a range of research projects related to global evidence and policy in this field (Box 13-1). These projects and the research program date back to the 1980s; at the initiation of research at Aga Khan University Hospital, diarrheal diseases, especially persistent and complicated diarrhea, were a major focus. Much of the research at that time related to optimizing dietary management strategies. Subsequently the team of investigators and research fellows at Aga Khan University Hospital, led by Dr Bhutta, played a key role in defining evidence-based interventions through robust systematic reviews and also in the important area of implementation research. Multiple projects in rural and urban Sindh focused on delivery strategies to the poorest sectors of the popula-

Box 13-1. Interventions Implemented by Aga Khan University Hospital

Interventions for Diarrhea

- Nutritional management in diarrhea
- Vitamin A supplementation
- Zinc supplementation for the prevention and management of diarrhea
- Micronutrient supplementation through micronutrient powders in children
- Community case management
- Solar water disinfection

Interventions for Pneumonia

- Zinc supplementation for respiratory infections
- Vitamin D supplementation for the prevention and management of pneumonia
- Community-based antibiotic treatment for pneumonia
- Vitamin A supplementation

tion through community health workers (CHWs) and delivery platforms. The team has worked on various domains in the prevention and treatment of diarrhea and pneumonia, including the support for enteral nutrition during diarrhea, and the work in this area includes evaluation of nutrient absorption and weight gain with consumption of traditional rice-lentil (khichri), yogurt, and milk diet with soy formula; promotion of use of zinc in diarrhea through co-packaging with ORS and promotion through CHWs; and solar disinfection at the point of use and delivery of care through CHWs. These projects generated some of the first evidence for scaling up zinc and low-osmolality ORS and also the feasibility of scaling up management of severe pneumonia in domiciliary settings using oral amoxicillin. More recently, in a significant breakthrough, the integration of diarrhea treatment and home-based water purification has also been demonstrated.

To expand the work to a global process, we secured funding from the Bill & Melinda Gates Foundation with an aim to plan and organize with multiple work groups a global consensus on research priorities and interventions to reduce childhood diarrhea morbidity and mortality and help develop an integrated action plan for diarrhea and pneumonia that can be implemented in various contexts and would make a difference in reducing equity gaps (Figure 13-2). As a first step, a strategic advisory group, which

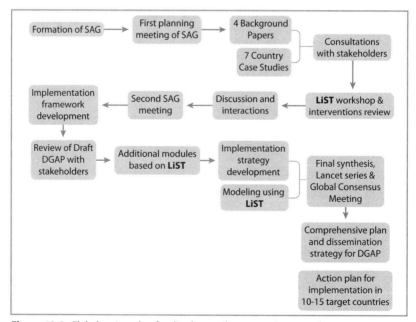

Figure 13-2. Global action plan for diarrhea and pneumonia—a road map.

involved eminent researchers representing lead institutions involved in key research and policy areas across countries, was constituted to steer and provide specific leadership to various streams of work. This project included a range of activities, from developing an inventory of all potential interventions relevant to childhood diarrhea and possible delivery platforms and estimating their effects to specific country case studies in 7 high-burden countries (India, Pakistan, Bangladesh, Vietnam, Kenya, Nigeria, Zambia) (Figure 13-3). A Child Health and Nutrition Research Initiative exercise, which involved various global experts, was also carried out to identify top research areas that would help reduce diarrhea and pneumonia burden (Box 13-2). The work involved all major UN agencies and collaboration with a range of academic partners (Johns Hopkins University; Boston University School of Public Health; the Hospital for Sick Children and Programme for Global Paediatric Research, Toronto) and organizations such as PATH, Clinton Health Access Initiative, and World Vision. Findings and recommendations that emerged from the range of

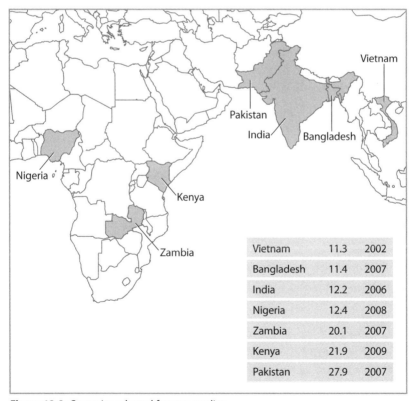

Vietnam	11.3	2002
Bangladesh	11.4	2007
India	12.2	2006
Nigeria	12.4	2008
Zambia	20.1	2007
Kenya	21.9	2009
Pakistan	27.9	2007

Figure 13-3. Countries selected for case studies.

Box 13-2. Research Priorities

We extensively evaluated research priorities using the Child Health and Nutrition Research Initiative method. For diarrhea, we expanded on previous efforts by identifying priorities to reduce morbidity and mortality caused by childhood diarrhea over the next 15 to 20 years; for pneumonia, we identified research priorities to reduce mortality caused by childhood pneumonia by 2015. Each research priority-setting exercise involved numerous global experts who generated the research priorities, which were then scored on the following criteria: 1) answerability; 2) likelihood of effectiveness; 3) likelihood of deliverability, affordability, and sustainability; 4) maximum potential effect on burden reduction; and 5) predicted impact on equity. The research priorities generated fell into 4 categories: description, discovery, development, and delivery.

Research priorities in development, which involve improving existing interventions, and research priorities in delivery, which include health policy and systems research, were seen as priorities in the pneumonia and diarrhea exercise. The top-ranked research questions within these 2 areas are displayed as follows in this box. Within these 2 areas, research priorities involving identifying barriers to health care access (including implementation barriers to increase coverage of existing, effective interventions) and identifying drivers of care-seeking behavior ranked highly. Additionally, the pneumonia and diarrhea exercise identified assessing the effect of Integrated Community Case Management (iCCM) or Integrated Management of Childhood Illness (IMCI) on early and equitable administration of appropriate treatment to be a priority. Furthermore, the pneumonia exercise identified a need to determine if community health workers or community volunteers can be trained to adequately assess, recognize danger signs, refer and treat acute respiratory infection (ARI), and effectively and safely administer antibiotics.

1. Identify the barriers to increasing coverage and ensure interventions that have already been proven to be effective (ie, oral rehydration solution, zinc, *Haemophilus influenzae* type b and pneumococcal vaccines, World Health Organization [WHO] 7-point plan, WHO ARI strategy) are reaching hard-to-reach populations.

2. Identify contextual or cultural factors that positively or negatively influence care-seeking behavior. Which factors most effectively drive care-seeking behavior?

3. Investigate the efficacy of the effect of culture-appropriate health education and public health messages on health-seeking behavior change, hospitalization, and mortality. Which communication strategies are best to spread knowledge and generate care-seeking behavior?

4. What are the main barriers to increasing demand for and compliance with vaccination schedules for available vaccines in different contexts and settings?

5. What is the added impact of iCCM or IMCI on early and equitable administration of appropriate treatment for acute diarrhea and pneumonia?

6. What are the best indicators for measuring uptake of interventions and effectiveness of communication strategies?

7. What is the effect of interventions to support mothers (eg, to reduce maternal depression, strengthen maternal coping, develop problem-solving skills for child health) on child health outcomes?

8. What is the capacity of health systems worldwide to correctly diagnose and manage childhood pneumonia, and what are obstacles to correct diagnosis and case management in a developing country setting?

9. How can we effectively train and sustain trained health workers? Can they be trained to adequately assess, recognize danger signs, and refer and treat ARI, including safe and effective administration of antibiotics?

10. What is the effectiveness of a community-led total sanitation approach?

interventions reviewed (Table 13-3) and country case studies (Table 13-4, showing specific findings from the Pakistan case study as an example) will form the development of additional modules for integration of the implementation framework with the Lives Saved Tool (LiST) for a concerted, broad-based strategy for decision-making and forming the core of the new integrated global action plan for diarrhea and pneumonia (and will also form the basis for a specific series in *The Lancet* devoted to the subject).

An important message emerging from this exercise is that attaining the MDGs will require universal coverage of key effective, affordable interventions complemented by strategies to enhance access. Given the shortage of human resources in some of the poorest areas of the world, this will require alternate strategies or platforms to accelerate the uptake and scale-up of proven interventions. One such strategy is reaching out to poor and difficult-to-reach families through CHWs. These CHWs offer a unique opportunity to address a range of preventive and promotive strategies for women and children (Box 13-3). Such outreach services and task shifting or sharing with physicians may offer a unique opportunity to address the MDGs as well as the challenge posed by noncommunicable diseases. Such delivery platforms also offer a unique opportunity for integrating services at the point of service delivery and enabling an implementation strategy in poor and difficult-to-reach populations. Access to essential drugs and technologies has become a priority for national governments, and removal of bottlenecks to address shortages of critical supplies and commodities, such as ORS and zinc for diarrhea and amoxicillin for pneumonia, have led to the recent creation of the UN Commission on Life-Saving Commodities to help improve the supply chain and insure their availability to countries at scale. The private sector also demands attention, as in many high-mortality

Table 13-3. Key Interventions for Diarrhea and Pneumonia and Potential Effects

Intervention	Effect Estimates
Water sanitation and hygiene	48%, 17%, and 36% risk reductions for diarrhea with hand washing with soap, improved water quality, and excreta disposal, respectively
Household air pollution reduction	Improved stove intervention reduces average exposure by 50% and results in a 16% reduction in physician-diagnosed pneumonia (although statistically nonsignificant).
Breastfeeding education and effects on breastfeeding patterns	Exclusive breastfeeding rates increase by 43% at 1 day, 30% until 1 month, and 79% from 1 to 6 months. Rates of no breastfeeding decrease by 32% at 1 day, 30% until 1 month, and 18% from 1 to 6 months.
Preventive zinc supplementation	18% reduction in diarrhea-related mortality
Vaccines for rotavirus	74% reduction in very severe rotavirus infection 47% reduction in rotavirus hospitalization
Vaccines for cholera	52% effective against cholera infection
Vaccines for *Haemophilus influenzae* type b	18% reduction in radiologically confirmed pneumonia 6% reduction in severe pneumonia
Vaccines for pneumococcal infections	29% reduction in radiologically confirmed pneumonia 11% reduction in severe pneumonia
Oral rehydration solution	69% reduction in diarrhea-specific mortality
Dietary management of diarrhea	Lactose-free diets reduce the duration of diarrhea treatment failure significantly—by 47%.
Therapeutic zinc supplementation	66% reduction in diarrhea-specific mortality 23% reduction in diarrhea hospitalization 19% reduction in diarrhea prevalence
Antibiotics for cholera	63% reduction in clinical failure rates 75% reduction in bacteriologic failure rates
Antibiotics for *Shigella*	82% reduction in clinical failure 96% reduction in bacteriologic failure rates
Antibiotics for cryptosporidiosis	52% reduction in clinical failure rates 38% reduction in parasitologic failure rates
Oxygen systems and diagnostics	35% reduction in severe pneumonia mortality
Community-based intervention platforms for prevention	160% increase in the use of oral rehydration solution 80% increase in the use of zinc in diarrhea 76% decline in the inappropriate use of antibiotics for diarrhea 13% increase in care seeking for pneumonia

Intervention	Effect Estimates
Community case management	63% reduction in diarrhea-related mortality 35% reduction in acute lower respiratory infection–related mortality
Financial support schemes	Conditional transfer programs: 14% increase in preventive health care use, 22% increase in the percentage of newborns receiving colostrum, and 16% increase the coverage of vitamin A supplementation

Table 13-4. Key Areas and Major Challenges Identified From Pakistan Country Case Study

Area	Challenges
Policy, strategy, and governance	Poor coordination Competing priorities
Funding and resource mobilization	Inadequate funds
Planning, management, and coordination	Poor coordination Poor and unstructured implementation practices Lack of public-private partnerships
Human resources	Poor knowledge and skills of health care workers Need for health care worker training Community health workers overburdened with tasks
Service delivery and referral	Poor coordination of government with producers and suppliers Poor procurement practices
Communication and social mobilization	Community engagement
Implementation of water, sanitation, and hygiene	Poor coordination
Supply chain management	Forecasting
Quality of care	Need for health care worker training Focus is on quantity, not quality.
Monitoring and evaluation	Data accuracy, completeness, and quality
Data in decision-making	Data accuracy, completeness, and quality
Public-private partnership	Partner coordination
Production and distribution of zinc and oral rehydration solution	Procurement and knowledge

Box 13-3. Role of Community Health Workers

- Home visitation
- Environmental sanitation
- Health education
- Nutrition education
- Nutrition supplementation
- Family planning
- Community development activities
- Growth monitoring
- Immunization
- First-line management of infectious diseases
- Antibiotic management of pneumonia
- Oral rehydration solution and zinc for diarrhea
- First aid
- Communicable disease control
- Referral
- Surveillance
- Record keeping
- Collection of data on vital events

countries a large proportion of care for childhood illnesses is provided by the private sector. Additionally, many families seek treatment for diarrhea and pneumonia from private retail outlets such as pharmacies and drug shops.

Of the various determinants of burden of diarrhea and pneumonia, poverty remains a major barrier impeding access to preventive and curative services. There is a clear need to overcome these barriers in enhancing uptake of services by provision of incentives as well as universal health coverage. It is notable that domestic health funding in 40 countdown countries is less than 10% of their gross domestic product, so measures are required to increase effective state ownership of public health through schemes such as national health insurance programs, which have been proven a success by a few programs and are being carried out in other lower-income countries like China, India, South Africa, and Colombia. This could prove to be a major scale-up of interventions to address childhood diarrhea and pneumonia and help achieve equity and efficient access to services. It is estimated that comparatively 6 times more lives could be saved in the poorest households by scaling up key pneumonia and diarrhea interventions to near-universal levels. Bangladesh provides a clear example of how this can be done for newborn health and other complex interventions, such as promotion of hand washing, sanitation, and clean water.

These targets of reducing the burden of childhood mortality are clearly in sight but require concerted efforts for ensuring implementation and sustainability. Trends do not represent the potential of new resources to accelerate the rate of decline in under-5 mortality. The major obstacles for the optimum use of resources to scale up the coverage of key interventions include health system bottlenecks such as the health workforce, health system infrastructure, management information systems, supply chain logistics, supervision, and monitoring and evaluation capacity. Progress is good for vaccines, as most countries have greater than 80% coverage, while great acceleration is required for other interventions to meet MDG 4. The key challenge remains delivering these interventions in an integrated manner at scale and to those hardest to reach. Apart from the emphasis on existing proven interventions, we also continue to focus on what is unknown, which includes areas like tropical enteropathy.

Only 22 of 75 countdown countries are on track to achieve MDG 4; 3 countries have made little or no progress. As we address the emerging global development agenda post-2015, it is important to underscore that child survival goals remain tenuous. The recent call for action by the United Nations Children's Fund and US Agency for International Development to reduce global child mortality to 20 or less per 1,000 live births by 2035 is a clear opportunity to keep the focus on saving lives and consonant with the overall goal of eliminating unnecessary diarrhea and pneumonia deaths. The fact that in many poor communities disorders have common risk factors and are frequently seen in the same children lends further credence to the need to integrate diarrhea and pneumonia strategies.

Given the close link with undernutrition and opportunity for integrating child survival and development interventions, a renewed global focus on eliminating childhood diarrhea and pneumonia deaths and reducing morbidity will yield many dividends beyond health. What is needed is the political will and partnerships to make this happen. The key challenge of delivering these integrated and cost-effective interventions to those in greatest need can only be met through concerted advocacy, contextual application of innovations, and robust monitoring and evaluation. We as individuals and members of the global fraternity have a role to play in ensuring that the tangible goal of eliminating diarrhea and pneumonia deaths is achieved and this global action plan for diarrhea and pneumonia can pave the way for reaching this goal in the near future in an organized, coherent, and efficient manner.

Chapter 14

Pneumonia Management: The World Health Organization Approach

Antonio Pio, MD
Harry Campbell, MD

Introduction

In the global health policies of the late 1970s, respiratory infections, with the exception of tuberculosis (TB), were still lost in obscurity.[1] In spite of the fact that pneumonia was one of the 3 major causes of child death in developing countries,[2] the main public and community resources for child health were invested in programs for the immunization and control of diarrheal diseases. The burden of childhood pneumonia morbidity and mortality, which was clearly apparent to frontline health staff in developing countries, was invisible to the advocates of child health in organizations and agencies for international cooperation. International public health policy to control respiratory disease was nonexistent.

The near-complete neglect by international agencies of the problem of childhood pneumonia in developing countries contrasted with available statistics. In those years, in many countries of Africa and in some countries of Asia and Latin America, about 50% of all deaths were in children younger than 5 years. Pneumonia was estimated to be the cause of between one-fourth and one-third of all these deaths, if neonatal pneumonia and pneumonia as a complication of measles and pertussis were taken into account.

The gap between countries located at opposite ends of the socioeconomic scale had extensively widened after the introduction of potent antimicrobials in the 1940s. While the mortality from pneumonia in infants in the United States and Canada decreased at an annual rate of 15%, in intermediate countries of Latin America such as Costa Rica, the mean annual decrease was of the order of 8%. In Paraguay, there was no decrease in mortality from pneumonia in infants between 1968 and 1977. In 1977, the rates of mortality from pneumonia in infants per 100,000 live-born were 30 times higher in Paraguay (1,519.6) than in the United States (50.6). Mortality from pneumonia in children 1 to 4 years of age was 200 to 300 times higher in developing countries than in developed countries.[3]

One did not need to be an epidemiologist to realize at that time that statistics were sufficiently compelling to support a legitimate call for international action to promote the establishment of control programs. However, it was an unforeseen fortuitous circumstance that led the World Health Organization (WHO) to start the development of an acute respiratory infection (ARI) program with the central objective of reducing mortality from pneumonia in young children in developing countries. The program was not put in motion by pediatricians or epidemiologists but by a pulmonologist who was mostly concerned with chronic respiratory diseases in adults.

As part of the debate about the TB program within the Sixth General Programme of Work for 1978 to 1983, the WHO Executive Board and later the World Health Assembly adopted the proposal put forward by the representative of France, Professor E. Aujaleu, that "the tuberculosis program will be extended to the control of communicable diseases of the respiratory system, which as a group form one of the principal causes of morbidity and mortality in many countries. The program should also include the chronic non-communicable lung diseases."[4]

This was an unexpected resolution to the WHO secretariat, in particular to the director of the Division of Communicable Disease Control, W. Charles Cockburn, MD, who was responsible for its implementation. Although the spirit of the WHO governing bodies' mandate was the control of respiratory communicable and noncommunicable diseases in adults, Dr Cockburn, who was a virologist, overlooked the intention of the legislator and correctly interpreted that the main global respiratory problem to be tackled was that of respiratory infections in young children. In consequence, he gave instructions to the TB unit to be the focal point for this activity and to develop an ARI program addressed at young children in collaboration with the WHO units for the control of viral and bacterial diseases.

Historical Review of Advocacy Within the World Health Organization Acute Respiratory Infection Program

From the start, it was clear to WHO staff that advocacy was critical to increase the visibility of the burden of pneumonia, particularly the high mortality, in children and enlist the support of those who could influence the allocation of resources for international cooperation and the ranking of priorities for fund allocation to support national health plans in developing countries.

Three distinct periods can be marked out in the history of global ARI program advocacy, each facing a different mixture of challenges, barriers, and favorable circumstances. Advocacy activities were tailored to highlight the main objectives of the ARI program of each particular period to create an environment that would encourage international agencies to assign high funding priority to the program.

- **Period 1: 1978 to 1982**

  Advocacy to raise awareness of the problem of pneumonia in young children in developing countries among public health authorities, academic institutions, and international cooperation agencies

- **Period 2: 1982 to 1988**

  Advocacy to promote collaboration for testing the technical validity and effectiveness of the case management strategy to reduce mortality from pneumonia in young children in developing countries

- **Period 3: 1988 to 1995**

  Advocacy to support the implementation and global expansion of the ARI program

After 1995, the WHO ARI program as such was disestablished and its activities were incorporated into the Integrated Management of Childhood Illness (IMCI).

Period 1: The Magnitude of the Problem: 1978 to 1982

The main focus of the advocacy activities between 1978 and 1982 was to raise awareness of the problem of pneumonia in young children in developing countries. The major activity of the new WHO ARI program was to compile and analyze information on the epidemiologic magnitude of the problem. The first report on morbidity and mortality from ARIs with singular emphasis on children was published in the *Bulletin of the World Health Organization* in 1978.[5] The wide dissemination of this report among ministries of health and international cooperation agencies contributed to the rapid development of an international recognition that childhood pneumonia, as documented, was a forgotten pandemic—the Cinderella of child health. A growing consensus was achieved that childhood pneumonia was as important a cause of severe morbidity and mortality as diarrheal diseases and that mortality from pneumonia in young children was the most important respiratory problem in the world.

However, no progress was made beyond that consensus for several years. While comprehensive global child health programs on immunization and for the control of diarrheal diseases were pursued actively, doubts and controversies created barriers to progress. Effective specific interventions for the prevention of pneumonia morbidity were limited to immunization against measles and pertussis. Effective vaccines against *Streptococcus pneumoniae* and *Haemophilus influenzae* were not yet available to incorporate within national child immunization programs. Some effect could be expected from prevention programs that included elements tackling low birth weight, malnutrition, and indoor air pollution, but those were long-term efforts. It appeared that only case management (ie, early diagnosis and treatment) could be the central strategy to produce a significant short-term impact on mortality from pneumonia in children, as developed countries had experienced in the previous decades after the introduction first of sulfonamides and later of penicillin and other antibiotics.[6] This analysis led to the next advocacy period in which research and development activities were promoted to establish the effectiveness of the case management strategy to overcome the initial barriers raised against its implementation as a public health program.

Period 2: Advocacy to Promote Research and Development: 1982 to 1988

In the search for a technical direction on case management, the incipient ARI program was hesitant and stalemated by contradictory advice on whether to put the emphasis on research or services.

On one side, the best available epidemiologic scholarship advised that a broad, long-term systematic case management research program was needed to find out the most effective ways to diagnose and treat childhood pneumonia and guide control efforts in developing countries. The arguments pointed out that it was improper and unwise to proceed with a case management program until the many uncertainties and gaps in knowledge were clarified.

- It was not possible to diagnose pneumonia in children without radiology.
- It was generally considered not wise to promote a widespread use of antibiotics in children without a better knowledge of the size, nature, etiology, and pathogenesis of the childhood pneumonia problem in developing countries.
- The legal, professional, and ethical frameworks with most developing countries did not support the prescription of antibiotics by community health workers and paramedical workers who provided primary health care (PHC) services to large sections of their populations.
- The effect of a case management program on the pattern and prevalence of respiratory bacteria resistance to standard antibiotics was not known.

On the other side, experts on public health management could not accept that nothing was known and everything had to be investigated before some control action could be taken. They argued that basic facts in support of a case management control program were well known.

- Bacteria were much more frequently involved in the etiology of pneumonia, as primary or secondary invaders, in developing countries than developed countries. Most severe cases of pneumonia in children were caused by 2 bacteria, *S pneumoniae* and *H influenzae*.
- There was some information on the value of objective clinical signs to identify and classify severity of pneumonia in children.
- There were neither clinical nor radiologic means to differentiate viral from bacterial causation of pneumonia in children.
- Empiric antibiotic treatment for clinical pneumonia was an acceptable practice everywhere. Effective and affordable antibiotics against the most common bacteria causing pneumonia were available.
- It was unjustified and unethical to deny antibiotic treatment to a child with clinical signs of pneumonia because the etiologic agent was unknown or could be resistant to the standard chemotherapy. Clinical experience could not be ignored.
- To resort only to research was not a socially or ethically acceptable response to the problem. Health managers had to act on the basis of what was already known.

This reflected the sentiments of Austin Bradford Hill, who stated, "All scientific work is incomplete—whether it be observational or experimental. All scientific work is liable to be upset or modified by advancing knowledge. That does not confer upon us a freedom to ignore the knowledge we already have or postpone the action that it appears to demand at a given time."[7]

The World Health Organization made a determined effort to work out a compromise to overcome disagreement among experts and proposed a comprehensive ARI program of phased implementation of services with strict monitoring of activities. This was linked to a research program focused on the 2 central questions to be answered.

- What is the validity of clinical signs (alone) for the diagnosis of childhood pneumonia in developing countries?
- How effective is a case management intervention to reduce mortality from childhood pneumonia in poor PHC settings?

This program was adopted by the World Health Assembly as an integral component of the Seventh General Programme of Work covering the period 1984 to 1989.[8] An important overarching consideration at that time was the general strategy aimed at providing PHC services to most of the world's population who had no access to any permanent form of health care. Because of the high morbidity and mortality of ARIs in children, the ARI program was seen as an essential component of the PHC system that was being expanded in many areas through peripheral health units staffed with nonmedical health workers and through community health workers.[9]

The first challenge was to define appropriate clinical guidelines to identify childhood pneumonia in the network of PHC services without radiologic facilities and to treat it by nonmedical health workers (the action by these health care providers having been deemed critical if a significant impact on case fatality was to be made). In 1984, WHO convened a meeting of experts in Geneva to define the technical content of this case management strategy. The invited participants were professors of pediatrics and experts in preventive medicine of developed and developing countries.

During the planning of this meeting, news reached WHO that a young Australian doctor working in Goroka, Papua New Guinea, had developed and tested very interesting new ideas on how to manage pneumonia in children in rural settings. Thus, Frank Shann was invited to the meeting despite his limited number of years of experience and relatively junior position to justify participation in a WHO expert group. This invitation was the most crucial decision taken during the developmental stages of the ARI program. His technical competence and directly relevant experience dispelled prevailing doubts and helped settle controversies. He put forward his innovative proposals with well-constructed arguments supported by the force of his clinical conviction, based on field experience, that pneumonia could reliably be diagnosed in young children presenting with cough or difficult breathing in outpatient facilities, even by community health workers, using 2 simple and objective signs: fast breathing (non-severe pneumonia) and chest indrawing (severe pneumonia).[10] The meeting attendees recommended that the Papua New Guinea clinical protocol had sufficient plausibility to merit further assessment of its validity and predictive value for the diagnosis of childhood pneumonia and evaluation. New controlled intervention trials to assess its feasibility, acceptability, and effectiveness as an approach to prevent mortality from childhood pneumonia in different settings of the developing world would be needed. These were the 2 main lines of research, which were then pursued by the ARI program. Thirty years later, in 2003, the *Bulletin of the World Health Organization* reproduced the 1984 paper by Frank Shann as a "Public Health Classic," ie, a groundbreaking contribution to public health.

The World Health Organization undertook an advocacy campaign targeted at ministries of health, university departments of pediatrics, and health research institutes of developing countries to highlight the critical need to further investigate the diagnostic value of the clinical protocol and determine its effectiveness through intervention studies. This research was to be conducted in rural areas where infant mortality was high, PHC depended on community health workers and nurses, and referral to a hospital was difficult.

The first line of research concerned the sensitivity of the clinical protocol to ensure that antimicrobial treatment be given to most children in the initial stages of pneumonia. Subsequent studies carried out in India (Vellore), the Gambia, Papua New Guinea, the Philippines, and Swaziland highlighted some shortcomings of a single definition of rapid breathing for all children younger than 5 years. These results led to the adoption of a modified definition of fast breathing that varied across 3 distinct age groups: younger than 2 months, 2 to 11 months, and 1 to 4 years.[11] These studies also led to a refinement of the clinical definition of chest indrawing such that only "lower chest wall indrawing" should be taken as a sign of severe pneumonia.[12]

While the technical strength of the case management strategy was being investigated, the WHO ARI team promoted the development of managerial instruments needed for the second line of research, ie, the implementation of this strategy in intervention trials. This comprised materials to train health workers (including videotapes to train them in counting the respiratory rate and identifying lower chest wall indrawing), supervision checklists, logistic guidelines for management of supplies, messages for educational activities and related visual materials, and methods of collection of data to measure selected indicators for monitoring and evaluation.

Institutions in 6 countries agreed to undertake intervention studies with WHO technical and financial support: India (Haryana), Indonesia, Pakistan, the Philippines, Nepal (Kathmandu Valley), and Tanzania. Other agencies supported studies in 3 other places: the Norwegian Agency for Development Cooperation and World University Service of Canada in Matlab, Bangladesh; the Ford Foundation and Johns Hopkins Bloomberg School of Public Health in Gadchiroli, India; and John Snow, Inc. under contract with the US Agency for International Development in Jumla, Nepal.[13]

Two of the 9 studies (Kathmandu Valley in Nepal and Indonesia) compared mortality in children before and after case management intervention was implemented. The other 7 studies compared child mortality in an intervention area with those in a concurrent control area. The trials provided strong evidence that this case management strategy was feasible even in the poorest rural areas. Health workers who were properly trained and supervised were able to recognize the key signs of childhood pneumonia and take appropriate decisions on referral or home treatment with antibiotics. The studies demonstrated that communities were actively involved and motivated to participate in the program.[14]

The trials also showed that the case management strategy resulted in a consistent and substantial effect on pneumonia-specific mortality in children younger than 5 years. This success was reflected in reduced overall childhood mortality, with a meta-analysis of the 9 studies indicating a reduction of 27% in neonates, 20% in infants, and 24% in children 0 to 4 years of age attributable to the pneumonia case management intervention. Pneumonia mortality was reduced by 42%, 36%, and 36%, respectively, in these 3 age groups. The impact was even found among low birth weight infants and in areas with a high prevalence of malnutrition.[15]

Therefore, these research results provided a solid basis from which WHO, and later the United Nations Children's Fund (UNICEF), promoted the case management strategy (after some further refinements) as the international strategy to reduce mortality from childhood pneumonia. In support of this strategy, both agencies funded projects for the development of sounding timers with which to count respiratory rates accurately and for the production of oxygen concentrators adapted to function properly in the adverse environment of small hospitals in tropical countries.[16]

Period 3: Advocacy to Support the Implementation and Global Expansion of the Acute Respiratory Infection Program: 1988 to 1995

The event that marked the start of this third period was the transfer of the ARI program within the WHO structure from the TB unit to the Division of Control for Diarrhoeal Diseases (CDD). This was a logical movement from a programmatic viewpoint as there was no scope for combined technical and managerial activities between the ARI and TB programs. In contrast, the similarities between ARI and CDD were many—same target population of children 0 to 4 years of age; same critical emphasis on a case management strategy delivered by health care providers dealing with children and their parents and other caregivers in the community; same surveillance of bacterial antimicrobial resistance; several common approaches for prevention (nutrition, prevention of low birth weight, personal hygiene); and the possibility of developing common managerial instruments for monitoring and evaluation—epidemiologic and operational household surveys, health facilities surveys, and program reviews.

By 1988, first reports of the intervention field studies in rural settings of developing countries were available. The results provided sufficient evidence to quell the prevailing objections and remove the reticence of the previous period. This led to the building of an advocacy coalition of institutions in support of the implementation of the ARI program with the participation of multilateral organizations (WHO, UNICEF, United Nations Development Programme [UNDP]), bilateral cooperation agencies (in particular from Italy, Japan, the Netherlands, Sweden, the United Kingdom, and the United States), and a number of international and national nongovernmental organizations.

The managerial experience of the CDD program was effectively applied in the development of ARI operational manuals, training modules, health education materials, evaluation surveys, and surveillance sentinel units. There was a close cooperation and also a sense of stimulating competition between the ARI and CDD programs during this period.

A single ARI and CDD program management review committee and single meeting of interested parties were established within WHO in 1988. The most important advocacy activity in support of the childhood pneumonia global program at that time was the First International Consultation on the Control of Acute Respiratory Infections, held in Washington, DC, in December 1991, jointly sponsored by WHO, UNICEF, and UNDP and attended by 405 participants from developing and developed countries (including 16 ministers of health and 27 other high-level health officials).

At the country level, advocacy played a major role in securing political and institutional commitment and the financial resources required for implementing the program. The World Health Organization promoted national seminars and workshops for health managers in which situation analyses were presented to identify possible obstacles to program implementation and advocacy tactics were proposed for removing these obstacles, enlisting the support of different institutions and mobilizing funds for the program such as media coverage, ARI program brochures, networking, and lobbying. A key element in advocacy efforts was the priority given to working with senior and influential pediatricians and other clinicians to convince them of the validity and effectiveness of the case management strategy and enlist their active support and participation.

The number of countries with ARI technical guidelines and plans of operations increased from 18 in 1986 to 82 in 1994, of which 67 had started implementation. At the end of 1994, the results of CDD/ARI household surveys were available in 8 countries and those of ARI health facility surveys in 11 countries.

In the early 1990s childhood pneumonia, the core of the ARI program, was at last given the level of priority in the global health agenda that was appropriate given its importance as the single largest cause of child mortality. However, rapid development of the program was constrained by insufficient international funding and the very scarce number of ARI consultants who could visit countries to help in developing national guidelines, planning operations, and evaluating program implementation. Acute respiratory infection program activities were disadvantaged in comparison with those of CDD because of the program's smaller budget and staff complement at all levels.

The last annual report of the ARI and CDD programs was issued in 1995.[17] In 1996 these programs were disestablished within the WHO structure and superseded by the IMCI program. Ten WHO programs and units had been involved since 1992 in developing the new approach, which at the beginning was cautiously called just an initiative.[18] All case management activities for the control of pneumonia and diarrheal diseases were integrated into the new approach together with those addressing other common and important child health problems.

Transition from disease-specific programs to integrated approaches had strong managerial bases and was welcomed by most public health managers. The most compelling reasons were those related to decentralization and the efficient use of limited resources in developing countries. However, in practice, the lack of focus on specific diseases also meant lack of visibility, diminished financial support, and slower progress in achieving epidemiologic goals.

Lessons on Advocacy From the Experience of the World Health Organization Acute Respiratory Infection Program

From its beginning, the WHO ARI program combined integrated and vertical managerial policies. The focus on a single disease, childhood pneumonia, was a vertical approach, but the delivery of the case management strategy was fully integrated into the PHC system. Diagnosis and treatment of pneumonia in children has been and always should be the responsibility of multipurpose health workers at outpatient services and small hospitals. In addition, managerial support at the district level is and should always remain a function of PHC administrators and supervisors. Thus, integration at health care delivery points and at the managerial district level was essential. However the specialized approach and visibility of the ARI program within the structure of WHO and at the central level of national ministries of health were crucial to develop effective advocacy in the 3 successive periods, as the focus was altered following the changing priorities as progress was being made. At the start, the objective was to create an awareness of the problem. Once the magnitude of the problem had been recognized, advocacy was directed at raising support for field research to test the technical strength of the case management strategy and its feasibility and effectiveness to reduce mortality in the most adverse socioeconomic settings of the developing world. Finally, advocacy was needed to promote the development of managerial tools (materials for training, logistics, health education, supervision, and evaluation) and to persuade national health authorities and cooperation agencies to implement the case management strategy through the PHC infrastructure.

The best advocacy plans, created and delivered perfectly, fail to have a health effect if the advocated strategy is technically incorrect or weak and its effectiveness not clearly established. At the height of the clamor for action when the magnitude of the childhood pneumonia problem was recognized in the early 1980s, there was some pressure to start implementation of the case management strategy urgently. However, the strategy lacked credibility and so its advocacy confronted serious objections, especially from UNICEF, which found it difficult to accept that community health workers would be able to identify and treat children with pneumonia. At that time a high-ranking UNICEF officer used to say that their child health plane could fly with 2 engines: diarrhea control and immunizations. In attempting to move fast, the ARI program risked overlooking weaknesses and oversimplifying complex elements of the strategy. The delay in implementing national control programs based on the novel case management guidelines caused some initial disappointment but ultimately provided time for the essential foundations of a solid and effective case management strategy to be put in place.

In retrospect, the use of the term *ARI program* was not ideal because it masked the central objective of the case management strategy, which was to prevent deaths from *pneumonia* in children. It would have been more appropriate to have adopted a name referring specifically to childhood pneumonia. This would have been more widely understood and would have resulted in fewer variations at local, national, and international level in the same way as "Stop TB" became the name of TB control everywhere, at international, national, and local levels. At present there is a tendency to use acronyms with some inspirational meaning, such as MPOWER (for "empower"), which is the prevailing name of tobacco control programs (*m*onitoring the problem, *p*rotecting nonsmokers, *o*ffering help to smokers, *w*arning on smoking habit risks, *e*nforcing legislation against tobacco advertising, and *r*aising tobacco taxes). A possible inspirational acronym for advocacy of the childhood pneumonia program would have been APPEAL, meaning *a*ction *p*rogram on *p*neumonia in *e*arly *l*ife, to reflect the need for many years to appeal to the international community to take this problem seriously and give it the priority it then deserved and continues to deserve today.

Acknowledgments

The promotion and development of the ARI program was the product of a considerable amount of innovative work by many gifted professionals in developed and developing countries with the support of a broad range of academic institutions and international cooperation agencies.

The program was particularly indebted to the directors of the Division of Diarrhoea and Acute Respiratory Disease Control, Michael Merson and James Tulloch, and to the members of the WHO staff who, collaborating with the authors of this chapter, made outstanding contributions to its rapid progress: Sandy Gove, for the coordination of research activities, refinement of the case management strategy, and development of evaluation guidelines; Adriano Cattaneo, for the field-testing of training materials and evaluation guidelines; Gretel Pelto, for the design and conduct of behavioral research, which generated ethnographic data on beliefs and practices of families related to pneumonia in children; and Robert Hogan, for the development and testing of the training course for program managers and supervisors.

The program was greatly benefitted by the professional input and help of external consultants, in addition to the contribution made by Frak Shann (Australia), which is mentioned in the text of the chapter: Robert Douglas (Australia), Juan Manuel Borgoño (Chili), and Alexander Muller (the Netherlands), for the chairmanship of the advisory technical group that provided technical guidance to the program; Felicity Savage King (United Kingdom), for the development and testing of the first training course for health care providers; and Stephen Berman (United States), for valuable advice and generous sharing of views on clinical guidelines and research priorities.

The achievements of the ARI program would not have been possible without the results of commissioned and noncommissioned critical studies carried out in many countries in the 1980s. The program owes a great deal to David Miller (United Kingdom), Ian Riley (Australia), Robert Black (United States), and Betty Kirkwood (United Kingdom) for epidemiologic research; Kim Mulholland (Australia), Eric Simoes (India), Thomas Cherian (India), Mark Steinhoff (United States), and Lulu Muhe (Ethiopia) for clinical research; and the principal investigators of the intervention studies that showed the feasibility and effectiveness of the case management strategy: Vijay Kumar (India), A. J. Khan (Pakistan), F. D. Mtango (Tanzania), Runisar Roesin (Indonesia), M. R. Pandey (Nepal), and Thelma Tupasi (Philippines).

References

1. Monto AS, Johnson KM. Respiratory infections in the American tropics. *Am J Trop Med Hyg.* 1968;17(6):867–874

2. Jellife D. Pediatrics. In: King M, ed. *Medical Care in Developing Countries: A Symposium From Makerere.* Nairobi: Oxford University Press; 1966

3. Pio A, Leowski J, Ten Dam HG. The magnitude of the problem of acute respiratory infections. In: Douglas R, ed. *Acute Respiratory Infections in Children: Proceedings of an International Workshop.* Adelaide, Australia: University of Adelaide; 1985:3–16

4. World Health Organization. *Sixth General Programme of Work Covering a Specific Period (1978–1983). Official Records of the World Health Organization.* No. 233, Annex 7. Geneva, Switzerland: World Health Organization; 1976

5. Bulla A, Hitze KL. Acute respiratory infections: a review. *Bull World Health Organ.* 1978;56(3):481–498

6. Clinical management of acute respiratory infections in children: a WHO memorandum. *Bull World Health Organ.* 1981;59(5):707–716

7. Hill AB. The environment and disease: association or causation? *Proc R Soc Med.* 1965;58:295–300

8. World Health Organization. *Seventh General Programme of Work Covering the Period 1984–1989.* Health for All Series No. 8. Geneva, Switzerland: World Health Organization; 1982

9. Pio A. Acute respiratory infections in children in developing countries: an international point of view. *Pediatr Infect Dis.* 1986;5(2):179–183

10. Shann F, Hart K, Thomas D. Acute lower tract respiratory infections in children: possible criteria for selection of patients for antibiotic therapy and hospital admission. *Bull World Health Organ.* 1984;62(5):749–753

11. WHO guidelines on detecting pneumonia in children. *Lancet.* 1991;338(8780):1453–1454

12. Pio A. Standard case management of pneumonia in children in developing countries: the cornerstone of the acute respiratory infection programme. *Bull World Health Organ.* 2003;81(4):298–300

13. Rasmussen Z, Pio A, Enarson P. Case management of childhood pneumonia in developing countries: recent relevant research and current initiatives. *Int J Tuberc Lung Dis.* 2000;4(9):807–826

14. Pio A. Public health implications of the results of intervention studies. *Bull Int Union Tuberc Lung Dis.* 1990;65(4):31–33

15. Sazawal S, Black RE; Pneumonia Case Management Trials Group. Effect of pneumonia case management on mortality in neonates, infants, and preschool children: a meta-analysis of community-based trials. *Lancet Infect Dis.* 2003;3(9):547–556

16. Pio A. Appropriate technology for the administration of oxygen to children at district hospitals in developing countries. *Int J Tuberc Lung Dis.* 2001;5(6):493–495

17. World Health Organization Division of Diarrhoeal and Acute Respiratory Disease Control. *1994-1995 Report, Including a Summary of Research and Development Achievements From 1980 to 1995 and Future Directions of the Division of Child Health and Development.* Geneva, Switzerland: World Health Organization; 1996

18. Integrated management of the sick child. *Bull World Health Organ.* 1995;73(6):735–740

Chapter 15

Preventing Diarrheal Diseases Through Sanitation in Peru

Claudio F. Lanata, MD, MPH

Introduction

Diarrheal diseases continue to be one of the most important public health problems affecting children younger than 5 years in developing countries. As documented by the Child Health Epidemiology Reference Group of the World Health Organization (WHO) and United Nations Children's Fund, the burden of acute diarrheal diseases has not changed despite an impressive reduction in the estimated number of worldwide child diarrheal deaths from 3.5 million in the 1980s to 712,000 in 2011.[1] This reduction in mortality is mostly attributable to oral rehydration solutions, the availability of antibiotics, and improved access to health services. Children younger than 5 years had an estimated rate of 2.2 episodes per child per year in 1980[2] (the low rate found in studies selected in this review used different surveillance methods from later studies), 3.0 episodes in 1990,[3] 3.2 episodes in 2001,[4] and 3.4 episodes per child per year in 2010.[5] It remains unclear why acute diarrhea rates have not decreased in the developing world during this time frame despite increased coverage of water, sanitation, and measles vaccine and improved nutritional status. Much of my career has been spent studying determinants of acute and persistent diarrhea, trying to understand what measures can overcome these determinants, and advocating for governmental policies that will implement measures to reduce this disease burden.

Determinants of Diarrhea in Lima, Peru

Background and Epidemiology

I began working in this area during my infectious diseases fellowship under the mentorship of Myron M. Levine, MD, at the Center for Vaccine Development at the University of Maryland. When I returned to Peru,

I joined the Instituto de Investigación Nutricional (IIN), a private, non-profit Peruvian nongovernmental research organization. My first project at the IIN was a study to identify causes of diarrhea in children younger than 5 years living in Canto Grande, a shantytown in the northern part of Lima, Peru. This study was a collaboration of Johns Hopkins University, Peruvian University Cayetano Heredia, and the IIN. Field-workers visited these households 3 times per week to identify and obtain a stool sample from children having a diarrheal episode. This was followed by a similar study in Canto Grande that focused on persistent diarrhea. These 2 studies influenced my subsequent research interests and child advocacy activities. We learned that children younger than 5 living in Canto Grande had a mean of 9 episodes of diarrhea per child per year from 6 to 18 months of age (Figure 15-1). The diarrhea rate was lower in the first 6 months of life and then later after 18 months of life.[6] The lower rate in infants younger than 6 months probably resulted from acquired maternal immunity and additional protection related to exclusive breastfeeding. Exclusive breast-feeding has been shown to prevent 30% to 50% of diarrhea in infants.[7] The peak rate of diarrhea between 6 to 18 months of age was associated with the introduction of weaning foods that were often heavily contaminated

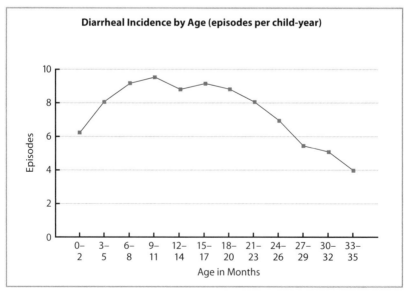

Figure 15-1. Incidence (episodes per child per year) of diarrhea in children 0 to 35 months of age in Canto Grande, a peri-urban of Lima, Peru, January 1985–March 1987.

with fecal coliforms. In this community the highest levels of fecal coliform contamination were found in food served to infants and young children. Milk-based products, rice, stews, and foods prepared at home and stored at room temperature for a prolonged period before serving had the highest amount of contamination.[8] Because these types of food did not appear or taste contaminated, they were often eaten without concern.

Sources of Bacterial Contamination

The sources of contamination varied. Kitchen utensils were almost always contaminated. Kitchen sponges were identified as an important contamination method. They usually remained wet, had repeated contact with food residues on contaminated surfaces, and were a very favorable environment for bacterial growth. These sponges contaminated the mothers' hands and therefore facilitated contamination to kitchen utensils and foods. Another common source of contamination for infants was the use of baby bottles. In the study 35% of baby bottles and rubber nipples were contaminated before any milk was added due to frequent reuse and poor cleaning techniques. Evaporated milk was also a source of contamination. While evaporated milk was sterile when first opened, 26% of samples became contaminated within 4 hours when left at room temperature.[8] Most households had free-range chickens in their houses. *Campylobacter jejuni* was isolated with high frequency in the cloaca of those chickens, and the bacteria survived up to 48 hours in chicken feces deposited in the household soil, particularly in soil kept humid in the shade.[9] Toddlers were observed touching chicken feces up to 3½ times per day when crawling, explaining in part why *C jejuni* was frequently isolated as a cause of diarrhea in these children. *Salmonella,* an organism associated with eggs and chicken meat processed at an industrial level, was rarely isolated in this community because eggs and chicken were purchased in local live markets. In the local market chickens were killed and processed in front of the purchaser in a way that caused heavy contamination of the meat with *C jejuni* from the chicken's intestines (Figure 15-2). Cutting chicken meat in their kitchen and then using the kitchen cloth or sponge to clean the cutting surface spread *Campylobacter* to other foods and containers.

Immunity

A child's immunity affected the frequency of diarrhea. Children who were anergic to antigens like *Candida, Trichophyton,* tuberculin, and others had the higher risk of diarrhea in the next 6 months compared with infants

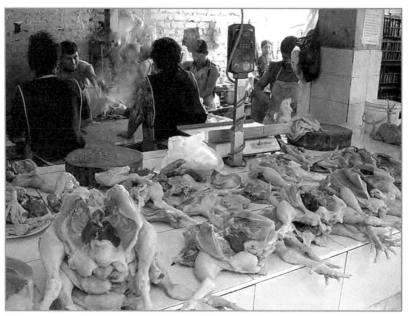

Figure 15-2. Chickens sold in a live market in Canto Grande, Lima, Peru.

who reacted.[10] When we applied the same antigens later, their newly developed ability to respond was correlated with their diarrhea risk. Cellular immunity was therefore identified as an important component in the host. Zinc deficiency has an adverse effect on cellular immunity. Zinc levels were very low in blood samples taken from these children— more than 80% were classified as being zinc deficient.[11] Consumption of foods with zinc highly bioavailable, like animal proteins or sea products, was very low in this population. Zinc has been identified as a very important risk factor for diarrheal diseases, particularly persistent diarrhea.[12]

Water and Sanitation

In Canto Grande, water was a very limited and expensive resource. It was purchased from cistern trucks and then stored in 200-L metal drums or small cement tanks. In a 12-hour in-house observation study,[13] we saw that families had a very elaborate scheme of water reutilization, starting with the "cleaner" uses and finishing with the step considered the "dirtiest." There were a mean of 8 to 10 water uses between the time it was taken from the tank or drum until it was finally discharged in the household floor. The greatest proportion of the water was used for laundry. Mean water consumption per person during the 12-hour observation period was only 10 L. Only 1 of the 10 L was used for personal hygiene, so the frequency and quality of hand-washing practices were very poor. In intra-household observation studies, we documented that mothers very infrequently washed their hands with water and soap after defecation.[13,14] In general, hand washing was usually done with only water, rubbing palms or tips of fingers. This was even less frequently done by infants and children. The importance of increasing household water availability to improve hygiene practices was clearly demonstrated by this work. Sanitation issues were also highlighted by our work. Although the majority of households had latrines, they were used mostly by adults as an emergency measure. Most adults preferred to defecate in open areas in the nearby hills. Latrines were considered "dirty" and dangerous for children to use. Feces of infants and young children were felt to be different and somehow cleaner, not considered "dirty."[15]

Giardia lamblia, enterotoxigenic *Escherichia coli,* and *C jejuni* were the most important organisms identified in stool samples obtained in mild diarrheal episodes, while rotavirus was the predominant agent in more severe diarrhea.[16] More than one pathogen was identified in a significant proportion of stool samples. When microbiologic studies were done in stools obtained from the same children when healthy, these same enteropathogens were also isolated. It was not possible to determine whether these positive cultures in healthy children indicated prolonged excretion once the diarrheal episode was terminated or asymptomatic infections due to the child's immunity.

Interventions

Improved Sanitation

Subsequent to these initial studies, we carried out many studies to document the effect of different interventions on reducing rates of diarrhea. Having identified the negative influences of poor hygiene practices, contaminated water at the household level, and free-range chicken in the houses in peri-urban Lima, we conducted an open randomized trial with 500 households to evaluate the efficacy of hand-washing promotion, avoiding water contamination, and corralling chickens in 500 households with children 6 to 35 months of age. These households had uncovered water reservoirs, dirt floors, and free-range chickens. We randomized 100 households to a personal hygiene intervention group that received a hand-washing education program. These homes had a hand-washing corner set up with a water container and free soap. Soap was weighed daily to document use (Figure 15-3A).[17] Another 100 households had a clean water intervention that covered the water reservoirs with a cement top and installed a faucet. Each family received a narrow-neck water container with

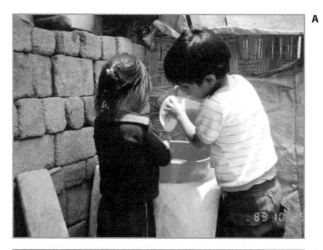

A

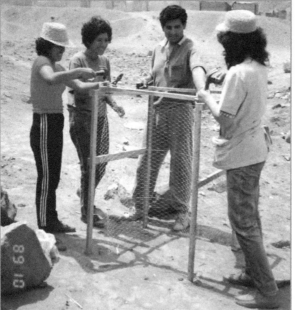

B

Figure 15-3. Interventions to control diarrheal diseases in peri-urban Lima: *A,* child helping sister wash her hands with soap and water in the household hand-washing corner; *B,* corral constructed to cage free-range chickens.

instructions not to use any other type of water reservoir. In another 100 households we corralled all chickens (Figure 15-3B) and implemented an education program focused on the need to keep household soil free of animal or human fecal material. We gave mothers a playpen and instructed them not to allow their children to crawl on the floor. In an additional 100 households we implemented all 3 interventions together to evaluate possible additive effects. Finally, in the remaining 100 control households, there were no interventions. The only intervention that reduced diarrhea episodes was the hand-washing intervention, but only when soap was adequately used. We did not see any effect of the water quality intervention or corralling of chicken and preventing infants from crawling on the floor.

Knowing the frequency of fecal contamination of household soil and the risk imposed to crawling toddlers,[18] further anthropologic studies determined that most mothers of toddlers wanted their children to use potties to avoid contaminating their households.[19] We developed an educational intervention to promote potty training. The program reduced diarrhea rates in a small pilot trial, but a larger trial done in collaboration with the Ministry of Health was compromised by the failure to properly carry out the training.[20]

Zinc

Understanding the importance of cellular immunity and zinc deficiency as risk factors for diarrhea and persistent diarrhea, we were part of the group evaluating the efficacy of zinc supplementation on diarrhea and growth. A placebo-controlled supplementation trial of zinc administered daily to young children demonstrated a 20% reduction of diarrhea and 50% prevention of persistent diarrhea, as compared with placebo.[21]

Infant Feeding Practices

Our group strongly promoted exclusive breastfeeding, and we successfully advocated with WHO and other agencies to incorporate this concept into the official policies of the Peruvian Ministry of Health. We also studied ways to improve food hygiene and home-based practices. We developed training programs to eliminate the use of baby bottles and instead offer a cup or glass. We carried out a trial done in rural Peru to expose kitchen cloths and sponges to the sun for disinfection (Figure 15-4) combined with sun exposure of drinking water and the installation of a kitchen sink with running water to promote hand washing.[22,23] The results demonstrated a reduction of diarrheal diseases in 250 households compared with 250 control households.

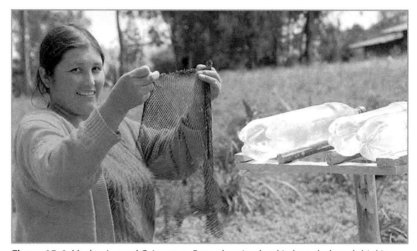

Figure 15-4. Mother in rural Cajamarca, Peru, showing her kitchen cloth and drinking water bottles exposed to solar disinfection.

Rotavirus Vaccine

Despite efforts to reduce environmental determinants of diarrhea, success in reducing the burden of diarrheal diseases has been elusive. Therefore, the development and introduction of rotavirus vaccine has been an important breakthrough. The development and testing of an effective rotavirus vaccine as the most important cause of severe diarrheal diseases began in the 1980s. Evaluation of the safety, immunogenicity, and efficacy of RIT 4237 bovine rotavirus vaccine[24] was our first vaccine trial. This vaccine was selected because it was found to be safe and protective in Finland. However, questions about its efficacy in developing countries were raised after disappointing initial findings of a study in Africa. After the first year of surveillance, the committee overseeing the vaccine development program at WHO decided to open the study code. Because the preliminary results of our trial after only 1 year showed low efficacy against rotavirus diarrhea, an alternative rhesus-based rotavirus vaccine was selected for development. When we published our final results, it became clear that the presence of mixed infections was not adequately considered in the first-year preliminary results. Our findings demonstrated that RIT 4237 rotavirus vaccine was protective against rotavirus-only diarrheal episodes (eliminating those with mixed infections) and most importantly, against severe rotavirus diarrhea and serotype 1 rotavirus.[24] The alternative rhesus-based rotavirus vaccine, developed by the National Institutes of Health,[25-27] had to be withdrawn due to a rare complication of intussusception in US children.[28] In my view, this complication, not seen in rotavirus strains that infect children, is really a side effect of the rhesus strain, which was known to be more virulent than human strains. All these problems were finally solved when 2 vaccine candidates were finally introduced into the market: the human-based attenuated rotavirus strain, which was proven to be safe, immunogenic, and effective against severe rotavirus diarrhea in a large multicenter rotavirus trial in which we participated by enrolling more than 12,000 infants in Lima (Figure 15-5),[29] and the reassortant penta-valent bovine-based rotavirus vaccine. If the RIT vaccine program had not been cancelled, the bovine rotavirus strain could have been used to produce human-bovine reassortant strains offering protection against the 4 human rotavirus strains 20 years earlier than the introduction of the current rotavirus vaccine by Merck. We became strong advocates for introducing rotavirus vaccine throughout Latin America by participating in many national and international forums, which helped to rapidly introduce this vaccine in public health programs in Peru and the majority of countries in America soon after becoming commercially available.

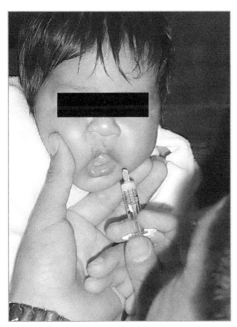

Figure 15-5. Infant receiving an experimental oral rotavirus vaccine in Lima, Peru.

Sewage Management

While the introduction of rotavirus vaccine has had a large impact on reducing severe diarrhea episodes, the burden of diarrheal disease related to bacterial pathogens remains a major problem. Sewage management plays an important role in preventing bacterial diarrhea. In developing countries, sewage systems dispose raw, untreated sewage into ocean or rivers (Figure 15-6A). Rivers are heavily contaminated by sewage, garbage, and industrial waste. We have documented how the Rimac River arrives in Lima from its uncontaminated headwaters with more than 1,000,000 fecal coliforms per cubic centimeter of water. While the Lima water treatment

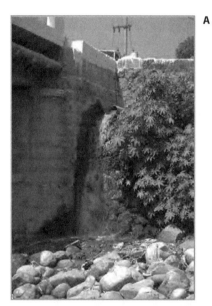
A

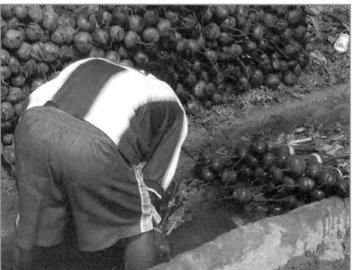
B

Figure 15-6. *A,* Raw sewage being discharged into the Rimac River. *B,* Farmer washing harvested beetroots in an irrigation channel with contaminated Rimac River water.

plant delivers high-quality drinking water to the city, the contaminated Rimac River is used to irrigate agricultural fields in the valley, where tomatoes, lettuce, and other produce are cultivated (Figure 15-6B). Washing tomatoes, lettuce, and cucumbers for 10 minutes with sterile water (water with chlorine or other antiseptics) does not change the amount of bacteria present in these vegetables because bacteria is located deeply, where washing is not effective. Santiago, Chile, with the fear of the 1991 cholera epidemic that affected Peru and many other countries in Latin America, decided finally to treat its sewage. The city not only eliminated typhoid fever but also reduced its rate of diarrheal diseases in children to those observed in the United States and other developed countries, eliminating hepatitis A and many other enteric diseases.

Why have Lima and other developing countries not followed the example of Santiago? First, treating sewage is expensive and complicated. Lima produces more than 40 cubic meters of sewage per second. Constructing sewage treatment plants and injecting that water into the water table would cost about US $2 billion. The water bill would need to be increased to cover the cost of operating not only water treatment plants but sewage treatment plants. Finally, people do not understand that simply piping sewage away from the home without sewage treatment is not enough to solve the diarrhea problem.

A Call to Action

In conclusion, after more than 30 years of doing research in diarrheal diseases, I feel blessed by seeing some effective interventions being implemented in the public health system, benefiting those most at need. The introduction of rotavirus vaccine, increased rates of exclusive and prolonged breastfeeding, less-frequent use of contaminated baby bottles, higher awareness of the value of hand washing with soap, use of zinc supplementation as part of diarrhea management guidelines, and higher proportion of commercially available foods fortified with iron and zinc all have promoted child health. We need to advocate for more effective ways to promote safe weaning foods in poor communities, and no one is seriously promoting sewage treatment plants in developing countries, at least in large cities. Until these issues are addressed, children and adults in developing countries will continue to eat bacteria-contaminated food as a regular part of their daily diet.

References

1. United Nations. *World Mortality Report 2011*. New York, NY: United Nations; 2012. http://www.un.org/esa/population/publications/worldmortalityreport2011/World%20 Mortality%20Report%202011.pdf. Accessed May 8, 2013

2. Snyder JD, Merson MH. The magnitude of the global problem of acute diarrhoeal disease: a review of active surveillance data. *Bull World Health Organ*. 1982;60(4): 605–613

3. Bern C, Martines J, de Zoysa I, Glass RI. The magnitude of the global problem of diarrhoeal diseases: a ten-year update. *Bull World Health Organ*. 1992;70(6):705–714

4. Kosek M, Bern C, Guerrant RL. The global burden of diarrhoeal disease, as estimated from studies published between 1992 and 2000. *Bull World Health Organ*. 2003;81(3):197–204

5. Fischer Walker CL, Perin J, Aryee MJ, Boschi-Pinto C, Black RE. Diarrhea incidence in low- and middle-income countries in 1990 and 2010: a systematic review. *BMC Public Health*. 2012;12:220

6. Lanata CF, Black RE, Gilman RH, Lazo F, Del Aquila R. Epidemiologic, clinical, and laboratory characteristics of acute vs. persistent diarrhea in periurban Lima, Peru. *J Pediatr Gastroenterol Nutr*. 1991;12(1):82–88

7. Bahl R, Frost C, Kirkwood BR, et al. Infant feeding patterns and risks of death and hospitalization in the first half of infancy: multicentre cohort study. *Bull World Health Organ*. 2005;83(6):418–426

8. Black RE, Lopez de Romaña G, Brown KH, Bravo N, Bazalar OG, Kanashiro HC. Incidence and etiology of infantile diarrhea and major routes of transmission in Huascar, Peru. *Am J Epidemiol*. 1989;129(4):785–799

9. Marquis GS, Ventura G, Gilman RH, et al. Fecal contamination of shanty town toddlers in households with non-corralled poultry, Lima, Peru. *Am J Public Health*. 1990;80(2):146–149

10. Black RE, Lanata CF, Lazo F. Delayed cutaneous hypersensitivity: epidemiologic factors affecting and usefulness in predicting diarrheal incidence in young Peruvian children. *Pediatr Infect Dis J*. 1989;8(4):210–215

11. Brown KH, Lanata CF, Yuen ML, Peerson JM, Butron B, Lönnerdal B. Potential magnitude of the misclassification of a population's trace element status due to infection: example from a survey of young Peruvian children. *Am J Clin Nutr*. 1993;58(4):549–554

12. Penny ME, Lanata CF. Zinc in the management of diarrhea in young children. *N Engl J Med*. 1995;333(13):873–874

13. Gilman RH, Marquis GS, Ventura G, Campos M, Spira W, Diaz F. Water cost and availability: key determinants of family hygiene in a Peruvian shantytown. *Am J Public Health*. 1993;83(11):1554–1558

14. Huttly SR, Lanata CF, Gonzales H, et al. Observations on handwashing and defecation practices in a shanty town of Lima, Peru. *J Diarrhoeal Dis Res*. 1994;12(1):14–18

15. Yeager BA, Huttly SR, Bartolini R, Rojas M, Lanata CF. Defecation practices of young children in a Peruvian shanty town. *Soc Sci Med*. 1999;49(4):531–541

16. Lanata CF, Black RE, Maúrtua D, et al. Etiologic agents in acute vs persistent diarrhea in children under three years of age in peri-urban Lima, Perú. *Acta Paediatr Suppl*. 1992;381:32–38

17. Lanata CF. Problems in measuring the impact of hygiene practices on diarrhoea in a hygiene intervention study. In: Cairncross S, Kochar V, eds. *Studying Hygiene Behaviour: Methods, Issues and Experiences.* London, United Kingdom: Sage Publications Ltd; 1994:127–134

18. Lanata CF, Huttly SR, Yeager BA. Diarrhea: whose feces matter? Reflections from studies in a Peruvian shanty town. *Pediatr Infect Dis J.* 1998;17(1):7–9

19. Huttly SR, Lanata CF, Yeager BA, Fukumoto M, del Aguila R, Kendall C. Feces, flies, and fetor: findings from a Peruvian shantytown. *Rev Panam Salud Publica.* 1998;4(2):75–79

20. Yeager BA, Huttly SR, Diaz J, Bartolini R, Marin M, Lanata CF. An intervention for the promotion of hygienic feces disposal behaviors in a shanty town of Lima, Peru. *Health Educ Res.* 2002;17(6):761–773

21. Penny ME, Peerson JM, Marin RM, et al. Randomized, community-based trial of the effect of zinc supplementation, with and without other micronutrients, on the duration of persistent childhood diarrhea in Lima, Peru. *J Pediatr.* 1999;135(2 Pt 1):208–217

22. Gil AI, Lanata CF, Hartinger SM, et al. Fecal contamination of food, water, hands, and kitchen utensils at household level in rural areas of Peru. *J Environ Health.* In press

23. Hartinger SM, Lanata CF, Hattendorf J, et al. A community randomised controlled trial evaluating a home-based environmental intervention package of improved stoves, solar water disinfection and kitchen sinks in rural Peru: rationale, trial design and baseline findings. *Contemp Clin Trials.* 2011;32(6):864–873

24. Lanata CF, Black RE, del Aguila R, et al. Protection of Peruvian children against rotavirus diarrhea of specific serotypes by one, two, or three doses of the RIT 4237 attenuated bovine rotavirus vaccine. *J Infect Dis.* 1989;159(3):452–459

25. Lanata CF, Black RE, Flores J, et al. Immunogenicity, safety and protective efficacy of one dose of the rhesus rotavirus vaccine and serotype 1 and 2 human-rhesus rotavirus reassortants in children from Lima, Peru. *Vaccine.* 1996;14(3):237–243

26. Lanata CF, Midthun K, Black RE, et al. Safety, immunogenicity and protective efficacy of one and three doses of the tetravalent rhesus rotavirus vaccine in infants in Lima, Peru. *J Infect Dis.* 1996;174(2):268–275

27. Linhares AC, Lanata CF, Hausdorff WP, Gabbay YB, Black RE. Reappraisal of the Peruvian and Brazilian lower titer tetravalent rhesus-human reassortant rotavirus vaccine efficacy trials: analysis by severity of diarrhea. *Pediatr Infect Dis J.* 1999;18(11):1001–1006

28. Centers for Disease Control and Prevention (CDC). Intussusception among recipients of rotavirus vaccine—United States, 1998-1999. *MMWR Morb Mortal Wkly Rep.* 1999;48(27):577–581

29. Ruiz-Palacios GM, Pérez-Schael I, Velázquez FR, et al. Safety and efficacy of an attenuated vaccine against severe rotavirus gastroenteritis. *N Engl J Med.* 2006;354(1):11–22

Chapter 16

Baylor International Pediatric AIDS Initiative

Mark W. Kline, MD, FAAP

Introduction and Scope of the Problem

The near elimination of new cases of HIV infection and AIDS among US children is a landmark public health success story. Routine screening of pregnant women for HIV infection and treatment of those found to be infected, together with the advent of pediatric highly active antiretroviral therapy (HAART), led to a greater than 90% decrease in the number of new US pediatric AIDS cases, from 945 in 1992 to just 48 in 2004.[1]

Unfortunately, the successes observed in the United States were not immediately replicated in the developing world, where children continued to be born with HIV infection and die from AIDS at astounding rates. Worldwide, about 700,000 children were newly infected with HIV in 2005 alone, and 570,000 died of AIDS.[2] In May 2005, it was estimated that between 15,000 and 25,000 children globally were receiving antiretroviral therapy,[3] fewer than 1% of the 2.3 million children who were living with HIV infection and only about 3% of all recipients of antiretroviral treatment.

Founded in 1996 to address the marked disparity in care and treatment access between children infected with HIV in the United States and the developing world, the Baylor International Pediatric AIDS Initiative (BIPAI) has been the recipient over the past 16 years of more than $180 million in external funding from the US government and a variety of private foundations. The Baylor initiative today provides care to more HIV-infected children and families than any other organization world-wide. Currently, BIPAI operates in Texas as a 501(c)(3) organization affiliated with Baylor College of Medicine (BCM) and Texas Children's Hospital (TCH). The Baylor initiative is able to function and employ staff in the countries in which it works through locally legalized foundations that it has established specifically for these purposes.

The Baylor International Pediatric AIDS Initiative has a wide variety of ongoing activities and programs in HIV/AIDS, including grants from the US Agency for International Development, National Institutes of Health, Centers for Disease Control and Prevention (CDC), and Department of State, and agreements with the United Nations Children's Fund, World Health Organization, and a number of governments to provide technical assistance in HIV/AIDS. The Baylor initiative produces *HIV Curriculum for the Health Professional*, which is used more widely than any other, as well as a number of technical manuals and materials pertaining to the care and treatment of HIV-infected children and families in resource-poor settings. Signature BIPAI elements are the Children's Clinical Centers of Excellence Network, currently comprised of clinical centers in Romania, Libya, Botswana, Lesotho, Swaziland, Malawi, Uganda, and Tanzania,[2] and the Pediatric AIDS Corps and Global Health Corps.

Needs Assessment and Program Implementation

Romania

The BIPAI program had its origins in a visit to TCH in fall 1995 by a small delegation of Romanian parliament members. A possible partnership around pediatric HIV/AIDS was discussed, and a reciprocal visit by a medical team from BCM/TCH was organized for February 1996.

By 2002, Romania had reported nearly 10,000 pediatric HIV/AIDS cases, representing more than half of all European pediatric HIV/AIDS cases.[4] Several disastrous policies of the communist government of Nicolae Ceaușescu had catalyzed the epidemic, including the use of whole human blood unscreened for HIV or other blood-borne pathogens and reuse of disposable needles. With support from the Sisters of Charity of the Incarnate Word, Abbott Fund, Open Society Institute, and Elton John AIDS Foundation, and in partnership with the Municipal Hospital Constanța and Romanian Ministry of Health and Family, BCM/TCH established a comprehensive pediatric HIV/AIDS care and treatment program in Constanța County, Romania.[5] Hundreds of Romanian health professionals were trained in the care and treatment of children with HIV/AIDS, an antiretroviral drug access and accountability program was established, more than 30,000 orphaned or abandoned children were tested for HIV and hepatitis B infection, and a computerized patient database was established to track health status and outcomes of infected children over time. A decrepit inpatient facility at the Municipal Hospital Constanța was extensively renovated, and a residential facility was established to house HIV-infected children who had been abandoned by their families.

In partnership with the Municipal Hospital Constanța, BIPAI opened the Romanian-American Children Center in April 2001. By August 2003, 452 HIV-infected children were receiving HAART in this center, more than in any other clinical center worldwide. The average daily census on the pediatric HIV/AIDS unit at the Municipal Hospital declined by almost 90% in just 3 years; the annual mortality rate declined from about 15% to just 1%. This was one of the earliest demonstrations that HAART could be administered safely and effectively to children in a resource-poor setting, with outcomes comparable to those observed in US settings.[5,6]

Africa and Children's Clinical Centers of Excellence Network
Based on the successful model BIPAI had implemented in Romania and with support from the Bristol-Myers Squibb Foundation, BIPAI entered into an agreement in 2002 with the government of Botswana to build, equip, furnish, and operate a Children's Clinical Center of Excellence on the campus of the Princess Marina Hospital in Gaborone. About 200 HIV-infected children began antiretroviral treatment in a small transitional facility operated by BIPAI while the main center was under construction, the very first children ever treated for HIV/AIDS in Botswana.

The Botswana-Baylor Children's Clinical Center of Excellence opened on June 20, 2003. In its first 2 years of existence, more than 4,400 children were brought to the center for testing and more than 1,400 HIV-infected children began HAART, more than in any other center worldwide at that time. The center became a focal point in Botswana for pediatric HIV/AIDS health professional training and community education. In partnership with the government of Botswana, the center catalyzed the establishment of Africa's first-ever national HIV/AIDS treatment program for children.

Expanding the Program Globally
Our experiences and lessons learned in Romania and Botswana led us to propose a 6-point plan for expanding access to lifesaving HIV/AIDS care and treatment for children and families worldwide.[7] One element of this plan was the creation of a Children's Clinical Centers of Excellence

Network designed to provide primary care and HIV/AIDS specialty care to tens of thousands of children and families and build critical mass of health professionals with the training and experience to manage HIV/AIDS and other serious or life-threatening medical conditions affecting the health and lives of children and families across Africa and around the world. With generous and sustained support from the Bristol-Myers Squibb Foundation, Abbott Fund, US government, and many others, this network came to fruition with the construction and opening of new clinical centers in Lesotho (2005), Swaziland (2006), Malawi (2006), Uganda (2009), and Tanzania (2 centers in 2011) (Figure 16-1).

Every BIPAI Children's Clinical Center of Excellence operates under a memorandum of agreement between BCM/TCH and the host government. Working side by side, American and local health professionals help to establish and exchange best practices for care and treatment of HIV-infected children and families, conduct research relevant and informative for local settings and needs, and educate whole communities on HIV/AIDS prevention and treatment. The network also has served to destigmatize HIV/AIDS, restoring hope to communities hard hit by the disease, and helped to curtail and reverse health professional brain drain by providing proper work environments and opportunities for professional advancement.

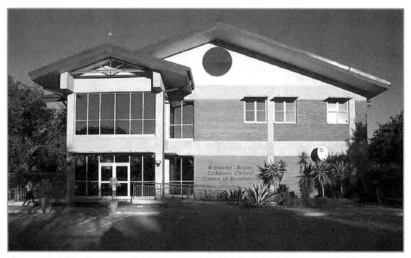

Figure 16-1. The Botswana-Baylor International Pediatric AIDS Initiative Children's Clinical Center of Excellence in Mbeya, Tanzania.

Pediatric AIDS Corps and Global Health Corps

Health professional capacity is severely limited across sub-Saharan Africa, where per-capita numbers of physicians and nurses are 1% to 2% of those in the United States. Pediatric health professional expertise is in particularly short supply. In Malawi, Lesotho, Swaziland, and Botswana, per-capita numbers of pediatricians range from 0.2 to 2.5 per 100,000 children (MWK, unpublished data), compared with a US figure of 106 per 100,000 children.[8]

A variety of strategies have been proposed for alleviating the African health professional resource crisis, including a US government-funded health service corps and task-shifting from more to less specialized health workers. Early in the development of our Children's Clinical Centers of Excellence Network, it became clear that local availability of health professionals would be rate-limiting in our ability to enroll children and families in care and treatment. We announced the Pediatric AIDS Corps in 2005 as an interim or emergency measure to scale up the care and treatment of HIV-infected children and families as local capacity for HIV/AIDS care and treatment was established.[9]

The Pediatric AIDS Corps and its successor, the Global Health Corps, recruit graduates of training programs in pediatrics, family medicine, internal medicine, and obstetrics/gynecology for long-term (1 year or greater) work assignments in Africa. Participants receive training at BCM/TCH in HIV/AIDS and tropical and travel medicine before departing for Africa. Participating physicians provide pediatric and family primary and specialty care in the Children's Clinical Centers of Excellence, numerous satellite health centers, and inpatient wards at affiliated public hospitals. They also participate in training programs to build local capacity for pediatric and family health care. Participants receive from the program a modest salary (about $45,000 per year) and full benefits, a housing allowance, and travel reimbursement, as well as ongoing supervision, training, and continuing education.

Between 2006 and 2012, the Pediatric AIDS Corps recruited, trained, and placed 161 physicians on long-term work assignments across sub-Saharan Africa. The average term of service for these physicians was about 2 years. The Pediatric AIDS Corps name was changed to Global Health Corps in 2012 to reflect a broader programmatic focus on a variety of conditions affecting the health and lives of children and families across sub-Saharan Africa, but the main objectives of the program, expanding access to life-saving medical care and treatment and building local health professional capacity, remain unchanged. As of September 2012, 40 Global Health Corps physicians were working at sites in Botswana, Lesotho, Swaziland, Malawi, Tanzania, Ethiopia, Angola, and Liberia.

Outcomes

As of December 2012, BIPAI had enrolled into care a total of 168,359 HIV-infected children; 101,437 of these children were receiving HAART (Figure 16-2). The overall mortality rate was 2.6 per 100 patient-years, a figure that compares favorably with that reported from other African studies.[10,11] More than 700 African health professionals receive training of some sort at the Children's Clinical Centers of Excellence each month; more than 500 professionals each quarter spend at least 1 week at one of the centers under the supervision of center staff. These mentoring activities have allowed BIPAI to establish defined standards of care and to "graduate" 52 individual health centers or district hospitals for care and treatment of HIV-infected children and families. The Baylor initiative has contributed substantially to the development of national HIV/AIDS treatment guidelines, prevention of mother-to-child HIV transmission, and care of thousands of HIV-exposed infants. The Baylor initiative also has assisted governments in preparing applications to the Global Fund to Fight AIDS, Tuberculosis and Malaria and provided technical assistance in the creation of local ethics committees and Good Clinical Practice training.

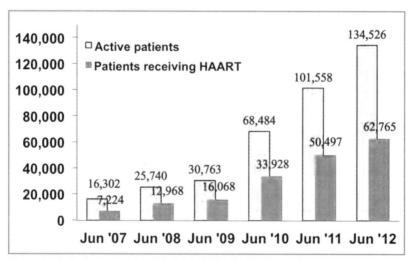

Figure 16-2. Baylor International Pediatric AIDS Initiative Network activity, 2007–2012.

Expanding Services to Treat Other Diseases

The network of clinical centers BIPAI has built and opened over the past decade in Romania and across sub-Saharan Africa today constitutes a platform and reservoir of health professional capacity unmatched by any other institution or organization worldwide. This network affords a unique opportunity to address in a meaningful way a host of serious and life-threatening diseases affecting the health and well-being of children globally, building on models developed in the fight against HIV/AIDS. Over the past 3 years, BIPAI and BCM/TCH have expanded and diversified their activities in global health in the following ways:

- Established a Residency Program in Global Child Health. This first-of-its-kind, 4-year residency program provides training domestically and at international sites for young physicians interested in global child health and the medical care of underserved patient populations here and abroad.
- Established new disease-specific initiatives, including a pediatric cancer care and treatment program in Botswana and Malawi, a pilot sickle cell infant screening and treatment program in Angola, and a global tuberculosis program. Each of these new initiatives leverages existing BIPAI infrastructure and human capacity.
- Established a new BCM National School of Tropical Medicine, Sabin Vaccine Institute, and TCH Sealy Center for Vaccine Development. Led by Peter Hotez, MD, the world's premier pediatric tropical diseases expert, this new initiative focuses on advocacy, prevention, and treatment of neglected tropical diseases affecting hundreds of millions of children worldwide.

Call to Action

For too long, children have been on the outside looking in. They have not had the same access to lifesaving medical care and treatment that their parents have had. Children residing in poor countries of the world have suffered unimaginably, still dying in large numbers from many diseases (eg, pneumonia, diarrhea, tuberculosis, sickle cell anemia) that are readily curable or manageable in the United States today.

To date, the world's reaction to millions of preventable child deaths each year largely has consisted of despair and a sense of hopelessness and inevitability. Nevertheless, the tragedy of the global HIV/AIDS pandemic has begun to shine a light on strategies that can be employed to control and manage even the most complex and serious medical conditions. Utilizing the know-how that has been developed in the fight against HIV/AIDS, we are on the cusp of an era in which millions of children and families worldwide will for the first time gain access to health-restoring, life-prolonging medical care and treatment. Pediatric health professionals, through their advocacy and actions, will be the catalysts that bring this dream to reality.

References

1. Centers for Disease Control and Prevention. *HIV/AIDS Surveillance Report: Cases of HIV Infection and AIDS in the United States, 2004.* Vol 16. Atlanta, GA: US Department of Health and Human Services, Centers for Disease Control and Prevention; 2005:13. http://www.cdc.gov/hiv/surveillance/resources/reports/2004report/pdf/2004SurveillanceReport.pdf. Accessed May 8, 2013

2. Joint United Nations Program on HIV/AIDS, World Health Organization. *AIDS Epidemic Update: December 2005.* Geneva, Switzerland: Joint United Nations Program on HIV/AIDS; 2005. http://www.unaids.org/en/media/unaids/contentassets/dataimport/publications/irc-pub06/epi_update2005_en.pdf. Accessed May 8, 2013

3. United Nations Children's Fund. UNICEF hails Clinton Foundation plan for children with AIDS. http://www.unicef.org/media/media_25964.html. Published April 11, 2004. Updated April 10, 2005. Accessed May 8, 2013

4. Romanian Ministry of Health and Family. HIV/AIDS update. *FORUM Newsl.* 2002;8

5. Kline MW, Matusa RF, Copaciu L, Calles NR, Kline NE, Schwarzwald HL. Comprehensive pediatric human immunodeficiency virus care and treatment in Constanta, Romania: implementation of a program of highly active antiretroviral therapy in a resource-poor setting. *Pediatr Infect Dis J.* 2004;23(8):695–700

6. Kline MW, Rugina S, Ilie M, et al. Long-term follow-up of 414 HIV-infected Romanian children and adolescents receiving lopinavir/ritonavir-containing highly active antiretroviral therapy. *Pediatrics.* 2007;119(5):e1116–e1120

7. Kline MW. Perspectives on the pediatric HIV/AIDS pandemic: catalyzing access of children to care and treatment. *Pediatrics.* 2006;117(4):1388–1393

8. Freed GL, Nahra TA, Wheeler JR; Research Advisory Committee of the American Board of Pediatrics. Relation of per capita income and gross domestic product to the supply and distribution of pediatricians in the United States. *J Pediatr.* 2004;144(6):723–728

9. Kline MW, Ferris MG, Jones DC, et al. The Pediatric AIDS Corps: responding to the African HIV/AIDS health professional resource crisis. *Pediatrics.* 2009;123(1):134–136

10. Damonti J, Doykos P, Wanless RS, Kline M. HIV/AIDS in African children: the Bristol-Myers Squibb Foundation and Baylor response. *Health Aff (Milwood).* 2012;31(7):1636–1642

11. Kabue MM, Buck WC, Wanless SR, et al. Mortality and clinical outcomes in HIV-infected children on antiretroviral therapy in Malawi, Lesotho, and Swaziland. *Pediatrics.* 2012;130(3):e591–e599

Chapter 17

HIV Advocacy in South Africa

Hoosen Coovida, MBBS, FCP, MSc, PhD

Understanding the Problem

HIV in South Africa is a high-prevalence condition, with 10.6% of the total population (ie, 5.58 million people) reported to be HIV positive in 2011.[1] Children between 0 and 18 years of age with HIV/AIDS accounted for 2.9% of the total population in 2008. This figure ranged from 3.3% at 0 to 4 years to 1.1% at 12 to 14 years.[2] In 2011, 137,113 children were receiving comprehensive HIV/AIDS treatment, and this accounted for 8.7% of all HIV/AIDS patients on treatment.[2] The mortality rate of children younger than 5 years, substantially due to HIV/AIDS, has recently decreased to about 52 per 1,000 live births.[1] Maternal-to-child transmission rates have been dramatically reduced to about 2.7%, and more than 90% of women who are pregnant and HIV positive are receiving adequate antenatal antiretroviral (ARV) therapy.[1] These changes have occurred recently under an enlightened health minister.

The harsh realities of the apartheid regime prior to 1994 created the conditions that allowed HIV to establish itself among the people, spreading like an unattended wildfire. In the postapartheid period, the misguided practices of the Mbeki government resulted in unbridled propagation of HIV. Doctors recognized that we needed to engage actively in advocacy to change health legislation and policies. We also needed to advocate for clinical approaches (eg, breastfeeding) that fit the reality of living conditions in South Africa.

Desperate Conditions Create a Breeding Ground for the HIV Epidemic

Before independence in 1994, a despotic racial oligarchy governed South Africa. The state employed authoritarian, oppressive, and often brutal means to deny basic human rights, including rights to health and development, to the majority nonwhite population.[3-6] There was visible and hidden violence of apartheid that directly affected the health of men, women, and children,[7–10] contributing to malnutrition, high rates of untreated infectious disease, and physical and emotional disability and death.

Those who recognized the detrimental health effects of apartheid knew that the root causes of serious health problems for South Africans must be addressed. To do this, we joined with those involved in the major political struggles representing the nonwhite majority (the Mass Democratic Movement). We were aware that we were taking extraordinary risks. Those who opposed the apartheid regime often lost their employment. There was a banning order restricting one to home or another location. People who spoke out against the government were routinely poisoned by state agents, assaulted, imprisoned, tortured, and murdered.

Despite this, in 1984, we established a specifically antiapartheid health organization, the National Medical and Dental Association (NAMDA), to engage actively in health struggles and eliminate racism in the health system. The National Medical and Dental Association raised funds for legal aid to political prisoners, brought psychosocial assistance to those tortured by the vicious Security Branch of the police, and advanced the development of health policies for the creation of a new South Africa. Figure 17-1 shows NAMDA and some of its supporters from the black hospital and medical school of the University of Natal, including nursing staff, professors, and lecturers at the medical school, and other health personnel and political activists leading a march in 1987 down the main

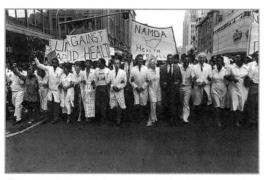

street of Durban, South Africa, to occupy the main whites-only hospital in Durban.

Figure 17-1. A march by progressive health personnel of the National Medical and Dental Association attached to the Durban Teaching Hospital and Medical School, University of Natal, down the main commercial street in Durban to occupy the whites-only Addington Hospital in 1987.

International Pressure and the Academic Boycott

International pressure was an essential constituent of the freedom struggle and so became a constituent of the NAMDA call for international support. Solidarity groups were established in the United States, United Kingdom, and Europe. The Committee for Health in South Africa in the United States became a leading supporter of health programs in South Africa. One of our more delicate tasks was to endorse and complement the overall boycott strategy of the liberation movement by devising an academic boycott without isolating South Africa from scientific advances.[11]

Implementation of the academic boycott restricted interaction with international pro-apartheid academics and involved close collaboration with our international solidarity groups. The academic boycott was one important strand in the rope that brought the apartheid regime to an end.

HIV Propagation

Once the formal struggle against apartheid was over, the extreme and highly visible dangers to life and liberty more or less faded. Great progress was made in a number of socioeconomic and political indicators for the black majority. Nonetheless, racial discrimination persisted with tenacious racial gradients in social determinants of health, opportunity, and wealth.[12]

Apartheid had created social conditions of abject poverty, lack of access to basic services, and persistent despair in which an epidemic like HIV could root. Unfortunately, the postapartheid government did not fully appreciate that HIV was affecting the entire society and was hitting the impoverished black population in a particularly devastating fashion. Preoccupied with moving the country beyond apartheid, the Mandela government could only pay limited attention to the foothold HIV/AIDS was gaining in the country.

In the mid-1990s, the African National Congress instituted an AIDS Advisory Committee, and I was appointed chair. The committee was widely representative of civil society with many members who had been part of the struggle against apartheid.[13] The committee undertook detailed analyses of issues to inform government policies about the impending AIDS crisis. Unfortunately, our work was all in vain. The government did not accept the recommendations of the committee. Rather, it offered a variety of spurious reasons for the refusal to implement a prevention of mother-to-child transmission of HIV program based on zidovudine. A government spokesperson, at a meeting between the author and

Department of Health senior staff, made the chilling comment that there was nothing to suggest that in impoverished rural areas, saving the life of a child would affect mortality statistics later on (HC, personal communication).

Prominent among government officials who stonewalled the recommendations of the committee was Deputy President Thabo Mbeki. He was largely responsible for a number of policy disasters related to HIV/AIDS. He supported a state-funded, exorbitantly financed, artistically weak, and educationally ineffective play "Sarafina 2" that premiered on World AIDS Day, 1995. Moreover, senior government figures, with Mbeki's encouragement, trumpeted an ostensible wonder drug for AIDS—Virodene—that turned out to be an industrial solvent (dimethylformamide).

As a result of the inaction and misdirected action of the government, by the late 1990s and early 2000s, HIV had taken hold with a vengeance in South Africa. The AIDS Advisory Committee continued to be at odds with the government and was particularly opposed to a government decision to make AIDS a notifiable disease, as it was believed to be counterproductive in a milieu where people with HIV were subjected to intense discrimination and occasional assaults. The committee was subsequently disbanded by the Department of Health.

Confronting Mbeki

Sadly, the second antiapartheid government with Mbeki as president directly thwarted scientific and health measures to address HIV and AIDS. As a result, the major issue for health advocacy in the late 1990s and early 2000s centered around the personalities, hubris, and lack of understanding of science and its methods by President Mbeki and his Minister of Health, Manto Tshabalala. President Mbeki continued to hold tenaciously to the astonishing notion that HIV is not the cause of AIDS. He famously said, "As I listened and heard the whole story told about our own country, it seemed to me that we could not blame everything on a single virus."[13]

The consequences of this challenge to the scientific method by a sitting president and minister of health are an extreme example of the resistance that existed throughout much of Africa and Asia to the acceptance of the reality of HIV facts during the early years of the worldwide epidemic. Mbeki's prominent position as Mandela's successor put him in a position of international moral authority, and his beliefs and statements reinforced the resisting voices in many parts of the globe.

A number of individuals with impeccable antiapartheid histories, including myself, were seriously concerned about the effect Mbeki's stance was having locally and worldwide. We wrote a private letter to President Mbeki urging him to reconsider the scientific advice he was being given. He sent back a rather long and rambling response that revealed a lack of understanding of how medical science works. To add insult to injury, he established a costly pseudoscientific Presidential AIDS Advisory Panel between "conventional scientists" and "dissidents" that was a colossal failure. The Mbeki panel prevented not only the delivery of evidence-based care for HIV but also rent the very fabric of the democratic society.

Advocacy and the AIDS 2000 Conference: Signing of the Durban Declaration

In 2000, for the first time, after 12 International AIDS Conferences in the rich world, the AIDS 2000 Conference was held in southern Africa, where the prevalence of HIV is the highest in the world. In a sense, the dramatic events at AIDS 2000 were the culmination of opposition, activism, and advocacy in the preceding 3 to 4 years against Mbeki's dangerous views on AIDS.

Governmental questioning of the cause of the epidemic escalated before the conference and Mbeki wrote to Kofi Annan, Secretary-General of the United Nations; President Bill Clinton of the United States; and other heads of states that the "assumption" of a link between HIV and AIDS by mainstream doctors, media, and others amounted to "intellectual intimidation and terrorism" and that the alleged link required further investigation; he wondered whether "…safe sex, condoms and anti-retroviral drugs [are] a sufficient response to the health catastrophe we face!"[13]

The viability of AIDS 2000 was threatened as scientists from other countries considered withdrawing from the event as a mark of their extreme disapproval of the misdirected opinions on HIV of the political leadership. One of the primary aims of the conference was, therefore, to provide information to the people of South Africa itself and to the world on the unchallengeable scientific evidence for the biological cause of AIDS and the need for national policies on measures for prevention.

The conference drew global attention to the incontestable epidemiologic evidence that southern Africa was in an HIV epidemic and the continent of Africa had the largest number of HIV infections. A predetermined goal of the conference was to challenge the exceedingly high cost of ARVs—about $20,000 per year per patient in industrialized countries—produced by the large research-based pharmaceuticals in Western countries.

AIDS 2000 served as a catalyst for the subsequent fall in the cost of ARVs—the price of 3 commonly used first-line ARVs for adults fell from $568 per month in 2000 to $51 per month in 5 years.[14] (See Figure 17-2.) Within 2 years of the conference, the number of people on ARVs for treatment had increased from 400,000 to 1 million.

"More than 5,000 scientists from around the world, including 12 Nobel Laureates, as well directors of leading research institutes, and presidents of academies and medical societies, were moved by these events to sign the Durban Declaration."[14] It affirmed, "The evidence that AIDS is caused by HIV-1 or HIV-2 is clear-cut, exhaustive and unambiguous, meeting the highest standards of science. The data fulfill exactly the same criteria as for other viral diseases, such as polio, measles, and smallpox." To "tackle the disease, everyone must first understand that HIV is the enemy. Research,

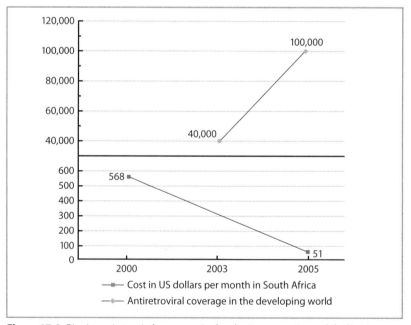

Figure 17-2. Rise in antiretroviral coverage in developing countries and decline in cost of HIV treatment. Adapted from Karim SS. Durban 2000 to Toronto 2006: the evolving challenges in implementing AIDS treatment in Africa. *AIDS.* 2006;20(15):N7–N9.

not myths, will lead to the development of more effective and cheaper treatments, and…a vaccine." It concluded on a note of optimism: "Science will one day triumph over AIDS, just as it did over smallpox. Curbing the spread of HIV will be the first step. Until then, reason, solidarity, political will and courage must be our partners."[15]

Many public health scientists and observers of the AIDS epidemic throughout the world consider the Durban meeting one of the most successful and significant AIDS conferences ever held. President Nelson Mandela ended the conference with these words: "This is not an academic conference. This is, as I understand it, a gathering of human beings concerned about turning around one of the greatest threats humankind has faced, and certainly the greatest after the end of the great wars of the previous century.…so much unnecessary attention around this conference had been directed towards a dispute that is unintentionally distracting from the real life and death issues we are confronted with as a country, a region, a continent and a world.…I am…old enough and have gone through sufficient conflicts and disputes in my lifetime to know that in all disputes a point is arrived at where no party, no matter how right or wrong it might have been at the start of that dispute, will any longer be totally in the right or totally in the wrong. Such a point, I believe, has been reached in this debate."[16] He received a rousing standing ovation from an exuberant audience of many thousands.

The Breastfeeding Saga

As we have seen, advocacy can play out at the governmental level. It also has a role in our clinical, scientific, and research experience. The centrality of advocacy in determining health policy is very well illustrated by the experience my colleagues and I had in the long, drawn-out disagreements with our peers in the field of child health on the question of breastfeeding by HIV-positive women in poor countries.

There is incontrovertible evidence that breastfeeding is the best form of infant feeding for all women everywhere, with very few and only marginal exceptions. This association between breastfeeding and child health and development has been known for centuries. The long-term effect of breastfeeding on education, learning, productivity, and adult morbidity and mortality from diseases associated with obesity, lack of exercise, and poor diets (noncommunicable diseases) are well documented.[17]

The HIV epidemic created an unprecedented dilemma for infant feeding because the virus was found to be transmitted by breastfeeding and could account for up to about 50% of the total transmission from mother to child. In the industrialized world, breastfeeding was discouraged in HIV-positive mothers and, with antiretroviral prevention, transmission rates fell substantially. In developing countries, avoidance of breastfeeding was not an option, as withdrawal of the protective properties of human milk to immature babies resulted in diseases and deaths. We have argued the scientific, biologic, social, cultural, economic, and political case for preserving breastfeeding through the HIV epidemic extensively.[18,19]

Based on our understanding of these factors, we decided to do the research to make breastfeeding by HIV-positive women as safe as possible; in this, we succeeded.[20–22] But opposition to the idea was widespread among the medicine regulatory body during President Mbeki`s government and scientists and health workers throughout Africa, the United States, and Europe. We were criticized and accused of lack of scientific plausibility, lack of hypotheses, poor study design, and finally experimenting with poor, vulnerable black children. Over a period of more than 10 years, evidence, which is now irrefutable, accumulated from many sources that breastfeeding could be made safe among HIV-positive women. World Health Organization policies[23] and national South African policies[24] on breastfeeding and infant feeding by HIV-positive women have changed as result of our research and advocacy.

National Planning Commission 2011 and the Future

Mbeki left office in fall 2008. With his departure, the political environment eased for civil servants and government ministers to speak a little more freely. I was asked to join the National Planning Commission (NPC) in 2010. The goal of the NPC was to "draft a vision and national development plan for consideration by Cabinet and the country."[25] Health and the prevention and care of HIV/AIDS is very much a part of the current plan.

The Diagnostic Report and the National Plan emphasized work and education as the highest priorities. South Africans from all walks of life welcomed the diagnostic as a frank, constructive assessment. The National Plan, released in November 2011, presented solutions or paths to resolve issues identified in the Diagnostic Report and added 4 thematic areas: rural economy, social protection, regional and world affairs, and community safety. After releasing the draft plan, the NPC held extensive consultations. Our public forums (physical and virtual) drew in thousands of people; we met with national departments, provincial governments, development finance institutions, state-owned entities, and local government formations, and we held talks with unions, business, and nonprofit organizations. The response to the draft plan has been overwhelmingly positive across the political, racial, and income spectrum. South Africans broadly support the plan and have expressed an interest in making it a success. Members of the public provided valuable suggestions on how the plan could be improved and how its implementation could be more effective. The NPC welcomed the input it received from thousands of people, which has informed the revised plan. Specialist and cognate groups formed the nuclei of discussions on each of the different themes and were responsible for writing up their contributions. I worked with a public health physician, Irwin Friedman, MBBS, with assistance from the secretariat, to draw up the health chapter. Plenary sessions ensured participation of each commissioner in every chapter. All 26 commissioners are therefore responsible for every part of the plan, which has a 20-year horizon to 2030.

This engagement in a national institution composed of independent-minded individuals across the racial divide is the end result of my cumulative and particular contributions to attaining health and development for all our people, as a member of the resistance and liberation movements in South Africa. The potential for contributing at scale to the uplifting of all South Africans, especially the poor, and bringing freedom, equity, solidarity, and dignity to all our citizens through the NPC makes this the apogee of my role in advocacy and the destination of a personal journey.

Call to Action

The sheer scale of serious HIV and health problems nationally (in South Africa), regionally (in southern Africa), and internationally can be so overwhelming as to imperil clear strategizing and paralyze actions for advocacy. This need not be so. The scope of international and internal communication through a wide choice of professional and social media puts information instantly in the hands of collaborators throughout most countries. Travel is generally much easier within national boundaries and across continents. At the AIDS 2012 XIX International AIDS Conference, July 22 through 27, in Washington, DC, the strength of new evidence on prevention and treatment of HIV generated a huge wave of hope for the future. The sense was that we had reached a critical threshold in the control of the AIDS epidemic. So there are multiple and uncharted avenues of advocacy to follow as governments, policy makers, activists, and funders traverse new ground in implementing large-scale HIV programs, determining priorities for scaling up, improving efficiencies so as to do more with less in a financially constrained global environment, redefining the role of nongovernmental organizations, and all the time monitoring and evaluating putative successes and failures. It seems to me that we may have to employ some or all of the measures I have described herein to facilitate advocacy for affected populations. Approaches to developing relevant HIV policies to lengthen survival, improve management of morbidities, improve care, strengthen health systems, and address social determinants of health and illness will include communicating the best of scientific evidence, mobilizing communities, engaging with governments, participating in state institutions that offer independent advice to governments, influencing policy makers, tracking global financial agencies, using legal channels and the courts, and adopting more robust public measures in the face of recalcitrant opposition to appropriate evidence-based recommendations depending on the circumstances within a country.

References

1. Mayosi BM, Lawn JE, van Niekerk A, et al. Health in South Africa: changes and challenges since 2009. *Lancet.* 2012;380(9858):2029–2043
2. Day C, Gray A, Budgell E. Health and related indicators. In: Health Systems Trust. *South African Health Review 2011.* Durban, South Africa: Health Systems Trust; 2011:119–248. http://www.hst.org.za/sites/default/files/sahr_2011.pdf. Accessed May 9, 2013
3. Coovadia H, Jewkes R, Barron P, Sanders D, McIntyre D. The health and health system of South Africa: historical roots of current public health challenges. *Lancet.* 2009;374(9692):817–834
4. World Health Organization. *Apartheid and Health.* Geneva, Switzerland: World Health Organization; 1983. http://whqlibdoc.who.int/publications/1983/9241560797.pdf. Accessed May 9, 2013
5. South African History Online. General South African history timeline: 1800s. http://www.sahistory.org.za/article/1800s. Accessed May 9, 2013
6. Mandela N. *Long Walk to Freedom: The Autobiography of Nelson Mandela.* New York, NY: Back Bay Books/Little, Brown and Company; 1995
7. Jinabhai CC, Coovadia HM, Abdool-Karim SS. Socio-medical indicators of health in South Africa. *Int J Health Serv.* 1986;16(1):163–176
8. Coovadia HM, Dean TSF, Solomons K. Violence against children in the cells, streets and schools: torture—the medical evidence. *Hum Rights Q.* 1988;10(1):22–30
9. Coovadia HM. Children in South Africa. In: *Children in the Front Line.* New York, NY: United Nations Children's Fund; 1989

10. Coovadia HM, Jinabhai CC. The pestilence of health care: black death and suffering under white rule. In: Cohen R, Muthien YG, Zegeye A, eds. *Repression and Resistance: Insider Accounts of Apartheid*. African Discourse vol 2. London, England: Hans Zell Publishers; 1990:86–116

11. Coovadia HM. Sanctions and the struggle for health in South Africa. *Am J Public Health*. 1999;89(10):1505–1508

12. National Planning Commission, Republic of South Africa. *Diagnostic Overview*. http://www.npconline.co.za/MediaLib/Downloads/Home/Tabs/Diagnostic/Diagnostic%20Overview.pdf. Accessed May 9, 2013

13. Coovadia H, Coovadia I. Science and society: the HIV epidemic and South African political responses. *Adv Exp Med Biol*. 2008;609:16–28

14. Karim SS. Durban 2000 to Toronto 2006: the evolving challenges in implementing AIDS treatment in Africa. *AIDS*. 2006;20(15):N7–N9

15. The Durban Declaration. *Nature*. 2000;406(6791):15–16

16. Nelson Mandela Foundation. Closing address by former president Nelson Mandela at the 13th International AIDS Conference, 14 July 2000, Durban. http://www.dirasengwe.org/Closing-Address-by-Nelson-Mandela/View-category.html. Accessed May 9, 2013

17. Coovadia HM, Bland RM. Preserving breastfeeding practice through the HIV pandemic. *Trop Med Int Health*. 2007;12(9):1116–1133

18. Coutsoudis A, Coovadia HM, Wilfert CM. HIV, infant feeding and more perils for poor people: new WHO guidelines encourage review of formula milk policies. *Bull World Health Organ*. 2008;86(3):210–214

19. Coovadia H. Breastfeeding by HIV positive women: do the benefits outweigh the risks? *Future Med*. 2007;1:1

20. Coutsoudis A, Pillay K, Spooner E, Kuhn L, Coovadia HM. Influence of infant-feeding patterns on early mother-to-child transmission of HIV-1 in Durban, South Africa: a prospective cohort study. South African Vitamin A Study Group. *Lancet*. 1999;354(9177):471–476

21. Coovadia HM, Rollins NC, Bland RM, et al. Mother-to-child transmission of HIV-1 infection during exclusive breastfeeding in the first 6 months of life: an intervention cohort study. *Lancet*. 2007;369(9567):1107–1116

22. Coovadia HM, Brown ER, Fowler MG, et al. Efficacy and safety of an extended nevirapine regimen in infant children of breastfeeding mothers with HIV-1 infection for prevention of postnatal HIV-1 transmission (HPTN 046): a randomised, double-blind, placebo-controlled trial. *Lancet*. 2012;379(9812):221–228

23. World Health Organization. *PMTCT Strategic Vision 2010–2015: Preventing Mother-to-Child Transmission of HIV to Reach the UNGASS and Millennium Development Goals*. Geneva, Switzerland: World Health Organization; 2010. http://www.who.int/hiv/pub/mtct/strategic_vision.pdf. Accessed May 9, 2013

24. The Tshwane declaration of support for breastfeeding in South Africa. *South Afr J Clin Nutr*. 2011;24(4):214

25. National Planning Commission. http://www.npconline.co.za. Accessed May 9, 2013

Chapter 18

Sickle Cell Disease: Creating a Global Network

Isaac Odame, MD

Understanding Sickle Cell Disease

Sickle cell disease (SCD) is one of the most common monogenetic diseases worldwide.[1] As a result of selection pressure due to heterozygote protection against severe forms of *Plasmodium falciparum* malaria, high frequencies of the disease are found in tropical countries and countries to which large populations have migrated from these regions.[2] Thus, SCD occurs widely in sub-Saharan Africa, regions of the Indian subcontinent, parts of the Middle East, and in some southern European populations, notably Greece and Italy. In most of these populations, heterozygote rates range between 5% and 25% but may reach as high as 40% in localized areas of Saudi Arabia and Uganda. Large population movements from Africa account for variable frequencies in the United States, Caribbean, Brazil, and Central America. Recently, economic migrations from Africa to Europe and North America have contributed to rises in disease frequency in these regions. In some areas of sub-Saharan Africa, up to 2% of all children are born with the disease. Sickle cell disease increasingly poses a major public health burden in many of these countries, a fact that has recently been acknowledged by the World Health Organization (WHO) and the United Nations.[3,4] The World Health Organization has estimated that more than 200,000 babies with SCD are born in sub-Saharan Africa every year.

Most children born with SCD in high-income countries, comprising only 10% of people living with the disease throughout the world, survive to adulthood as a result of interventions including newborn/neonatal screening, prophylactic penicillin, widespread pneumococcal vaccination, and better quality medical care. In contrast, it is estimated that 50% to 80% of babies born with SCD in sub-Saharan Africa, where the disease is common, die before the age of 5 years. Five percent of all deaths of children younger than 5 years in Africa and up to 16% in West Africa are related to SCD.[3] The causes of mortality include infectious complications such as malaria, pneumonia, and pneumococcal sepsis and severe anemia.

The public health implications of SCD are significant as evidenced by the associated high mortality of children younger than 5 years. Also, survivors may suffer from recurrent, unpredictable, severe, painful episodes; anemia; respiratory failure from acute chest syndrome (pneumonia/pulmonary infarction); stroke; avascular necrosis of bones; osteomyelitis; leg ulcers; renal failure; and priapism. With scaled-up implementation of primary health care programs such as immunization and nutritional programs and use of antibiotics, under-5 mortality rates in children with SCD have started to fall, particularly among populations in the upper quintiles of socioeconomic strata with relatively better access to these interventions. As result, increasingly more early childhood survivors of SCD will need to be diagnosed and treated for SCD in poorly resourced health systems.[5] Furthermore, without definitive policies to ensure universal access to care, inequities underlying access to known interventions that affect SCD outcomes are likely to widen.

To improve control and management of SCD, a number of challenges must be overcome. First, public education and awareness of the underlying genetic cause of SCD are crucial in combating the social stigma and erroneous cultural beliefs associated with the disease. Misunderstandings about the disease and its manifestations can pose barriers to seeking appropriate care even when available within the local setting. Second, national governments and health policy makers need to acknowledge that SCD poses a public health problem and develop the political will to craft systematic plans to combat it. Third, long-term partnerships between clinicians and researchers in rich and poor countries have tremendous potential in building clinical care and research capacity in low-income counties with the highest disease burden. Such partnerships need to be broadened to include international donor and development agencies, governments, nongovernmental organizations (NGOs), and industry to build sustainable programs for care and study of patients in low-resource settings. Fourth, solutions to the problem of SCD in poor countries have to be evidence-based and cost-effective and should consist of interventions that can be integrated into already existing health care systems at the primary, secondary, and tertiary levels. These solutions, rather than simply being delivered as transferred strategies that work in rich countries, must be studied and implemented by trained professionals within the poor countries.

There is evidence that neonatal screening for SCD, when linked to timely diagnostic testing, parental education, penicillin prophylaxis, appropriate immunization, and comprehensive care, markedly reduces SCD-related morbidity and mortality in infancy and early childhood.[6-9] Pilot programs of well-organized clinical care that include easy access to designated centers no matter the patient's ability to pay have demonstrated significantly improved outcomes for children with SCD in low-income countries.[10-12] Yet in most countries where SCD is a public health problem, disease management is inadequate, national control programs do not exist, basic diagnostic and treatment facilities are lacking, and systematic screening is not common practice. In these countries, simple, affordable, and cost-effective procedures, such as penicillin prophylaxis to prevent life-threatening pneumococcal infections, are not widely available. The need for coordinated advocacy to mobilize a concerted global effort to address these deficiencies inspired the formation of the Global Sickle Cell Disease Network (GSCDN). The case has been made that to further research and advance clinical care for SCD, global, long-term partnerships need to be established between SCD clinicians and researchers in rich and poor countries. The GSCDN would act as a catalyst in promoting advocacy for SCD on a global scale and foster collaborations between SCD professionals in rich and poor countries with a goal to help reduce the disease burden globally. Further, the GSCDN would seek to promote broader partnerships among organizations including governments, NGOs, international donor/development agencies, health care institutions, academic societies, industry, philanthropic organizations, patient/family organizations, and civil society to help find and deliver sustainable solutions where they are most needed.

Appropriate Interventions

Early Screening

In many high-income countries, survival rates of about 95% at 18 years of age have been achieved for children born with SCD.[6,7] Similar results have been achieved in middle-income countries such as Jamaica and Brazil.[8,9] This increased survival of children can be attributed to neonatal screening, early diagnosis, and implementation of penicillin prophylaxis and pneumococcal immunizations, as well as education of caregivers. Successful pilot projects in low-income countries such as Ghana, Benin, and the Democratic Republic of the Congo have demonstrated that such screening programs are feasible and can achieve similar results as in middle- and high-income countries.[12,13]

Prevention and Treatment of Bacterial Infections

Reduced splenic function is one of the hallmarks of SCD. This accounts for the high incidence of invasive infections in SCD from encapsulated bacteria. One study in Kenya reported that the pooled odds ratio for *Streptococcus pneumoniae* in SCD was 36 times higher compared with the non-SCD population. The same odds ratio for *Haemophilus influenzae* type b (Hib) was 13 times higher in SCD.[13]

These findings provide support for early screening and initiation of penicillin prophylaxis and pneumococcal immunization in this patient population. Current global efforts to include Hib and pneumococcal protein conjugate vaccines into primary immunization programs, if fully implemented, will provide universal coverage for all children, with incremental benefit to children with SCD at higher risk for these infections.

Malaria

Several studies have shown a lower risk of malaria infection and a lower prevalence of high-density parasitemia in people with SCD. However, malaria is associated with higher mortality in children with SCD because of malaria-associated severe anemia.[14,15] Strategies such as use of insecticide-impregnated nets, antimalaria prophylaxis during seasons of high infection transmission, and early treatment of febrile illness would be effective in reducing malaria-associated mortality in SCD.

Hydroxyurea Therapy

Clinical trials of hydroxyurea in the United States and Europe have demonstrated efficacy in reducing acute painful episodes, acute chest syndrome, the need for blood transfusions, and hospitalizations. Furthermore, reports from the United States, Greece, and Brazil have shown that hydroxyurea therapy improves survival in adults with SCD.[16,17] In low-income countries, major barriers including limited clinical and laboratory resources, the effect of nutritional and other infectious comorbidities, cost of medication, and acceptability of treatment to patients and families precludes widespread implementation of this efficacious treatment. Implementation research studies exploring the effectiveness of hydroxyurea therapy in low-income settings are needed. Improved access to hydroxyurea at a reduced cost will require partnerships among clinician investigators in low- and high-income countries, funding agencies, and the pharmaceutical industry.

Strategy for Action

In 2007, I arrived at the Hospital for Sick Children (SickKids) in Toronto, Canada, to take up the position of codirector of the hemoglobinopathy program. Prior to that, I had played a leading role in the design, development, and implementation of universal newborn screening for SCD in the province of Ontario, Canada. At SickKids, I became aware of the Programme for Global Paediatric Research (PGPR) headed by Alvin Zipursky, MD. The programme had been established by Dr Zipursky following his tenure as editor of the *Pediatric Research* journal to mobilize the international community of pediatric researchers to focus on major health problems affecting children and adolescents in the developing world. Sickle cell disease, I believed, represented a perfect fit for this model—a major health problem affecting children predominantly in sub-Saharan Africa, regions of India, the Middle East, Caribbean, and Brazil. I approached Dr Zipursky to explore how PGPR might be engaged in helping to initiate efforts to establish a global network for SCD. The programme fully embraced the vision of building a global community of SCD clinicians and researchers to focus on reducing the global burden of SCD through North-South partnerships to promote research and advance clinical care, particularly in low-income countries with the highest disease burden. We consulted with David Weatherall, MD, who had made a compelling case in an article in the journal *Blood* for establishment of long-term partnerships between research groups in rich and poor countries to reduce the burden of SCD globally.[18]

Birth of the Global Sickle Cell Disease Network

The first major step to mobilize action occurred at the 21st annual meeting of the American Society of Pediatric Hematology/Oncology (ASPHO) in Cincinnati, OH, where Dr Zipursky and I organized a symposium and workshop, "Sickle Cell Disease: Global Impact and the Case for Partnerships between Research Groups in Rich and Poor Countries." There was hardly any standing room for symposium participants—evidence that many ASPHO members were ready to embrace the vision. In a follow-up workshop for a smaller group of participants, a proposal was tabled to organize a conference in Cotonou, Republic of Benin, in conjunction with the official opening of a newly expanded SCD center directed by Cherif Rahimy, MBBS. The Cotonou meeting in 2009, attended by 80 SCD experts from 25 countries, considered clinical and research needs in SCD, particularly in low-income countries. Four working groups on natural history and newborn screening, infectious diseases in SCD, hydroxyurea therapy in low-income regions, and the genetic/environmental factors that govern phenotypic diversity presented findings of their deliberations. The conference concluded with an enthusiastic decision to forge ahead with the formation of the GSCDN.[19] Dr Zipursky and I received an endorsement from the leadership of SickKids to move forward with proposing SickKids as the coordinating center of the newly formed GSCDN.

The American Society of Pediatric Hematology/Oncology provided the opportunity for the 2008 symposium and workshop that mobilized SCD experts in North America to embrace the idea to establish the GSCDN. The American Society of Hematology (ASH), in line with its strategic focus on SCD, has provided needed support to enable GSCDN participants to meet at annual ASH meetings. The limitations and accomplishments in SCD, particularly in low-income countries, was a focus of a special educational program on international hematology at the 2012 ASH meeting in Atlanta, GA. The World Health Organization, through its release of a special report on SCD in 2006 and the 2010 release of a strategy for Africa by its Regional Committee for Africa, has provided indirect support for enhanced global partnership to combat the disease.[3,20] A direct partnership between the GSCDN and WHO could do more to strengthen advocacy aimed at persuading national governments to craft and develop plans for the control and management of SCD.

Communication Strategy

Having secured the support of key SCD clinicians to establish a global network to advocate and promote collaboration for enhanced clinical care and research aimed at finding evidence-based solutions, the major challenge we faced was to develop an efficient communication strategy for the network. To create better opportunities for collaborative research, ways to reduce the cost of connection and increase the speed of interaction between experts in rich and poor countries had to be found. We retained the services of a Web strategy consultant to guide us through the process of developing communication tools to meet the needs of a full range of GSCDN constituents in low-, middle-, and high-income countries. This culminated in the development of 2 complementary online offerings, a social networking site using a customizable infrastructure (www.globalscd.ning.com) and the GSCDN Web site (www.globalsicklecelldisease.org).

Challenges and Difficulties

The major initial obstacle that had to be overcome to get the GSCDN initiative started was persuading SCD clinicians and scientists from developed countries of the value in creating long-term partnerships with counterparts in low-income countries. Many SCD experts in North America and Europe viewed themselves as relatively disadvantaged compared with colleagues in other fields of hematology and oncology with regard to access to research funding and clinical care resources. Sickle cell disease research remains in dire need of extra funding support, while clinical care for SCD patients, even in rich countries, needs further resource enhancement for better outcomes. The partnerships being proposed by the GSCDN concept would put further strains on the limited funding available for SCD. A strong and compelling case had to be made in emphasizing that global partnerships would likely result in mutual benefits—reduced SCD-related morbidity and mortality through improved clinical and diagnostic facilities and better disease control and management in low-income countries—while providing abundant opportunities to discover more reliable predictors of end-organ damage and new therapies to improve outcomes in low- and high-income countries.

Having persuaded stakeholders of the value of a global network, backing and funding support had to be sought to establish a coordinating office as an engine to run the network. The executive leadership of SickKids embraced the challenge and positioned the GSCDN initiative as an institutional funding priority. This enabled the design and development of the GSCDN Web site and social networking infrastructure.

The social networking tool has not created as much interaction between the GSCDN constituents in low-income countries as it has in high-income settings. This may be a reflection of the lack of comfort with social networking medium and challenges with reliable Internet access in low-income countries. However, recent expansion of wireless phone facilities for Internet access in low-income countries could bridge these gaps and improve interactions via social networking in these regions.

Organizational Structure of the Global Sickle Cell Disease Network

An international advisory council made up of 7 world SCD leaders provides strategic direction, guides the network in fostering partnerships, and supports SCD advocacy globally. Five working groups led by 2 cochairpersons (one from a low-income country; the other from a high-income country) have been mandated to define specific questions and challenges that need to be addressed within their subject areas: newborn screening and surveillance, infections in SCD, hydroxyurea therapy in low-income regions, genetic/environmental factors involved in phenotypic diversity of SCD, and laboratory/data management. The GSCDN Coordinating Office, funded by SickKids and staffed with a medical director, executive director, senior communications specialist, project manager, and administrative assistant, provides overall leadership and ensures that the GSCDN vision is supported and a strategy for funding is in place.

Outcomes

Advocacy efforts within the GSCDN are spurring development of regional SCD networks in East/Central Africa, the Middle East, and India as SCD professionals embrace the idea of fostering collaboration to seek evidence-based solutions within their regions. The GSCDN is in a position to disseminate best practices in developing newborn screening programs and establishing clinical care programs in low-income settings. Safety and effectiveness pilot studies of hydroxyurea therapy are about to be launched. There is the realization that reliable epidemiologic data is required to strengthen advocacy if governments, policy makers, and international donor agencies are going to place SCD high on their agenda.

While SCD is associated with high mortality in children younger than 5 years in sub-Saharan Africa and manifests as a chronic, debilitating lifelong disorder in many high-, middle-, and low-income countries, coordinated global effort by big funders in global health to combat this disease remains elusive. The GSCDN faces a major challenge in quantifying the contribution of SCD to under-5 mortality due to the weak clinical care and data-capture infrastructure in the countries with highest disease burden. Yet such valuable data are actively sought by international global health funders as a justification to include SCD in their programs.

Call to Action

Sickle cell disease advocacy needs further strengthening to mobilize a broad partnership including SCD professionals, patient and family groups, academic health institutions, national governments, NGOs, international donor agencies, and philanthropic groups including industry, WHO, and the UN Educational, Scientific and Cultural Organization. The reports generated by the WHO Secretariat in 2006 and the superbly crafted strategy by the WHO Regional Committee for Africa should serve as reference points for developing a global action plan. These documents recommend the implementation of priority interventions including improvements and accessibility of health care, screening of newborns, training of health professionals, genetic counseling, public awareness, and advocacy. To translate these laudable goals into actionable steps, governments in countries with high disease burden must develop an in-depth understanding of the scale of the problem as an impetus for crafting needed strategies for solutions. The action plan must take into account limited resources and competing priorities for health care financing. The solutions must be evidence-based and cost-effective if they are going to be sustainable. Furthermore, the interventions should be integrated into existing health care systems at the primary, secondary, and tertiary levels. Newborn screening, nutrition, immunization, antibacterial and malarial prophylaxis, and SCD education are all interventions that lend themselves to integration into the primary care system.

Sickle cell disease professionals, patients, families, and organizations should embark on concerted efforts aimed at raising public awareness through education, coupled with well-informed and coordinated advocacy efforts to help place SCD issues high on the agenda of government officials and health policy makers within countries. On the global front, global health funders should consider supporting efforts needed to further quantify the burden of SCD and its contribution to under-5 mortality. In doing so, there should be an awareness of the epidemiologic shift that has already began in certain regions, with consequent increase in the population of children who have survived in early life and are in need of long-term care. It is time to include SCD on the list of chronic noncommunicable diseases needing a coordinated global effort to tackle.

References

1. Modell B, Darlison M. Global epidemiology of haemoglobin disorders and derived service indicators. *Bull World Health Organ.* 2008;86(6):480–487

2. Weatherall DJ. Genetic variation and susceptibility to infection: the red cell and malaria. *Br J Haematol.* 2008;141(3):276–286

3. World Health Organization. Sickle-cell anemia. In: *Fifty-Ninth World Health Assembly, Geneva, 22-27 May 2006, Summary Records of Committees and Reports of Committees.* Geneva, Switzerland: World Health Organization; 2006:87–91

4. United Nations General Assembly. Recognition of sickle cell anaemia as a public health priority. December 2008. http://www.un.org/ga/search/view_doc.asp?symbol=A/63/PV.73&Lang=E. Accessed May 9, 2013

5. Aygun B, Odame I. A global perspective on sickle cell disease. *Pediatr Blood Cancer.* 2012;59(2):386–390

6. Quinn CT, Rogers ZR, McCavit TL, Buchanan GR. Improved survival of children and adolescents with sickle cell disease. *Blood.* 2010;115(17):3447–3452

7. Telfer P, Coen P, Chakravorty S, et al. Clinical outcomes in children with sickle cell disease living in England: a neonatal cohort in East London. *Haematologica.* 2007;92(7):905–912

8. King L, Fraser R, Forbes M, Grindley M, Ali S, Reid M. Newborn sickle cell disease screening: the Jamaican experience (1995-2006). *J Med Screen.* 2007;14(3):117–122

9. Fernandes AP, Januário JN, Cangussu CB, Macedo DL, Viana MB. Mortality of children with sickle cell disease: a population study. *J Pediatr (Rio J).* 2010;86(4):279–284

10. Odunvbun ME, Okolo AA, Rahimy CM. Newborn screening for sickle cell disease in a Nigerian hospital. *Public Health.* 2008;122(10):1111–1116

11. Rahimy MC, Gangbo A, Ahouignan G, Alihonou E. Newborn screening for sickle cell disease in the Republic of Benin. *J Clin Pathol.* 2009;62(1):46–48

12. Tshilolo L, Aissi LM, Lukusa D, et al. Neonatal screening for sickle cell anaemia in the Democratic Republic of the Congo: experience from a pioneer project on 31 204 newborns. *J Clin Pathol.* 2009;62(1):35–38

13. Williams TN, Uyoga S, Macharia A, et al. Bacteraemia in Kenyan children with sickle-cell anaemia: a retrospective cohort and case-control study. *Lancet.* 2009;374(9698):1364–1370

14. Makani J, Komba AN, Cox SE, et al. Malaria in patients with sickle cell anemia: burden, risk factors, and outcome at the outpatient clinic and during hospitalization. *Blood.* 2010;115(2):215–220

15. McAuley CF, Webb C, Makani J, et al. High mortality from Plasmodium falciparum malaria in children with sickle cell anemia on the coast of Kenya. *Blood.* 2010;116(10):1663–1668

16. Charache S, Terrin ML, Moore RD, et al. Effect of hydroxyurea on the frequency of painful crises in sickle cell anemia. Investigators of the Multicenter Study of Hydroxyurea in Sickle Cell Anemia. *N Engl J Med.* 1995;332(20):1317–1322

17. Voskaridou E, Christoulas D, Bilalis A, et al. The effect of prolonged administration of hydroxyurea on morbidity and mortality in adult patients with sickle cell syndromes: results of a 17-year, single-center trial (LaSHS). *Blood.* 2010;115(12):2354–2363

18. Weatherall D, Hofman K, Rodgers G, Ruffin J, Hrynkow S. A case for developing North-South partnerships for research in sickle cell disease. *Blood.* 2005;105(3):921–923

19. Odame I, Kulkarni R, Ohene-Frempong K. Concerted global effort to combat sickle cell disease: the first global congress on sickle cell disease in Accra, Ghana. *Am J Prev Med.* 2011;41(6 Suppl 4):S417–S421

20. World Health Organization Regional Office for Africa. Sickle cell disease: a strategy for the WHO African region. June 2010. http://www.afro.who.int/index.php?option=com_docman&task=doc_download&gid=6638. Accessed May 9, 2013

Section 5

Maternal and Newborn Health

Chapter 19

Newborn Survival

Joy Lawn, MBBS, MRCP(Paeds), MPH, PhD
Mary Kinney, MSc
Zulfiqar Bhutta, MBBS, FRCP, FRCPCH, FAAP(Hon), PhD
Peter Waiswa, MBChB, MPH, PhD
Elizabeth Bocaletti, MD, MPH
Charles Mwansambo, MBChB, BSc, DCH, MRCP, FRCPCH(UK)
Kate J. Kerber, MPH

Rising Importance of Newborn Survival

The pace of progress toward Millennium Development Goal (MDG) 4 for child survival is accelerating as the 2015 target draws nearer. Mortality in children younger than 5 years has almost halved in a generation, with breakthroughs even in the poorest countries. While fewer newborns are dying each year, progress remains much slower than for children after the first month of life. Neonatal deaths decreased from 4.4 million in 1990 to 3.0 million in 2011. As a result, newborn deaths now account for 43% of deaths among children younger than 5 years—up from 36% in 1990 (Figure 19-1).[1,2] More investment in health care for women and children contributed to greater progress for the survival of mothers (3.2% per year) and children after the neonatal period (3.0% per year) than for newborn survival (1.8% per year).[1] While some countries are on track to achieve the MDG 4 target for child survival by 2015, many others, particularly in sub-Saharan Africa, are not yet making sufficient progress.

Rising Voice for Newborns at the Global and Regional Levels

There were many reasons for the lack of visibility of newborn deaths. Primary among these was the fact that the vast majority of these deaths occurred at home, uncounted, as well as the perception that addressing such deaths without intensive care was impossible. Taboos and seclusion around the time of birth contributed to social invisibility. Yet the lack of

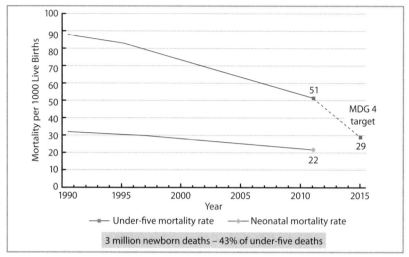

Figure 19-1. Under-5 mortality rate versus neonatal mortality rate, linked to Millennium Development Goal 4 progress. Adapted from Lawn JE, Kinney MV, Black RE, et al. Newborn survival: a multi-country analysis of a decade of change. *Health Policy Plan.* 2012;27(Suppl 3):iii6–iii28, with permission from Oxford University Press.

public mourning for newborn deaths does not equal a lack of pain for the families who lose these babies. Another reason was the perceived complexity of managing sick newborns that was thought to be only possible in tertiary institutions with pediatricians and neonatologists. Over the last decade, strategic shifts in the availability of data about the problem and solutions, as well as a widespread movement for change, have helped to bring these millions of newborn deaths to wider attention.

Prior to *The Lancet* "Neonatal Survival Series" in 2005,[3] there were no globally or nationally comparable estimates for causes of neonatal deaths. An important methodologic shift published in *The Lancet* "Neonatal Survival Series" and in the World Health Organization (WHO) *World Health Report 2005* was to classify neonatal deaths into programmatically relevant categories instead of a single "perinatal causes" category (Figure 19-2).[6] This adjustment clearly demonstrated the high proportion of under-5 deaths in the neonatal period, which were previously hidden in the categories of "perinatal causes" and "other," notably neonatal infections.

National estimates for cause of death and mortality rates were developed for more than 190 countries using data from vital registration and studies.[3,7] These methods are now used for UN annual mortality rate estimates and biennial cause-of-death updates and trend projections.[5] Data now clearly show that 3 causes of death account for more than 85% of the

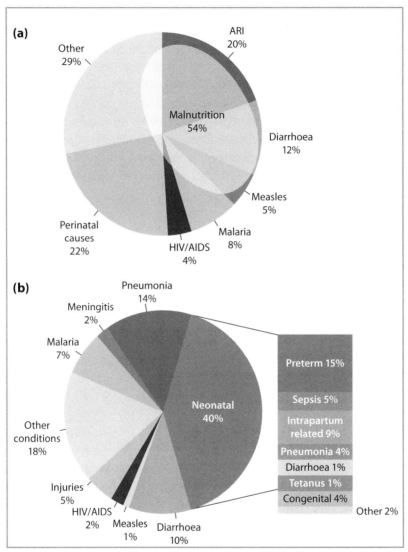

Figure 19-2. Improved visibility in causes of newborn death shows 3 leading killers of newborns: preterm birth, intrapartum complications, and infections, all with effective and feasible programmatic solutions. *a,* Child and neonatal causes of death globally in 2000 show neonatal deaths comprised 36% of under-5 deaths but were not visible being split across "perinatal causes" and other causes.[4] *b,* Child and neonatal causes of death global estimates for 193 countries for 2010 show increased visibility for deaths in the neonatal period.[5] Adapted from Lawn JE, Kinney MV, Black RE, et al. Newborn survival: a multi-country analysis of a decade of change. *Health Policy Plan.* 2012;(Suppl 3):iii6–iii28, with permission from Oxford University Press.

world's neonatal deaths: complications of preterm birth, infections, and intrapartum-related causes (birth asphyxia). The proportionate burden of single causes of death has shifted over time, with preterm complications now contributing a larger share. More than 1 million babies born too soon die shortly after birth; countless others suffer some type of lifelong physical, neurologic, or educational disability, often at great cost to families and society. Highlighting the 3 main causes of death helped to move from an overwhelming number of deaths that seemed intractable to specific causes with linked solutions. Robust and programmatically relevant data enabled effective advocacy efforts to gain traction in policy and program change.

Pediatricians working in partnership with other professionals have been at the center of the movements to improve numbers and knowledge and catalyze this change for newborns. A number of key products have been developed with and for policy makers, program managers, and health professionals and have brought increasing global attention to newborn survival (Table 19-1). *The Lancet* "Neonatal Survival Series" was developed by an informal network of experts, including pediatricians, and galvanized attention for newborn health at global and country levels. It came as the result of several years of efforts building on advances in data as well as rational health system planning guidance with evidence for cost-effective interventions.[3,15] Regional and country-specific guidance followed through multi-partner products, such as *Opportunities for Africa's Newborns,*[8] the Pan American Health Organization strategy for reducing neonatal mortality,[9] and national newborn health situation analyses.[11] These publications raised awareness of the number and causes of newborn deaths; identified context-relevant, evidence-based interventions that could be delivered within the existing health system; strengthened regional and national coalitions; and often led to change in national policies and programs.

Global movements have been critical to increased attention to newborn survival and integration into maternal, newborn, and child health packages, and the importance of small, informal networks across countries and organizations was especially critical.[15] The informal network of global health professionals working for the promotion of newborn survival was a powerful and influential group for change. This group, consisting of motivated and like-minded professionals, was instrumental in changing the landscape and reducing the sense of fatalism around neonatal mortality. Shiffman found that the success of this group resulted from a clearly defined goal to reduce neonatal mortality; the small size of the group; the existence of Saving Newborn Lives (SNL), an initiative of Save the

Table 19-1. Products and Messaging That Built a Movement for Change for Newborn Survival

Product	Focus
The Lancet "Neonatal Survival Series"[3]	First national and global estimates of numbers of newborn deaths, causes, lives saved, and cost for feasible interventions *Message: 4 million newborn deaths each year are critical to address for MDG 4 progress and have specific causes and solutions possible at the community level.*
Opportunities for Africa's Newborns[8]	Context-specific consensus-building on practical opportunities to integrate and scale up newborn care with political commitment through launch at Pan-African Parliament *Message: Stakeholders in African countries can maximize opportunities in existing programs and resources for newborn survival and transform Africa's next generation.*
Pan American Health Organization *Reducing Neonatal Mortality and Morbidity in Latin America and the Caribbean: An Interagency Strategic Consensus*[9]	Wide consensus building on evidence-based interventions for newborn care in communities and through health services, with a focus on the most marginalized population groups *Message: Many Latin American countries are on track for MDG 4, but newborn survival remains an issue for the poorest and requires action.*
Countdown to 2015: Maternal, Newborn & Child Survival[10]	At the first countdown meeting in 2005, the focus was mainly on child survival. The movement has since widened to include reproductive, maternal, newborn, and child health. Data profiles for 75 high-priority countries are the core product and are now produced annually and include some newborn care indicators. *Message: Accountability for action for maternal, newborn, and child health is a priority, and data for newborn survival is being increasingly incorporated in global tracking systems.*
Save the Children country situation analyses for newborn survival[11]: Afghanistan, Bangladesh, Bolivia, India, Malawi, Mali, Nepal, Nigeria, Pakistan, Tanzania, Uganda, Vietnam	Multiple countries have developed situation analyses to plan action to reduce their newborn deaths. Each is unique and several have led to implementation plans with subnational investments and accountability. *Message: The problem, solutions, and recommended actions are context-specific and national governments, partners, and champions can and must drive change.*

Table 19-1. Products and Messaging That Built a Movement for Change for Newborn Survival *(continued)*

Research on community-based newborn care culminating in WHO/UNICEF joint statement on home visits for newborn care[12]	Proof of concept trials showing that community-based mechanisms to delivering care during pregnancy and the postnatal period is effective and feasible. *Message: There is consensus on the importance and approach for home visits for maternal and newborn care; the specific package and cadres will vary by setting.*
Lawn et al, *International Journal of Gynaecology and Obstetrics*[4]	First systematic review of evidence-based intervention to reduce intrapartum-related deaths *Message: 2 million deaths at birth and 60 million home births each year require urgent attention, action, and innovation for the sake of women and their babies.*
The Lancet "Stillbirth Series"[13]	First country-cleared estimates of stillbirth numbers and rates as well as effect and cost of interventions linked to maternal and newborn care *Message: Stillbirths do count and are a loss to women, families, and communities. Care at birth gives a triple return on investment.*
Born Too Soon: The Global Action Report on Preterm Birth[14]	First national estimates of preterm birth rates and consensus on actions to reduce deaths and disability due to preterm birth, with more than 50 organizations involved and foreword by UN Secretary General *Message: 15 million babies are born too soon, and 1 million newborns die due to complications of preterm birth each year, with rates rising in most countries. Premature babies can be saved now with feasible, cost-effective solutions, especially kangaroo mother care and antenatal steroids. Everyone has a role to play and parents are especially powerful.*
Helping Babies Breathe training program and devices	Simplified algorithm for newborn resuscitation with training package and lower-cost robust devices involving targeted advocacy and developing global and national champions *Message: Improving care at birth through practical skills and lower-cost equipment saves lives and is feasible.*

Abbreviations: MDG, Millennium Development Goal; UNICEF, United Nations Children's Fund; WHO, World Health Organization.

Children funded by the Bill & Melinda Gates Foundation, to facilitate interactions and link to change in countries; the lack of division on technical issues; and a teamwork approach. *The Lancet* "Neonatal Survival Series" solidified this informal network and enabled the group to move the agenda forward. In addition, SNL provided technical guidance and advocacy for newborn survival globally, to global health organizations (eg, WHO, United Nations Children's Fund [UNICEF]), and in the countries where they work. Also, the gap in research for newborn survival, particularly on solutions at a community-based level, allowed the informal group with SNL to encourage academia to invest further in relevant research (Box 19-1).

The first formal global newborn network was the Healthy Newborn Partnership. This group began in 2000 and grew to more than 30 organizations by 2005, with SNL serving as the secretariat. The maternal and child health communities had had similar networks, the Safe Motherhood Initiative and the Child Survival Partnership, respectively. Thus, to unify these communities, the Partnership for Maternal, Newborn & Child Health (PMNCH) was established in 2005.[23] Pediatricians, including representatives from the International Pediatric Association, continue to serve on the PMNCH advisory group. The PMNCH has made significant strides in advancing maternal, newborn, and child health issues, including the UN Secretary General Global Strategy for Women's and Children's Health and the Commission on Information and Accountability for Women's and Children's Health. In 2010, a Web community was launched called Healthy Newborn Network, and this has widened the community to include powerful parent groups and civil society, including more than 70 organizations and 3,000 individual members.

Over the last decade, a number of products addressing specific accountability and knowledge gaps were associated with a wide consensus process involving formal and informal networks and represent more than just publications. Countdown to 2015: Maternal, Newborn & Child Survival, established in 2005 as a multidisciplinary, multi-institutional collaboration, increasingly incorporated newborn data into its tracking mechanisms and reports.[10] Pediatricians led research on community-based newborn survival interventions, particularly in South Asia (Box 19-1),[17-21] resulting in a WHO/UNICEF joint statement on home visits for newborn care.[12] Peer-reviewed academic supplements on stillbirths and intrapartum-related deaths received widespread media attention and emphasized the need to improve care during pregnancy and birth and in the first days of life.[4,13,24] Pediatricians have also been at the forefront of efforts to address specific

Box 19-1. Example of Building the Evidence Base for Community-Based Newborn Care

Increasing advocacy was paired with the initiation of community-based projects and research trials to generate local evidence on solutions to improve newborn survival. In 1999, published results from the home-based neonatal care program developed by the Society for Education Action and Research in Community Health in Gadchiroli, India, influenced several community-based initiatives for newborn survival in other countries.[16] From 1999 to 2008, trials on behavior change and communication activities for newborn health including women's groups, testing home visits for preventive and care seeking, as well as community-based curative care took place in South Asia, primarily in rural settings, where female literacy was 40% or lower, the majority of births took place at home, and research studies were mainly outside the public sector health care systems. Studies in Bangladesh, India, Pakistan, and Nepal found that a major effect on neonatal mortality is achievable through community-based intervention packages.[17-21] The evidence base has been further reviewed systematically and in depth with support from the International Initiative for Impact Evaluation[22] and Cochrane Collaboration[22] and extensive analysis of findings from 18 trials that evaluated community-based intervention packages. Systematic reviews demonstrated that these packages of care could reduce neonatal and perinatal mortality by as much as 24% and 20%, respectively. The evidence base of these community platforms played a significant role in moving newborn survival from implausible to plausible, resulting in a policy shift toward a more community-based approach in these settings.

Trials and implementation research are completed or underway in 7 African countries using models adapted from the Asian studies, including cluster randomized trials in Ethiopia, Ghana, South Africa, Tanzania, and Uganda—collectively known as the Africa Newborn Network. In most African countries, approximately half of all births take place in a health facility, making the continuum of care between the home and health facility and the quality of facility care critical; these have been an explicit part of most of the African trials. Nationally, adaptation and testing of these packages involved government and local stakeholders, including health care professionals, and the process and results have already begun to inform integrated newborn care in these countries and across the continent.

Linking studies as a research network provides collective value for building the evidence, including

- Comparable results allowing for pooling—common definitions and tools to define and measure mortality, cause of death, intervention coverage, human resource capacity, and cost.

- A health system implementation approach to assessing cost and human resources has been key, using a standard approach called the Cost of Integrated Newborn Care tool.

- Country-to-country sharing—a series of workshops and site visits have provided opportunities for investigators to share experiences, tools, findings, and methodologic challenges as well as to interact with other newborn health experts.

- Capacity building for research—health and research professionals are linked into the settings in which research is taking place. Many network members are in the process or have finished postgraduate education linked to the research.

causes of newborn deaths and interventions, through Helping Babies Breathe[25] and the *Born Too Soon* report.[14] Continuous leadership in the movement for newborn health has continued to be provided by the small informal network of actors, several of whom are pediatricians.[15]

Rising Momentum for Change in Countries

There is no "one size fits all" solution for newborn health and survival. In each country, the numbers and causes of neonatal deaths, capacity of the health system, and obstacles faced differ, as do stewardship from policy makers and availability of resources, including health professionals. Effective planning involves a participatory political process that identifies and engages key stakeholders, promotes an enabling policy environment, and results in ownership of a plan and identification of the resources needed for implementation.

In countries there have been various mechanisms to convene national stakeholders on policies, implementation strategies, and monitoring of newborn survival initiatives. For example, informal partnerships in Bangladesh among the Ministry of Health, partner organizations, and high-profile newborn health champions have resulted in policy and programmatic change for newborn survival.[26] In Uganda, the national Newborn Steering Committee (NSC) was established as a formal advisory arm to the Ministry of Health on newborn health issues (Box 19-2).[27] The NSC, together with groups independent from government such as professional organizations, the media, and academia, has worked to establish newborn health as national policy. In addition, the NSC mobilized the Ministry of Health and partners for Uganda to spearhead survival of preterm babies as a champion country under *Born Too Soon*. The National Neonatology Forum in India, led by pediatricians, has worked closely with partners on a wide range of initiatives to improve newborn health through policy, training, education, and research since 1980, including publishing the quarterly *Journal of Neonatology* and organizing fellowships.[28] Nepal and Bangladesh also have vibrant perinatal societies led by senior pediatricians. Similarly, the Nigerian Society for Neonatal Medicine, founded in 2008 by concerned national pediatricians, was among the first neonatal societies in sub-Saharan Africa. In addition to annual meetings and skills training, the group has sought to strengthen links between tertiary care and primary- and community-level care through outreach and mentorship opportunities, particularly related to neonatal sepsis prevention and treatment.

Box 19-2. Example From Uganda of a Network of Champions for Newborn Survival

Following the publication of *The Lancet* "Neonatal Survival Series" in 2005, Ministry of Health representatives and health professionals in Uganda identified newborn survival as a gap requiring specific technical expertise to transform policy and scale up interventions. Consequently, the national Newborn Steering Committee (NSC) was established in 2006 as an advisory arm to the Ugandan Ministry of Health.

The NSC provides a forum for champions, implementers, researchers, academics, and policy makers to regularly meet and share best practices as well as coordinate efforts and outputs for newborn survival. The multidisciplinary NSC comprises approximately 20 members from different backgrounds, portfolios, institutions, and organizations. Professional organizations including pediatricians are active members.

Key outputs of the NSC include conducting and launching the first ever *Situation Analysis of Newborn Health in Uganda* in 2008, developing a component of the National Child Survival Strategy pertaining to a framework for newborn health implementation as well as specific norms and standards for newborn services at each level of the health system, and providing technical expertise to the creation of job aids for newborn care. The NSC continues to link with training institutions and health professional associations to bring together upcoming champions for newborn health. It also spearheaded the Uganda Newborn Survival Study (UNEST), the early experiences of which were used to inform the national village health team (community health worker) strategy that is being scaled up. An effective advocacy strategy used by UNEST was to develop an advocacy video to engage the Ministry of Health, partners, and the public.

With greater attention on newborn health at a national level, the committee is shifting focus toward ensuring district-level planning and financing of newborn health programs within the current 5-year Health Sector Strategic & Investment Plan.[27] Currently the NSC is spearheading efforts for Uganda to become one of the African examples in scaling up preterm prevention and care. It works closely with the media to achieve this.

In addition to the participatory political process, effective planning for newborn care requires a systematic management and prioritization process, such as the 4-step approach proposed in *The Lancet* "Neonatal Survival Series."[29]

The first step involves using data and evidence to assess the newborn health situation in the context of maternal, newborn, and child health. Where and why are newborns dying, and what is the coverage of lifesaving care? Which existing policies provide a platform for saving newborn lives? Are there missed opportunities that can be addressed, for example, due to inadequate staff or the need to change policies to allow midwives, nurses, or community health workers to be equipped and enabled to perform lifesaving tasks? Are basic commodities available? The UN Commission on Life-Saving Commodities for Women and Children has included 4 high-priority commodities for newborn survival—a great opportunity to accelerate the scale-up of these interventions.

Advances in evidence for community-based care have been critical, especially to focus on reaching the poorest and in showing "do-ability" for saving newborn lives even for the 54 million born at home (Box 19-2). *The Lancet* "Newborn Survival Series" paper on evidence-based, cost-effective interventions remains one of the most cited and influential papers on newborn care over the last decade and a basis for many subsequent efforts at defining intervention platforms and packages for care.[30] The evidence synthesized at the time recognized 16 cost-effective and feasible interventions with the potential to save lives at scale. The paper suggested that almost two-thirds of all neonatal deaths could be prevented each year if high coverage was achieved for packages of proven, cost-effective interventions that are delivered through 3 service delivery models (outreach, family-community, and facility-based clinical care) at different points along the continuum of care (preconception and antenatal, intrapartum, and postnatal care).

The second step requires the identification of solutions within the constraints of the existing situation and implementing phased approaches to maximize the number of lives saved now as well as overall health system strengthening over time. In a weak health system, improving community care and outreach services might be the first priority. Up to one-third of newborn deaths can be prevented through healthy family behaviors, and home care is feasible in almost all health systems.[12] The first week is the riskiest week of life, yet many countries are only just beginning postnatal care programs to reach mothers and babies at this critical time.[26] Now is the time to ensure the inclusion of newborn health interventions in community packages that are being scaled up in a number of low- and middle-income countries as part of the second primary health care revolution. To succeed, however, we need to learn from the past and have a focused set of tasks, with adequate training, supervision, incentives, and referral links. Addressing missed opportunities in health facilities will improve quality of care for those able to access services. Epidemiology is a key driver; for example, in Malawi, with the highest estimated rate of preterm birth in the world, this is a political and programmatic priority. Indeed, Malawi has made significant progress in scaling up kangaroo mother care and using various cadres to provide this care. Several other African countries have come on learning visits to Malawi, and this illustrates a general principle that as well as published evidence and products, seeing program reality is very important.

A number of country teams have also undertaken visits to Nepal to see female community workers providing home-based management of neonatal sepsis; this experience has been influential, for example, for a team of Ethiopians who have visited twice.

The third step is to implement interventions and strengthen the health system overall, with particular attention to human resources. Comprehensive human resource plans must focus not only on training but also on retaining and sustaining existing staff. While staffing remains a major challenge, lack of key supplies and drugs also contributes to lives lost. This gap has led to the creation of the UN Commission on Life-Saving Commodities for Women and Children, which aims to increase access to medicines and health supplies including those needed for newborn survival. Systematically scaling up newborn care also requires increasing demand for services and overcoming access bottlenecks, particularly for

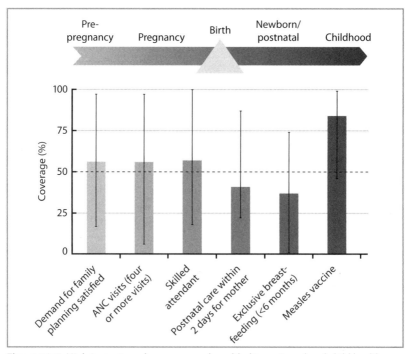

Figure 19-3. High-impact newborn care can be added to maternal and child health care along the continuum of care, but coverage remains low, especially for the poorest countries.[14] Note that many specific, high-impact newborn care interventions lack coverage data, eg, kangaroo mother care, neonatal resuscitation.[10] *Note:* Median for 75 countdown priority countries with available data; bars refer to ranges between countries.

the poorest families. Coverage of newborn care is currently the weakest contact point in the continuum of care (Figure 19-3), with only 41% of women reached with postnatal care within 2 days after delivery.

The final step in the program cycle is to monitor coverage and measure the effect and cost of services. Quality of data, frequency of data collection, and use of data for decision-making are crucial. Ongoing advancements to mortality and cause-of-death data have informed program planning, but key gaps remain in coverage data for high-impact interventions and process data for tracking the strength of implementation limit capacity for health systems evaluation. More effort is needed to improve national vital registration systems as well as to generate comparable cost analyses and data for health system planning, and for prioritizing implementation research gaps. A major research gap being explored is how to reach mothers and babies at birth and the early postnatal period in settings where the majority of births occur at home. There are promising community-based service delivery models that have been tested mainly in research studies in Asia that are now being adapted and evaluated at scale and tested through a network of African implementation research trials (Box 19-1).

Accelerating Change, Strengthening Champions

Improved data and evidence for action as well as implementation strategies and resources for newborn survival alone are not enough to tackle the high burden of deaths globally. Greater change requires coalitions. While pediatricians have been leaders of change, institutionalizing the newborn care agenda will require a team of champions for all health care professional groups. Neonatologists often lead newborn care efforts in high-income countries; however, there are few, if any, neonatologists in most African countries and also a limited number of pediatricians. The benchmark set by WHO for physicians, nurses, and midwives is 23 per 10,000 people, a level met by only 20% of countries in the high-burden regions of sub-Saharan Africa and Southern Asia.[31] In contrast, the density of these health workers in Norway is 361 per 10,000 people.

Different cadres of health care professionals have complementary roles in advancing newborn survival (Box 19-3). Health care professionals, including pediatricians, can take specific action to *advocate, act,* and *amplify* change for newborns.

Box 19-3. Newborn Survival: A Test of Health Care Professional Teamwork

A baby's survival is dependent on the mother's health and care at birth and immediately after. This care depends on a team of health workers.[32]

- Midwives, who care for the women, ensure safe birth and essential newborn care, and if necessary, resuscitate the baby

- Obstetricians, who provide care to the woman, especially for complications during pregnancy and childbirth, although in many countries the numbers are limited and more likely to be in urban centers

- Pediatricians, who undertake advanced resuscitation and ongoing care if needed, though where most newborns are born and die, there are few pediatricians and almost no neonatologists

- Neonatal nurses, who have specific skills in newborn care, such as resuscitation, kangaroo mother care, caring for preterm and sick newborns, and support for well babies including breastfeeding and counseling on healthy behaviors

- Community health workers, who educate women on identifying danger signs in pregnancy and conduct postnatal care visits, and other primary health care workers such as those involved in immunization and nutrition programs

This team approach will save lives because there is no one cadre solely responsible for newborn care. If each of these groups does not take collective responsibility, speak up, and work together for newborns, more babies will continue to die. For millions of babies worldwide, nurses, midwives, and community health workers are the main frontline workers. Thus, it is essential that physicians facilitate an effective team response based on context. The gap for neonatal nurses is especially acute, with almost no accredited neonatal nurse training programs in Africa and South Asia. Pediatricians can choose to be promoters of change to enable skills in other team members and support the system to reach the poorest families.

Task shifting for emergency obstetric care and care for newborns to nonphysician clinicians, including nurses and midwives, has been widely embraced and is yielding positive results in some countries where physician density is low. For example, Malawi is on track for Millennium Development Goal 4 despite only having 16 obstetricians and 8 pediatricians nationwide. Nurses provide much of the inpatient care for newborns, and clinical officers perform the bulk of emergency obstetric operations in Malawi district hospitals.[33] Home visits to mothers and newborns are provided by the community-based health cadre called Health Surveillance Assistants.

Advocate for Appropriate Policies and Financing Across the Continuum of Care for Maternal, Newborn, and Child Health

Invest time and resources to train more health workers, including health care professionals as well as community health workers. This includes preservice training, upgrading of skills, and provision of competency-based education as defined by the specific professional association.

Act to Improve Service Delivery, Audit, and Accountability

- Set standards for care. Health care professionals need to be aware of, maintain competency in, and adhere to standard care protocols, including correct assessment of patients and lifesaving skills, especially during labor, childbirth (eg, neonatal resuscitation), and management of childhood illness. Move beyond survival toward improving quality of care.
- Adapt to new evidence and changing technology; develop and introduce improved tools and treatments.

Amplify Change Through Other Networks and Partnerships and Developing Champions

- Partner with other professional bodies, research institutions, and government. Identify proven, effective interventions and make them known to association members; promote links with academic institutions to undertake research, education, and monitoring through existing networks.
- Improve the performance and capacity of frontline workers, including neonatal nurses and community health workers, as well as all mothers and community members, to care for newborns.

There is great potential for accelerated progress in reducing newborn deaths around the world and improving the health of the next generation. The key ingredients are in place with effective interventions, more investment in commodities, and increasing partnership and leadership from professional organizations. The final push toward the MDG deadline of 2015 presents an opportunity and also the threat of loss of momentum after the deadline. Ensuring ongoing progress and programmatic action is critical for the future of maternal, newborn, and child health.

References

1. Lawn JE, Kinney MV, Black RE, et al. Newborn survival: a multi-country analysis of a decade of change. *Health Policy Plan.* 2012;27(Suppl 3):iii6–iii28
2. United Nations Children's Fund. *Levels & Trends in Child Mortality Report 2012: Estimates Developed by the UN Inter-agency Group for Child Mortality Estimation.* New York, NY: United Nations Children's Fund; 2012. http://www.unicef.org.uk/Documents/Publications/UNICEF_2012_IGME_child_mortality_report.pdf. Accessed May 9, 2013
3. Lawn JE, Cousens S, Zupan J; Lancet Neonatal Survival Steering Team. 4 million neonatal deaths: when? Where? Why? *Lancet.* 2005;365(9462):891–900
4. Lawn JE, Lee AC, Kinney M, et al. Two million intrapartum-related stillbirths and neonatal deaths: where, why, and what can be done? *Int J Gynaecol Obstet.* 2009;107(Suppl 1):S5–S19

5. Liu L, Johnson HL, Cousens S, et al. Global, regional, and national causes of child mortality: an updated systematic analysis for 2010 with time trends since 2000. *Lancet.* 2012;379(9832):2151–2161

6. Lawn JE, Osrin D, Adler A, Cousens S. Four million neonatal deaths: counting and attribution of cause of death. *Paediatr Perinat Epidemiol.* 2008;22(5):410–416

7. Lawn JE, Wilczynska-Ketende K, Cousens SN. Estimating the causes of 4 million neonatal deaths in the year 2000. *Int J Epidemiol.* 2006;35(3):706–718

8. The Partnership for Maternal, Newborn & Child Health. *Opportunities for Africa's Newborns: Practical Data, Policy and Programmatic Support for Newborn Care in Africa.* Cape Town, South Africa: The Partnership for Maternal, Newborn & Child Health; 2006. http://www.who.int/pmnch/media/publications/oanfullreport.pdf. Accessed May 9, 2013

9. Benguigui Y, Fescina R, Camacho V, et al. *Reducing Neonatal Mortality and Morbidity in Latin America and The Caribbean: An Interagency Strategic Consensus.* Guatemala: Pan American Health Organization; 2007

10. Countdown to 2015: Maternal, Newborn & Child Survival. http://www.countdown2015mnch.org. Accessed May 9, 2013

11. Healthy Newborn Network. Countries. http://www.healthynewbornnetwork.org/page/countries. Accessed May 9, 2013

12. World Health Organization, United Nations Children's Fund. *Home Visits for the Newborn Child: A Strategy to Improve Survival.* Geneva, Switzerland: World Health Organization; 2009. http://www.unicef.org/health/files/WHO_FCH_CAH_09.02_eng.pdf. Accessed May 9, 2013

13. Lawn JE, Blencowe H, Pattinson R, et al. Stillbirths: where? When? Why? How to make the data count? *Lancet.* 2011;377(9775):1448–1463

14. March of Dimes; The Partnership for Maternal, Newborn & Child Health; Save the Children; World Health Organization. *Born Too Soon: The Global Action Report on Preterm Birth.* Geneva, Switzerland: World Health Organization; 2012. http://www.who.int/pmnch/media/news/2012/201204_borntoosoon-report.pdf. Accessed May 9, 2013

15. Shiffman J. Issue attention in global health: the case of newborn survival. *Lancet.* 2010;375(9730):2045–2049

16. Bang AT, Bang RA, Baitule SB, Reddy MH, Deshmukh MD. Effect of home-based neonatal care and management of sepsis on neonatal mortality: field trial in rural India. *Lancet.* 1999;354(9194):1955–1961

17. Bang AT, Reddy HM, Deshmukh MD, Baitule SB, Bang RA. Neonatal and infant mortality in the ten years (1993 to 2003) of the Gadchiroli field trial: effect of home-based neonatal care. *J Perinatol.* 2005;25(Suppl 1):S92–S107

18. Baqui AH, Arifeen SE, Rosen HE, et al. Community-based validation of assessment of newborn illnesses by trained community health workers in Sylhet district of Bangladesh. *Trop Med Int Health.* 2009;14(12)1448–1456

19. Bhutta ZA, Memon ZA, Soofi S, Salat MS, Cousens S, Martines J. Implementing community-based perinatal care: results from a pilot study in rural Pakistan. *Bull World Health Organ.* 2008;86(6):452–459

20. Manandhar DS, Osrin D, Shrestha BP, et al. Effect of a participatory intervention with women's groups on birth outcomes in Nepal: cluster-randomised controlled trial. *Lancet.* 2004;364(9438):970–979

21. Kumar V, Mohanty S, Kumar A, et al. Effect of community-based behaviour change management on neonatal mortality in Shivgarh, Uttar Pradesh, India: a cluster-randomised controlled trial. *Lancet.* 2008;372(9644):1151–1162

22. Lassi ZS, Haider BA, Bhutta ZA. Community-based intervention packages for reducing maternal and neonatal morbidity and mortality and improving neonatal outcomes. *Cochrane Database Syst Rev.* 2010;(11):CD007754

23. Bustreo F, Requejo JH, Merialdi M, Presern C, Songane F. From safe motherhood, newborn, and child survival partnerships to the continuum of care and accountability: moving fast forward to 2015. *Int J Gynaecol Obstet.* 2012;119(Suppl 1):S6–S8

24. Rubens CE, Gravett MG, Victora CG, Nunes TM; GAPPS Review Group. Global report on preterm birth and stillbirth (7 of 7): mobilizing resources to accelerate innovative solutions (Global Action Agenda). *BMC Pregnancy Childbirth.* 2010;10(Suppl 1):S7

25. American Academy of Pediatrics, Helping Babies Breathe. Guides. http://www. helpingbabiesbreathe.org/guides.html. Accessed May 9, 2013

26. Rubayet S, Shahidullah M, Hossain A, et al. Newborn survival in Bangladesh: a decade of change and future implications. *Health Policy Plan.* 2012;27(Suppl 3):iii40–iii56

27. Mbonye AK, Sentongo M, Mukasa GK, et al. Newborn survival in Uganda: a decade of change and future implications. *Health Policy Plan.* 2012;27(Suppl 3):iii104–iii117

28. National Neonatology Forum of India. http://www.nnfi.org. Accessed May 9, 2013

29. Knippenberg R, Lawn JE, Darmstadt GL, et al. Systematic scaling up of neonatal care in countries. *Lancet.* 2005;365(9464):1087–1098

30. Darmstadt GL, Bhutta ZA, Cousens S, et al. Evidence-based, cost-effective interventions: how many newborn babies can we save? *Lancet.* 2005;365(9463):977–988

31. World Health Organization. Welcome to the WHO Global Atlas of the Health Workforce. http://apps.who.int/globalatlas/default.asp. Accessed May 9, 2013

32. Kinney M, Davidge R, Lawn J. 15 million born too soon: what neonatal nurses can do. *J Neonatal Nurs.* In press

33. Chilopora G, Pereira C, Kamwendo F, Chimbiri A, Malunga E, Bergström S. Postoperative outcome of caesarean sections and other major emergency obstetric surgery by clinical officers and medical officers in Malawi. *Hum Resour Health.* 2007;5:17

Chapter 20

Helping Babies Breathe

Susan Niermeyer, MD, MPH, FAAP
William J. Keenan, MD, FAAP

Introduction: Problem/Issue Identification

The day of birth is also a day when many babies and mothers die. Globally, every year, 3 million newborns die in the first month of life and a similar number are stillborn.[1,2] *Asphyxia,* the failure to breathe or sustain effective breathing, is a leading cause of death on the day of birth. Intrapartum-related events, or perinatal asphyxia, account for an estimated one-third of all stillbirths. Prematurity/low birth weight also result in early death from respiratory distress, hypothermia, and inability to feed effectively. Serious infection, including sepsis and pneumonia, is the third major cause of death in the first 28 days of life.[1] Birth carries a high risk of maternal death as well, primarily due to postpartum hemorrhage, preeclampsia/eclampsia, obstructed labor, and infection.[3] Every year 350,000 women die of such pregnancy-related causes globally, and their deaths directly or indirectly jeopardize survival of the fetus or newborn. Although the loss of a baby or mother is an especially tragic event anywhere, the burden of neonatal and maternal mortality is disproportionately borne by low- and middle-income countries, where more than 98% of neonatal and maternal deaths occur.[4]

In the 1930s Ethyl Dunham, MD, the director of the US Children's Bureau and a noted maternal and child health advocate, oversaw a series of studies documenting that the majority of child deaths occurred within the neonatal period and most of these deaths occurred in the first 24 hours following birth. Dr Dunham initiated a series of publications, *Standards and Recommendations for Hospital Care of Newborn Infants,* which was then sponsored by the American Academy of Pediatrics (AAP). In industrialized countries, such changes in perinatal care in the first half of the 20th century made uncomplicated birth a clean and safe passage for mother and baby. When complications do occur, a host of interventions and sophisticated medical technology generally are readily accessible—cesarean delivery in the case of obstructed labor or evidence of intrapartum hypoxia; strict infection-control practices and antibiotic treatment when infection is suspected; and support in the delivery room and neonatal intensive care unit for babies who need help to breathe at birth or who need specialized care for multiple medical problems. Despite this heightened focus during the 1950s to 1970 on the newborn's transition to extrauterine life, asphyxia still ranked as the sixth leading cause of infant death in 1979.[5]

In 1956 the Medical Society of New York published a report that pointed out that improvements in neonatal resuscitation were critical but required investments in appropriate equipment, trained personnel, and ongoing education and research.[6]

In the 1970s William Tooley, MD, and James Sutherland, MD, were tasked to write a neonatal resuscitation chapter for the AAP Committee on Fetus and Newborn. They documented general lack of consensus on neonatal resuscitation and influenced the National Institute of Child Health and Human Development (NICHD) to support innovative neonatal educational projects. One of these projects was the curriculum developed at the Charles Drew Postgraduate Medical School in Los Angeles, which served as the basis of the Neonatal Resuscitation Program (NRP) curriculum. Leadership in the AAP and American Heart Association (William Keenan, Errol Alden, John Raye, George Peckham, Leon Chameides) came together with the principal investigators, Ron Bloom and Catherine Cropley, to publish a professional educational program, the NRP. Beginning in 1987, dissemination proceeded through AAP districts in a cascade from national faculty to regional trainers, hospital-based instructors, and providers. The explicit goal of NRP was to have a trained provider at every delivery who is capable of initiating neonatal resuscitation. Neonatal Resuscitation Program completion quickly became the de facto standard for credentialing of physicians in delivery and newborn nursery settings and demonstrating age-specific competencies among nursing staff. The NRP emphasized psychomotor skills and interprofessional teamwork developed through hands-on practice with mannequins. The NRP resulted in demonstrable changes in practice and improvement in short- and long-term outcomes.[7,8] The rate of asphyxia-specific mortality in the United States fell by nearly 75% from 1979 to 1996.[5]

International dissemination of NRP began very rapidly after the program's introduction in the United States. Pediatricians in other countries who were confronting high rates of neonatal mortality sought out training and, in many countries, established comprehensive national programs to reach professionals attending in-facility births. American Academy of Pediatrics leadership, staff in the AAP Division of Life Support Programs, members of the NRP Steering Committee, and many volunteer trainers from the United States worked with foreign professional organizations (pediatricians and neonatologists), medical universities, and ministries of health to spread training to more than 130 countries. Official translations of NRP educational materials exist in 24 languages (www.aap.org/nrp/global. html). The NRP also established a competitive research support program to help strengthen the evidence base for effective neonatal resuscitation.

Formal implementation research evaluating neonatal resuscitation has been limited, and a conventional randomized, controlled trial would be unethical. Numerous observational before-and-after studies from many different regions of the world support the effectiveness of neonatal resuscitation educational approaches. A systematic review and Delphi estimate of the effect of neonatal resuscitation with studies from China, India, Macedonia, Bulgaria, and Zambia concluded that neonatal resuscitation training in health facilities can avert 30% of intrapartum-related neonatal deaths.[9] A national program of neonatal resuscitation training in Malaysia from 1996 to 2004 coincided with a decline in neonatal and perinatal mortality rates.[10] A nationwide NRP in China showed that in 20 target provinces, the proportion of infants with low Apgar scores (<7 at 1 minute) decreased and intrapartum-related deaths in the delivery room fell by more than half by 4 years after implementation.[11]

International collaboration also strengthened the scientific evidence base for neonatal resuscitation. United States resuscitation experts joined with their counterparts from resuscitation councils in Canada, Latin America, Europe, Australia/New Zealand, South Africa, and Asia through the International Liaison Committee on Resuscitation (ILCOR) (www.ilcor. org). Committee panels work collaboratively to identify important questions in resuscitation, then evaluate and debate the scientific evidence to produce a consensus on neonatal resuscitation science every 5 years. This consensus forms the basis of guidelines produced by regional resuscitation councils. In this way, important research findings from all over the world are quickly incorporated into the evidence base, and the global consensus on science and practice guidelines rapidly transmit the latest recommendations to all parts of the world through open-access electronic publishing. Questions which have central importance in regions with limited medical resources, such as use of air versus oxygen in resuscitation and management of neonates born through meconium-stained amniotic fluid, have quickly come to the forefront. As a result, air rather than 100% oxygen is now recommended globally for initiation of positive-pressure ventilation in term newborns, and there has been a shift away from routine intubation and suctioning of all babies with meconium-stained amniotic fluid.[12] Obstacles to the implementation of practices widely accepted in the developed world have accelerated reexamination and revision of these practices globally.

Problem/Issue Analysis

Despite widespread implementation of NRP and evidence-based guidelines in hospitals around the world, it became obvious that neonatal mortality—especially death from asphyxia or intrapartum-related events—continued to account for a huge burden of mortality in areas with very limited medical resources. The Millennium Development Goals (MDGs), adopted in 2000, aimed at reducing the global impact of poverty and set measurable objectives for reducing maternal and child mortality by 2015. Millennium Development Goal 4 aimed specifically to reduce deaths of children younger than 5 years by two-thirds of 1990 levels by 2015. As the midpoint of the 15-year period passed, a series of scholarly analyses in the medical literature[2,13,14] pointed out the gaps between achieved reductions and 2015 targets for child and maternal mortality. Furthermore, they emphasized the growing proportion of under-5 child mortality due to deaths in the neonatal period. Programs to reduce childhood deaths from acute respiratory infection and diarrhea were saving the lives of older infants and children, but there were few targeted interventions to address the causes of death in the first 28 days of life. As a result, neonates came to account for 40% or more of under-5 child deaths in many countries.

Newborns die of different causes than older infants and children, and thus different interventions are needed. Prematurity and low birth weight, serious infection, and asphyxia account for most deaths in the first month of life (Table 20-1). Among existing interventions for neonates, kangaroo mother care addressed some of the needs of low-weight and premature newborns. Use of clean delivery kits, availability of antibiotic therapy in the community, and exclusive breastfeeding helped to prevent and treat serious infections. However, no simple, low-cost, and effective intervention against asphyxia existed outside of hospitals. The NRP was inappropriate

Table 20-1. Causes of Neonatal Death, Global Data

Cause of Death	Percent of Newborn Deaths
Intrapartum-related complications	23
Complications from preterm birth	35
Severe infections	23
Sepsis/meningitis	13
Pneumonia	11
Tetanus	2
Diarrhea	2
Congenital	9
Other	6

Source: Adapted from Liu L, Johnson HL, Cousens S, et al. Global, regional, and national causes of child mortality: an updated systematic analysis for 2010 with time trends since 2000. *Lancet.* 2012;379(9832):2151–2161

because much of its content dealt with proper use of oxygen and medications and advanced interventions such as chest compressions and intubation. The NRP educational materials were sophisticated, including a comprehensive textbook, multimedia platforms, and relatively costly neonatal mannequins and simulators for skills training. Most of the world viewed neonatal resuscitation as part of intensive care and beyond the scope of primary care.

Further challenges limiting intervention to reduce mortality from intrapartum-related events lay in the scarcity of workforce to provide care at birth. In many MDG 4 and 5 countries, rates of in-facility birth were below 50% and even among the births taking place in medical facilities, the proportion of attendants with appropriate training in neonatal care and equipment to carry out a resuscitation was very small (Figure 20-1). When a birth was attended, usually a single person was present to care for mother and baby. The birth attendant in most cases was not a doctor; in some settings qualified midwives might be present, but more often the training of birth attendants was limited and highly variable from one country to another and even one region to another within a given country.[15,16] Controversy over the most effective devices to provide neonatal resuscitation (mouth-to-mouth or mouth-to-mask, mouth-to-tube-and-mask, bag and mask) created confusion among public health authorities. Supply chain issues, especially in Africa, limited the availability of any devices.

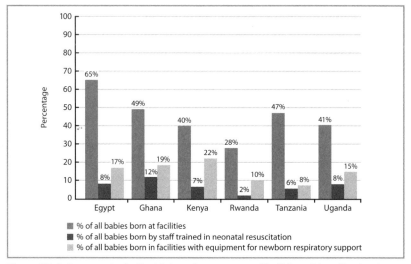

Figure 20-1. Access to in-facility birth and percentage of facilities with staff trained in neonatal resuscitation and equipped with bag and mask. Source: Wall SN, Lee AC, Niermeyer S, et al. Neonatal resuscitation in low-resource settings: what, who, and how to overcome challenges to scale up? *Int J Gynaecol Obstet.* 2009;107(Suppl 1):S47–S64

The relatively high cost of teaching mannequins—often imported with attendant shipping costs, duties, and fees—restricted the spread of training and simultaneous delivery of training and clinical equipment to carry out resuscitation.[17] Once trained, birth attendants who experienced a limited volume of births might lose critical skills rapidly.

The critical problem disproportionally affecting babies born to the poor needed a new approach. In 2006, a group of pediatricians organized the Global Implementation Task Force (GITF) under the auspices of the AAP to design a new educational program that would emphasize basic interventions known to help newborns not breathing at birth. The desired result was to be evidence based, transportable, acceptable across cultures, low cost, and readily disseminated. The advocacy approach of the GITF addressed resuscitation preparation for all birth attendants, development of educational approaches effective in low-resource circumstances, development of high-quality education, wide availability of commodities to assist education and deliver resuscitation, and continuing research. From the beginning, representatives of the World Health Organization (WHO) were involved in program development and coordinated the new curriculum with revision of the WHO *Guidelines on Basic Newborn Resuscitation.* American Academy of Pediatrics volunteers who had taught NRP extensively in international settings and participated in the ILCOR scientific evidence-evaluation process provided the core of experience, along with medical volunteers from LDS Charities who had created an abridged NRP curriculum (excluding intubation and medications) for use in resource-limited settings. Early advice from the Hesperian Health Guides infused the design of the program with an emphasis on empowerment of the first-level health care provider. The GITF saw as its mission the creation of an educational program that would allow birth attendants to help babies breathe wherever they were born. The guiding principle was that all babies in the world deserve the benefit of a birth attended by a person who can help them breathe.

The AAP and members of the GITF began to identify stakeholders in global neonatal survival and collect from them perspective and information about the problem/issue and potential solutions. The AAP had entered into a strategic alliance with Laerdal Medical for joint development of educational strategies incorporating video-guided instruction and basic to advanced simulation. As manufacturers of products for emergency lifesaving and training in life support, Laerdal committed to production of economical training materials and addressing gaps in the clinical equipment available in resource-limited regions. Save the Children Saving Newborn Lives brought a strong policy and advocacy perspective and a focus on documenting the evidence and potential action steps to prevent intrapartum-related deaths. In addition, data from its own field trials supported the potential of basic neonatal resuscitation to save lives.[18] Save the Children programs in several countries expressed interest in implementing a basic neonatal resuscitation training program. Field research underway in the Global Network for Women's and Children's Health Research of the National Institutes of Health[19] informed the content and pictorial style of the curriculum under development and emphasized the importance of forging links with Essential Newborn Care (ENC). The US Agency for International Development (USAID) was seeking a simple, effective resuscitation intervention for programs in maternal and child health.

The Laerdal Foundation for Acute Medicine funded early development of educational materials, as did LDS Charities. Tore Laerdal, MSc, a globally recognized leader in the field of resuscitation, provided crucial analysis of the chain of survival for mother and baby on the day of birth, emphasizing the potential to save as many as 1 million lives each year through improved attention in that crucial 24-hour period. Further in-kind grants made available educational and graphic designs that spurred development of a learner-centered educational program with a focus on active, hands-on learning and skills mastery. Simultaneous engineering and product design advances resulted in the creation of a high-fidelity, low-cost neonatal simulator that was custom-built to display the cardinal evaluation signs for neonatal resuscitation: crying, breathing (spontaneous and assisted), and heart rate (Figure 20-2). The simulator extended the concept of a simple air-filled plastic body mold with highly realistic facial/airway features that had been developed for teaching CPR in the home.[20] When filled with warm water, the simulator had the weight of a 2-kg baby, the warmth of a newborn, and the tone of one who urgently needed resuscitation—a startlingly realistic simulator produced at a cost of around $50, in contrast with other less-functional mannequins at 10 times the cost. Availability of such a low-cost training tool allowed the development of an educational program that focused on continuous active learning with a pair of participants interacting with their own neonatal simulator. Furthermore, participants would leave the training with their simulator and the equipment necessary for resuscitation, so that refresher training and further dissemination could continue at their workplace. Simplification of the self-inflating bag to provide positive-pressure ventilation made it possible to distribute materials for training and highly disinfect or sterilize them for patient use. Design of a reusable bulb suction device that could be opened for cleaning/disinfection and boiled for sterilization overcame another deficiency in equipment; disposable supplies meant for single patient use were often reused without adequate cleaning, leading to potential unintentional contamination and infection. Further improvements in the bag-and-mask system to deliver resuscitation breaths are underway. Special advocacy efforts have resulted in the addition of neonatal resuscitation equipment as part of international health commodities for the first time.[21]

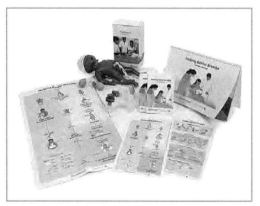

Figure 20-2. Helping Babies Breathe educational materials.

Development of the training program, titled Helping Babies Breathe (HBB), proceeded through successive phases of formative evaluation. Members of the GITF identified key elements of the curriculum and drafted the first outline of content. Rather than begin with abstract concepts of physiology, the program led off with preparation for birth and planning for routine and emergency circumstances. Essential practices of thermal stability, cleanliness, and early and exclusive breastfeeding formed the core components of routine care, giving strong emphasis to the idea that these practices are critical and lifesaving in their own right. For babies who need help to breathe, thorough drying, clearing the airway if necessary, and specific stimulation to breathe constituted a triad of initial steps that were often effective and sufficient if applied in a timely manner. Positive-pressure ventilation with bag and mask using air followed immediately if the initial steps did not result in spontaneous breathing. Chest compressions, included in many previous curricula for first-level settings, were omitted, but assessment of heart rate as an indicator of adequacy of ventilation was included, as were explicit steps to improve positive-pressure ventilation. The HBB editorial board honed the resuscitation algorithm, or Action Plan, and worked closely with educational and graphic designers to create a set of pictorial learning materials supported by limited text but abundant practice of skills and case scenario exercises. Content and draft materials for learner and facilitator underwent 2 cycles of review by a Delphi panel of outside experts in neonatal resuscitation and child survival. Task force members critically reviewed the draft materials and Delphi comments, resulting in strengthening of the concept of immediate attention at birth, or The Golden Minute, recognizing that all too often, resuscitation was being delayed while the birth attendant focused on the third stage of labor. Experimentation with various structures for practice revealed clear advantages of paired learning with the neonatal simulator. Field trials demonstrated that when participants experienced the roles of learner and teacher, knowledge translation was enhanced and the stage was set for ongoing learning in the workplace.[22] A third round of expert review took place at a technical expert consultation organized by WHO; with experts from each WHO region, materials and content were harmonized with existing WHO guidelines and perinatal care protocols.

Field-testing of the educational package in Kenya, Pakistan, and India refined the instructional methodology and materials themselves.[22] Providers and facilitators rated the materials highly, and knowledge and skills increased among participants. However, participants universally requested more opportunities for practice, so additional exercises and case scenarios were added. Evaluation materials were also revised to make the written/verbal evaluation a straightforward check of fundamental concepts and to emphasize mastery of the skill of bag-and-mask ventilation. Knowledge and skill checks were preparatory to objective structured clinical evaluations that examined integrated decision-making as well as skills in basic and advanced scenarios. Field-testing also highlighted the need to provide reinforcement of skills through low-dose, high-frequency practice in the workplace. The portability, low cost, and technology independence of the neonatal simulator and educational materials, as well as the model of learning and teaching in pairs, facilitated this goal.

A third phase of evaluation consisted of larger-scale field trials to examine implementation and clinical effect. Trials in Tanzania, Bangladesh, and Belgaum, India, were initiated prior to public release of the educational materials in 2010. Initial data on early neonatal mortality and stillbirth rates showed promising trends; however, demand for the materials and a sense of urgency to put them in the hands of birth attendants as quickly as possible prompted the program's launch before complete data were available. Additional data now available confirm a reduction in the fresh stillbirth rate with no increase in neonatal mortality in India[23] and a reduction in mortality at 24 hours among babies not breathing at birth in Tanzania.[24]

Action Planning/Implementation

A Global Development Alliance (GDA) for HBB coordinated launch and implementation of the program. The US Agency for International Development, with the leadership of Lily Kak, PhD, organized 5 principal stakeholders who had shaped early development of HBB into a public-private alliance for its implementation and dissemination. The founding partners of the GDA included USAID, the AAP, Laerdal Medical, the NICHD, and Save the Children Saving Newborn Lives. The official launch of the program took place in conjunction with the 2010 Global Health Council conference in Washington, DC. Members of the GITF and investigators from the field trials trained nearly 100 master trainers and presented data from educational and implementation field trials. The chief executives of the GDA member organizations formally signed the alliance agreement and pledged to support the goal, principles, and objectives of the GDA. The national advocacy office of the AAP arranged a congressional briefing on Capitol Hill and informational visits to legislators' offices in connection with the launch.

Goal, Principles, and Objectives of the Global Development Alliance for Helping Babies Breathe

- Goal: to reduce mortality from birth asphyxia (intrapartum-related events)
- Principles
  - Inclusiveness and collaboration
  - Country-owned and -led initiatives
  - Integration
  - Shared goal, results, and recognition
  - Brand non-exclusivity
- Objectives
  - Increase international, regional, and national commitment and resources for newborn resuscitation as part of essential newborn care.
  - Improve availability of high-quality, appropriate, affordable resuscitation devices and training materials.
  - Improve resuscitation capabilities of birth attendants with an emphasis on skilled birth attendants.
  - Strengthen supply chain logistics for resuscitation devices.
  - Evaluate effect of resuscitation programs at scale.

Partners in the GDA also used the media to highlight the issue of global neonatal mortality and their responses, including HBB. The AAP and USAID implementing agency K4Health created public and internal Web sites to answer frequently asked questions, publicize and report training workshops, and make available resources for facilitators, master trainers, program managers, and policy makers. Opinion leaders from the GDA posted blogs on USAID sites and the Save the Children Healthy Newborn Network (www.healthynewbornnetwork.org) to explain the work of the GDA and showcase stories from the field. The CORE Group of USAID-affiliated organizations featured HBB at its annual meetings and encouraged member organizations to contribute their expertise in support of the initiative. Laerdal Medical exhibited the neonatal simulator and HBB training package in its commercial booth at medical and professional conferences around the world. Additional workshops for master trainers were held across the United States, in Canada under the auspices of the Canadian Paediatric Society, in South Africa at the International Pediatric Association congress, and in Panama with the ALAPE meetings. Task force members and investigators for field trials not only presented papers and posters at scientific meetings but also presented informational sessions at Women Deliver, the International Confederation of Midwives congress, and the annual meetings of the American College of Nurse-Midwives; Association of Women's Health, Obstetric and Neonatal Nurses; and International Federation of Gynecology and Obstetrics.

Momentum among GDA partners built quickly. Just 2 years after the HBB launch, the program had spread to 48 countries, and 10 countries had completed a plan for national dissemination. This cooperative effort has supported the training of approximately 80,000 health providers. Almost 82,000 ventilation bag-and-mask devices and 93,000 reusable suction bulbs had been sold at cost, and 27,000 neonatal simulators had been distributed. The educational materials became available in official Spanish and French translations and translated into 19 additional national and regional languages. An implementation guide, published online in English and Spanish, offered strategic advice for policy makers and program managers as well as tools for master trainers. A video for facilitators, also available freely on the HBB Web site, illustrated learning methodology and key resuscitation skills. The GDA membership has recently expanded to include LDS Charities, Johnson & Johnson, and the International Pediatric Association.

Implementation and dissemination also confronted challenges. Many countries that had committed to training in ENC waited for a clear message from WHO that HBB could serve as the neonatal resuscitation component of ENC training. In some countries, differences in practice from that taught in HBB resulted in confusion or opposition to the new training program. A 2012 revision of the WHO *Guidelines on Basic Newborn Resuscitation* closely aligned this document with HBB and specifically mentioned HBB as a means of putting the new guidelines into practice, helping to resolve potential confusion. While some countries have emulated the partnerships of the GDA at a national level, others have not successfully achieved a strong joint effort among governmental, nongovernmental, professional, academic, and private enterprise partners.

Where rivalries or conflicts continue among stakeholders, less progress has been achieved. The AAP has responded by creating a cadre of mentors, master trainers in HBB who have leadership skills and credentials that qualify them to serve in particular countries as advisors to HBB implementation efforts.

Measuring Outcomes and Success and Modifying the Plan

Ultimately, the success of the HBB initiative will be measured in rates of neonatal and under-5 child mortality. To track progress toward the ultimate goal, partners of the HBB GDA developed a logic model that defines outputs, outcomes, and impact. *Outputs* refer to measures of coverage—numbers and percentages of birth attendants trained, numbers and percentages of birth facilities with trained staff and equipment for resuscitation, and proportion of deliveries attended by trained personnel. *Outcomes* track application of the resuscitation algorithm. A specific short-term outcome measure for resuscitation is the proportion of babies not breathing at birth who are breathing by 1 minute (spontaneously or with positive-pressure ventilation). Finally, *impact* is measured by reduction in fresh stillbirths and neonatal deaths at 24 hours, 7 days (early neonatal mortality), and 28 days (neonatal mortality). Because the HBB Action Plan initiates resuscitation for every baby who is not crying at birth, with the exception of obviously macerated newborns, those babies who might previously have been classified as stillborn (no breathing, no movement) have resuscitation initiated promptly and generally respond to stimulation and positive-pressure ventilation. This fluidity between fresh stillbirth and neonatal depression at birth confounds conventional demographic statistics and requires crosscutting measures to capture the true reduction in burden of mortality.

Large-scale trials to measure the effect of HBB training on perinatal mortality are underway in Kenya, India, Tanzania, Bangladesh, and Malawi. Three sites in the NICHD Global Network for Women's and Children's Health Research (Eldoret, Kenya; Belgaum; Nagpur, India) are conducting regional trials in areas where robust community baseline data exist from neonatal mortality registries. In Tanzania, Bangladesh, and Malawi, national-level data collection is underway. Experiences in these counties are shaping modifications to public health data sets to permit more accurate monitoring and reporting of neonatal deaths.

More than 2 years after the HBB launch, the major advocacy foci remain personnel, equipment, education, and research. The HBB working group remains devoted to sustainability of practices and integration of the initiative with efforts aimed at improved prenatal/intrapartum care and postnatal care. Maintenance of fidelity and quality of training is an essential component of every national training plan, and again, collaboration among stakeholders has been essential. In many cases, pediatric professional organizations or academic centers have assumed this role. Continued practice after initial training is also key to maintenance of skills. Low-dose, high-frequency practice has been demonstrated to be very effective in maintaining and even improving resuscitation skills. Setting the expectation of sustainability from the very beginning, making training and renewal of training routine, and incorporating resuscitation training into policies and procedures are all steps to help ensure sustainability. While resuscitation gives a newborn an improved chance of survival immediately after birth, appropriate care must continue throughout the neonatal period to affect 28-day mortality. Initial data suggest that babies who receive resuscitation at birth go on to be generally healthy survivors. However, the sequelae of severe asphyxia, infection/sepsis, and problems associated with prematurity and low birth weight take their toll throughout the first weeks. Similarly, care received intrapartum influences the incidence of asphyxia directly. Improved access to timely caesarean delivery and prevention and management of obstetric hemorrhage, intrapartum infection, and preeclampsia/eclampsia are critical to reducing the rate of intrapartum-related events. Educational programs that build on the HBB approach are currently under development for prevention and management of postpartum hemorrhage (Helping Mothers Survive) and essential newborn care (Helping Babies Survive and Thrive). Helping Babies Breathe is also recognized as an important element in combating mortality from prematurity, but there is opportunity to develop more extensive educational materials aimed at this globally important cause of neonatal mortality.

Reflections

What did the advocacy work mean for us? Helping Babies Breathe provided an opportunity to apply the latest and best science worldwide and at last target areas of the world where 98% of global neonatal deaths are occurring. As neonatal intensive care in the developed world turns to more sophisticated and complicated interventions such as fetal surgery, ex utero intrapartum treatment–extracorporeal membrane oxygenation, and fetal stem cell therapy, the possibility to save hundreds of thousands of lives each year through very basic interventions is a moral imperative. When these sustainable and scalable interventions are carried on by empowered birth attendants and local health authorities whose decisions are informed by evidence of positive effect, there is the potential for just, equitable, and lasting change.

Did it change how we viewed our work? The AAP tagline, "Dedicated to the health of all children," effectively became, "Dedicated to the health of all the world's children." Many members of the GITF had a clear memory of being called "dreamers" when they proposed that every birth in the United States should be attended by a person trained in neonatal resuscitation. Those same people are now daring to dream of a day when every baby in the world shares this advantage.

Did it provide us with a new direction? The NRP and HBB have propelled the AAP to a new level of leadership on the global stage. The AAP was awarded the 2010 Summit Award from the American Society of Association Executives, and the HBB GDA was named the outstanding global development alliance for 2011 by USAID. Development and involvement with NRP and HBB by many pediatric physicians and nurses have enhanced global neonatal survival as a career focus and serve as a bridge between intensive care medicine and public health. Increased collaboration among governmental, nongovernmental, and professional and private enterprise organizations has been stimulating, hopeful, and likely to serve as a blueprint for further advances in child health.

What is next? Examples of successful implementation and positive impact need to be analyzed so that lessons learned can be applied in regions where difficulties have slowed progress. Hopefully, the change created around neonatal resuscitation will serve as a catalyst for broader change and improvement in the entire continuum of perinatal care. Important challenges of prematurity and maternal mortality still are inadequately met. Ultimately, addressing issues of access to education for girls and women and to effective family planning will further improve maternal survival, enhance child health, and bring greater prosperity.

References

1. Liu L, Johnson HL, Cousens S, et al. Global, regional, and national causes of child mortality: an updated systematic analysis for 2010 with time trends since 2000. *Lancet.* 2012;379(9832):2151–2161

2. Lawn JE, Gravett MG, Nunes TM, Rubens CE, Stanton C; GAPPS Review Group. Global report on preterm birth and stillbirth (1 of 7): definitions, description of the burden and opportunities to improve data. *BMC Pregnancy Childbirth.* 2010;10(Suppl 1):S1

3. Thaddeus S, Maine D. Too far to walk: maternal mortality in context. *Soc Sci Med.* 1994;38(8):1091–1110

4. World Health Organization, United Nations Children's Fund, United Nations Population Fund, World Bank. *Trends in Maternal Mortality: 1990 to 2008.* Geneva, Switzerland: World Health Organization; 2010. http://whqlibdoc.who.int/ publications/2010/9789241500265_eng.pdf. Accessed May 9, 2013

5. Guyer B, Martin JA, MacDorman MF, Anderson RN, Strobino DM. Annual summary of vital statistics—1996. *Pediatrics.* 1997;100(6):905–918

6. Resuscitation of newborn infants: a report by the Special Committee on Infant Mortality of the Medical Society of the County of New York. *Obstet Gynecol.* 1956;8(3):336–363

7. Singhal N, McMillan DD, Yee WH, Akierman AR, Yee YJ. Evaluation of the effectiveness of the standardized neonatal resuscitation program. *J Perinatol.* 2001;21(6):388–392

8. Patel D, Piotrowski ZH, Nelson MR, Sabich R. Effect of a statewide neonatal resuscitation training program on Apgar scores among high-risk neonates in Illinois. *Pediatrics.* 2001;107(4):648–655

9. Lee AC, Cousens S, Wall SN, et al. Neonatal resuscitation and immediate newborn assessment and stimulation for the prevention of neonatal deaths: a systematic review, meta-analysis and Delphi estimation of mortality effect. *BMC Public Health.* 2011;11(Suppl 3):S12

10. Boo NY. Neonatal resuscitation programme in Malaysia: an eight-year experience. *Singapore Med J.* 2009;50(2):152–159

11. Xu T, Wang HS, Ye HM, et al. Impact of a nationwide training program for neonatal resuscitation in China. *Chin Med J (Engl).* 2012;125(8):1448–1456

12. Perlman JM, Wyllie J, Kattwinkel J, et al. Part 11: neonatal resuscitation: 2010 International Consensus on Cardiopulmonary Resuscitation and Emergency Cardiovascular Care Science With Treatment Recommendations. *Circulation.* 2010;122(16 Suppl 2):S516–S538

13. Ronsmans C, Graham WJ; Lancet Maternal Survival Series steering group. Maternal mortality: who, when, where, and why. *Lancet.* 2006;368(9542):1189–1200

14. Lawn JE, Lee AC, Kinney M, et al. Two million intrapartum-related stillbirths and neonatal deaths: where, why, and what can be done? *Int J Gynaecol Obstet.* 2009;107(Suppl 1):S5–S19

15. Ariff S, Soofi SB, Sadiq K, et al. Evaluation of health workforce competence in maternal and neonatal issues in public health sector of Pakistan: an assessment of their training needs. *BMC Health Serv Res.* 2010;10:319

16. Harvey SA, Blandón YC, McCaw-Binns A, et al. Are skilled birth attendants really skilled? A measurement method, some disturbing results and a potential way forward. *Bull World Health Organ.* 2007;85(10):783–790

17. Coffey P, Kak L, Narayanan I, et al. *Case Study: Newborn Resuscitation Devices.* Prepared for the United Nations Commission on Life-Saving Commodities for Women and Children. Seattle, WA: Program for Appropriate Technology in Health; 2012

18. Program for Appropriate Technology in Health. *Reducing Birth Asphyxia Through the Bidan di Desa Program in Cirebon, Indonesia: Final Report Submitted by Program for Appropriate Technology in Health (PATH) to Save the Children US.* Jakarta, Indonesia: Program for Appropriate Technology in Health; 2006

19. Carlo WA, Goudar SS, Jehan I, et al. Newborn-care training and perinatal mortality in developing countries. *N Engl J Med.* 2010;362(7):614–623

20. Pierick TA, Van Waning N, Patel SS, Atkins DL. Self-instructional CPR training for parents of high risk infants. *Resuscitation.* 2012;83(9):1140–1144

21. The Partnership for Maternal, Newborn & Child Health. *Essential Interventions, Commodities and Guidelines for Reproductive, Maternal, Newborn and Child Health: A Global Review of the Key Interventions Related to Reproductive, Maternal, Newborn and Child Health.* Geneva, Switzerland: The Partnership for Maternal, Newborn & Child Health; 2011. http://www.who.int/pmnch/topics/part_publications/essential_interventions_18_01_2012.pdf. Accessed May 9, 2013

22. Singhal N, Lockyer J, Fidler H, et al. Helping Babies Breathe: global neonatal resuscitation program development and formative educational evaluation. *Resuscitation.* 2012;83(1):90–96

23. Goudar SS, Somannavar MS, Clark R, et al. Stillbirth and newborn mortality in India after Helping Babies Breathe training. *Pediatrics.* 2013;131(2):e344–e352

24. Msemo G, Massawe A, Mmbando D, et al. Newborn mortality and fresh stillbirth rates in Tanzania after Helping Babies Breathe training. *Pediatrics.* 2013;131(2):e353–e360

Chapter 21

Reducing Maternal and Neonatal Mortality in Rural China

Zonghan Zhu, MD

The primary role of a pediatrician is caring for children in hospitals and clinics. However, this is not enough. When we leave our clinical settings to learn about the living conditions of our patients and better understand the assets and problems of their communities, we can more effectively advocate for their health and well-being. Pediatricians in China and throughout the world have a responsibility to speak out on behalf of those who have no political voice. Children have no voice and no choice. Children cannot explain their situation and needs by themselves. They need us to speak for them. Great improvements can be made when we communicate how children have been treated.

Foundation

In China there is wide variability in maternal and neonatal mortality rates. In 2004, infant mortality and mortality of children younger than 5 years were 21.5 per 1,000 and 25 per 1,000, respectively. Based on a rough estimation of 16 million births per year, this means that about 344,000 babies died before they reached their first year of life and about 400,000 children died before their fifth birthday. However, mortality rates varied greatly by region. In more developed regions, such as Beijing, Shanghai, and other cities where infants and children had access to good medical care and adequate nutrition, child mortality rates were as low as 6 per 1,000. Therefore, about 300,000 of the 400,000 child deaths could have been avoided. According to an analysis of the causes of death, about 70,000 or 20% of infants died of pneumonia. Yet there was no outcry about these excessive deaths. Compare this with the outcry associated with the Chinese severe acute respiratory syndrome epidemic in 2003, when there were 5,326 cases with 347 deaths. While this was treated as a national crisis, our Chinese society was silent and insensitive to the fact that every year, 70,000 babies died from treatable pneumonia.

Based on additional data from 1998, there were 16 provinces that had a maternal mortality rate higher than the national average level, 7 of which had a maternal mortality rate above 100 per 100,000; all were located in the western regions. These regions are predominately rural and poor with very limited health care facilities. To identify risk factors and possible solutions to the problem of high maternal and neonatal mortality, a survey was conducted, with support from the Ministry of Health and United Nations Children's Fund (UNICEF), in 40 counties in 6 western provinces. From the survey, more than 70% of maternal deaths occurred with home deliveries, and the main cause of death was obstetric hemorrhage. Additional causes included hypertension during pregnancy, heart disease during pregnancy, amniotic fluid embolism, and infections. Together these constituted 68.7% of maternal mortality. The survey found that 60% to 70% of the deaths of children younger than 5 years were neonatal deaths. Among neonatal deaths, birth asphyxia and premature birth were the 2 main causes. The survey also found that neonatal tetanus was still occurring in some rural areas. These findings suggested that shifting deliveries from the home to the hospital would reduce maternal and neonatal mortality. Furthermore, more than 90% of the women responded in the survey that "if there is financial support, they would be willing to go to the hospital for delivery." This finding was encouraging because promoting hospital delivery with subsidies would be a simpler and easier intervention than trying to change cultural and traditional practices. However, in some ethnic minority areas, such as Guangxi, we would later discover that even with subsidies, women still did not go to the hospital to give birth because of traditional cultural practices.

Based on the findings of this initial survey, the Safe Motherhood Project (SMP) was initiated in 1998, with support from the Ministry of Health and UNICEF. Our interventions were based on the technical expertise of international organizations such as the World Health Organization and UNICEF, from whom we also received financial support. While our interventions had a strong evidence base in other settings, we had to prove their effectiveness and feasibility in our own Chinese settings. The main intervention involved providing subsidies to encourage hospital delivery in 11 counties from 6 western provinces (Gansu, Qinghai, Ningxia,

Guizhou, Tibet, Xinjiang). In the year after implementation, monitoring and evaluation documented that the hospital delivery rate increased from 20% to 30% to 60% to 70%. This pilot program demonstrated the need for a more comprehensive approach that included giving hospital delivery subsidies; establishing a maternal referral system; shifting functions of the village midwife to providing prenatal care and encouraging the community to support hospital delivery; training grassroots obstetricians; and improving the infrastructure of delivery services in hospitals. It was also recognized that social mobilization was needed to gain support from local governments.

Based on experience from the first stage of SMP implementation, an integrated package of interventions to reduce maternal and neonatal mortality was developed based on the comprehensive approach described previously. Community engagement was a core part of the program. For example, in Guangxi mountainous areas where ethnic minority people live, traditional beliefs hamper women from institutional delivery. After social mobilization, a volunteer stretcher team was organized to escort pregnant women to the hospital in case of emergency (figures 21-1 and 21-2). This comprehensive approach involved establishing maternal social

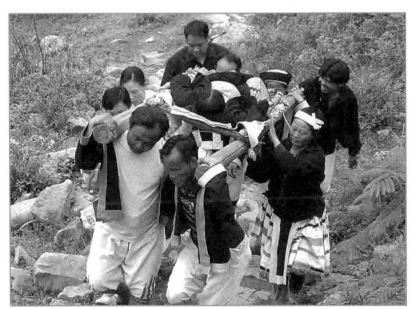

Figure 21-1. Volunteer stretcher team. A pregnant woman with dystocia was urgently transferred from a village to the township hospital by the village health worker and volunteer team in an ethnic minority area, Guangxi. Photo provided by Lili Cheng, MD, chief of maternal and child health, Guangxi Provincial Health Department.

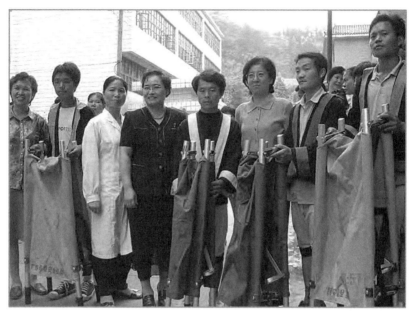

Figure 21-2. Volunteer stretcher teams, Guangxi.

support mechanisms, particularly in remote areas; defining responsibility and leadership roles within the local government; and integrating a system to monitor maternal and infant mortality rates into the local socioeconomic development planning to ensure funding for the program. This more comprehensive intervention package became the cornerstone for future expansion.

Beginning in 2000, under the support of the National Working Committee on Children and Women under the State Council, the Ministry of Health, and the Ministry of Finance, SMP was expanded to 378 poverty-stricken counties in central and western regions. This was the first maternal and child health project that received financial support from the central government. The main components are listed in Box 21-1.

The program was gradually scaled up. From 2000 to 2001, SMP was implemented in 378 poor counties with maternal mortality rate above 80 per 100,000 from 12 provinces (Inner Mongolia, Jiangxi, Hunan, Chongqing, Sichuan, Guizhou, Yunnan, Tibet, Gansu, Qinghai, Ningxia, Xinjiang). The central government allocated 50 million yuan (approximately US $8 million) annually, and provincial government matched funds by a certain percentage. From 2002 to 2004, the project expanded to an additional 440 counties in 16 provinces (Inner Mongolia, Jilin, Jiangxi,

Box 21-1. Components of the Safe Motherhood Project

- Encourage and subsidize hospital delivery.
- Train obstetric professionals and technical staffs to improve service and build capacity to manage obstetric emergencies.
- Carry out neonatal resuscitation training.
- Allocate maternal and child experts to county levels to train local staff and help facilitate implementation of the project.
- Train doctors in rural areas to carry out prenatal care, high-risk pregnancy screening, and neonatal visits.
- Carry out health education to distribute knowledge on maternal health care and safe delivery and to build community support mechanisms.
- Equip county and township hospitals with obstetric and neonatal resuscitation and other basic equipment.
- Subsidize poor pregnant women with 200 to 400 yuan (approximately US $30–$50) per childbirth for hospital delivery.

Hubei, Hunan, Guangxi, Chongqing, Sichuan, Guizhou, Yunnan, Tibet, Shaanxi, Gansu, Qinghai, Ningxia, Xinjiang), covering a population of 150 million people. From 2005 to 2007, the project further involved 6 more provinces (Hebei, Shanxi, Heilongjiang, Anhui, Henan, Hainan) and covered a total of 1,000 counties in 22 central and western provinces and a population of 4.2 million people.

In 2008, the project included an additional 200 counties in the central and western regions. In 2010, the project was operational in 2,000 counties in rural areas throughout the country.

Effectiveness of the Safe Motherhood Project

The project resulted in major improvements of maternal and child health indicators.

- The hospitalized delivery rate improved significantly. In 2007, the hospital delivery rate was 86.8% in the project area, which was 47.6% higher than 2001.
- The maternal mortality rate decreased significantly, dropping to 39.4 per 100,000 in 2007, a decrease of 48.2% compared with 2001.
- Neonatal mortality decreased significantly. Neonatal mortality rate in the project areas in 2007 dropped to 8.4%, a decrease of 45.1% compared with 2001.
- Neonatal tetanus incidence declined markedly. Incidence of neonatal tetanus in 2007 was reduced to 0.06% in the project areas.

Our strategy has been implemented in 3 phases.

- In an initial phase, we carried out a research project to identify the efficacy and effectiveness of proposed interventions.
- Next, we expanded the project to pilot study areas so we could test implementation feasibility and outcomes in communities with different conditions and cultures.
- Finally, we took successful interventions to scale through their inclusion in government child health policy.
- The maternal neonatal project promoted the overall level of maternal and child health in the project areas. Millions of mothers had safe deliveries with good outcomes, and lives of thousands of endangered mothers and their babies were saved.

During all 3 phases we needed a process to engage the community and media as well as our pediatric society and governmental organizations. We had to build an analytic evidence base through our research to successfully educate the community and advocate for our solutions. Families needed to understand that their concerns and problems related to the health of their children had solutions and that together we could get the governmental and civic support to implement these solutions. Pediatricians and pediatric associations circulate scientific data within our professional societies, but we often fail to recognize the importance of transmitting the data to more people through mass media. Success ultimately depends on our ability to engage the community to help obtain support for and participation in our solutions. We have to learn the art of advocacy, the way to most effectively tell our story with powerful pictures and video. When we effectively tell our story, many will join us and the program will be taken to scale throughout the country.

Chapter 22

Reducing Neonatal Mortality in Chile

Juan Pablo Beca, MD
Jaime Burrows, MD, PhD

Introduction

In Chile the rates of infant mortality and undernourishment in the 1960s were high. At the beginning of that decade, the former reached 120 in 1,000 live births and the latter reached almost 60% of the population younger than 6 years. After finishing my fellowship in pediatrics at Hospital Dr Luis Calvo Mackenna in Santiago in 1968, I became particularly interested in kwashiorkor and neurodevelopmental disorders as a consequence of malnourishment. These were not exceptional cases. Malnutrition was the underlying condition of most children admitted to the hospital with acute diarrhea and dehydration in summertime and respiratory infections in winter.

During that decade new public policies to prevent and treat infant malnutrition were implemented. These included special primary care–related programs such as distribution of powdered milk for all children younger than 2 years, immunizations, and medical leave for mothers with a sick child younger than 1 year. These programs were developed together with efforts to promote breastfeeding. In 1975, infant mortality was reduced to 65 per 1,000 (Figure 22-1).[1,2]

By agreement between the Ministry of Health (MOH) and universities, some residents had financial support during their training period. For those who obtained this support, it was compulsory to work in a public hospital in a province outside of a metropolitan area of Santiago for at least 2 years. Under that commitment and with the purpose of working to prevent and treat infant malnutrition, I was appointed as a pediatrician in the Regional Hospital of Antofagasta. This is a city located 1,300 km north from Santiago, close to the desert of Atacama. In those years, Antofagasta

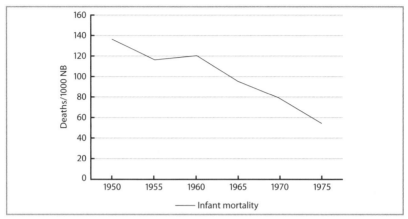

Figure 22-1. Infant mortality rates in Chile, 1950 to 1975.

counted about 300,000 dwellers; although it was the main port for copper-mining companies and a hub for the fishing industry, the city had high rates of poverty.

My duties as a pediatrician were divided half-time with inpatients in the infant wards and outpatients in the hospital and a community clinic. I expected and saw high levels of malnutrition—but was astonished by how many children with cerebral palsy received no monitoring or follow-up care. I asked my superiors if I could dedicate at least some time to caring for children with neurologic damage, mainly epilepsy and cerebral palsy. This was accomplished with the assistance of some pediatric neurologists from Santiago.

Before long, I realized that most neurologic damage could have been prevented through better neonatal care and more effective management of perinatal asphyxia. I then asked to work in the neonatal unit of the hospital, where intensive care was quite limited. I committed myself to neonatal care with the purpose of preventing neurologic damage. I applied to the Pan American Health Organization (PAHO) for a fellowship in neonatology at Hammersmith Hospital in London under the direction of Professor Peter Tizard. At Hammersmith Hospital I learned about preventing and managing birth asphyxia, cardiorespiratory resuscitation, mechanical ventilation, cardiac and respiratory monitoring, and other aspects of neonatal intensive care in practice at that time. When the fellowship finished, I returned to Chile, organizing Chile's first neonatal intensive care unit (NICU).

In 1972, I started work at the Premature Center of the Hospital Dr Luis Calvo Mackenna under the direction of Clara Roman, MD. This center was created in 1958 thanks to a United Nations Educational, Scientific and Cultural Organization grant to develop good neonatal care for premature babies. Newer neonatal intensive care techniques and technologies had not been introduced, so we proposed a new project called "Innovations in Neonatal Care." In 1975, we set up the first NICU in Chile, for 4 babies, as a pilot program (Figure 22-2). We had a central system for oxygen distribution, monitoring equipment, transport incubator, infusion pumps, a Gregory box continuous positive airway pressure (CPAP) system (Figure 22-3), and a neonatal mechanical ventilator.

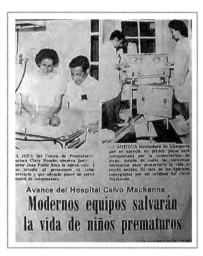

Figure 22-2. Newspaper article about new equipment for the Premature Center at Hospital Dr Luis Calvo Mackenna.

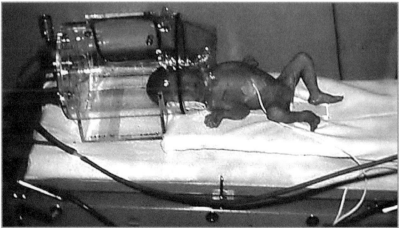

Figure 22-3. The Gregory box, a neonatal continuous positive airway pressure system at Hospital Dr Luis Calvo Mackenna.

The same year our NICU opened, 2 other public hospitals inaugurated similar units in Santiago. All 3 units were funded with private donations because the budget of the National Healthcare Service was focused on other priorities. The Pinochet government was progressively reducing expenditures in health care and applying a decentralization policy that affected the National Healthcare Service.

In the final months of 1975 the Chilean Pediatric Society held a course in neonatal intensive care for pediatricians who were developing NICUs. Although we had not worked together before, we organized a working group to prove that providing neonatal intensive care was not only possible but necessary despite the limited resources of our country. Our aim was to advocate for a national policy to reduce neonatal mortality and prevent neurologic sequelae in children by improving neonatal intensive care.

The working group began to meet every week, starting with 12 neonatologists of different hospitals. Eight left the group, doubting that our effort would ever succeed, leaving the task to only 4: Mario Ferreiro, Juan Pablo Beca, Sergio Vaisman, and Ruben Maler. Each of us worked in a different public hospital in Santiago. We were all motivated by a moral duty to attempt to influence child health public policy regardless of the difficulty in getting the government to respond.

We first carried out an analysis of the effect of nutrition programs on infant mortality rates. While there was a dramatic fall in postneonatal infant mortality from 1960 to 1975, neonatal mortality had not improved. In fact, the neonatal component of infant mortality had increased in relative terms from 30% of infant mortality in 1960 to 50% in 1975 (Figure 22-4). Data showed that further substantial reductions in infant mortality would require improvements in neonatal mortality. Achieving these improvements would only be possible with a new national neonatal care policy.[3] Analysis also showed that this new policy was needed to reduce the high frequency of neurologic-development problems related to birth asphyxia and sequelae of prematurity.

The literature and our working group submitted a proposal to the MOH to establish a national program to reduce neonatal mortality and prevent neurologic sequelae. Our preliminary proposal was well received and we were designated as a national advisory committee charged with writing a formal and detailed proposal for the government. We identified the chief issues that needed to be included in the national policy: prenatal care;

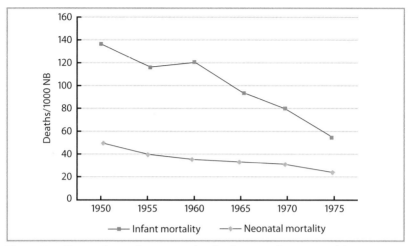

Figure 22-4. Neonatal mortality compared with infant mortality rates in Chile, 1950 to 1975.

detection and management of high-risk pregnancies; professional assistance of all deliveries; rationalization and regionalization of the care of ill term and preterm newborns; good ambulatory follow-up for all newborns during their first months of life; and social education on the need for special care of pregnant women and newborns.

In 1975 the infant mortality rate was 55.4 per 1,000 live births, and neonatal mortality was 24.8 per 1,000 (45% of infant mortality). Although there were no data on the frequency of neurologic damage, it was estimated that there were 3,200 cases of severe or moderate damage per year.[4] Studies showed that good obstetric and neonatal care was an effective prevention of neurologic damage and cerebral palsy, with a rate of cerebral palsy of 10% among newborns less than 1,500 g who survived.[4,5]

In 1976, the committee presented to the MOH a formal proposal, "National program for the reduction of neonatal mortality and the prevention of neurological damage." The objectives of such a program were to achieve a 30% reduction of neonatal mortality in 5 years and to decrease the number of severe neurologic sequelae. The proposal outlined a regionally coordinated system, as well as providing basic resuscitation and heating equipment for small rural hospitals with a training program. The plan was to install this program during a 3-year period, with an estimated cost of 5 million dollars a year for equipment.

Unfortunately, our plan was rejected by the MOH, which was opposed to any expansion of the central government's role in health care. Our proposal was counter to the Pinochet government decentralization policy and was considered too socialistic.

We were shocked by this response and requested an interview with the minister, which was denied. Our committee was dismissed, saying we were no longer needed. We presented our work to the Chilean Medical College and published it in a pediatric journal. We had no further communication with the MOH for 4 months, until we were called the last day of the fiscal year (December 31). The MOH had unallocated funds in its annual budget and because the neonatal project was the only one available with a detailed cost analysis, it received funding. By chance and luck the program was approved and our committee was reactivated to assume responsibility for implementing the program with a budget administrator assigned by the MOH.

We analyzed population and hospital delivery data throughout the country to define the criteria for resource allocation. We identified 25 hospitals needing NICUs, 90 hospitals requiring the necessary equipment to function as intermediate care units, and 300 facilities with less than 500 deliveries per year that should receive basic equipment such as a basic heating system, aspiration pipettes, neonatal Ambu bags, and communication systems with regional hospitals. The NICUs were designated for all main hospitals having the highest number of deliveries, from the city of Arica in the northern end of Chile to the city of Punta Arenas in the southern end. Each NICU was designed to coordinate with selected intermediate care units in each region. This partnership ranged from regions with only one intermediate care unit such as the desert of Atacama in the north to more than 20 intermediate care units in the region of Araucanía.

Intermediate units received standard incubators, phototherapy equipment, neonatal resuscitation equipment, and transport incubators to transfer the most ill babies to NICUs in larger hospitals in the same area. Neonatal intensive care units received intensive care incubators, radiation heaters, cardiac and apnea monitors, CPAP boxes, mechanical ventilators, phototherapy equipment, portable x-ray equipment, bilirubinometers, and blood-gas determination equipment.

The installation of equipment began in 1978 and finished in 1981. It was necessary to modify the physical structure of many neonatal units, with the installation of central oxygen and air for ventilation, isolation spaces, and other facilities. One of the first new units was established at Hospital del

Salvador in Santiago in 1978, where we had to work with oxygen and air bottles (Figure 22-5).

At the same time the neonatal care program was being implemented, obstetric care improved as the MOH acquired ultrasound equipment and fetal monitoring for all larger obstetric units in the public health system. Although there was no financial support for training, we organized seminars and workshops for pediatricians, midwives, and nurses on neonatal care techniques and use of the new equipment. These were carried out in all regional centers and NICUs. By 1981 all units were established and functioning. However, the global economic crisis and government cutbacks on health care spending led to the dismissal of our committee and the end of federal support for the program. It was not until 1990, under a new government, that the national neonatal program was again funded to provide new equipment, more staff, and pulmonary surfactant.

Outcomes

Despite the end of federal support, neonatal mortality was dramatically reduced from 18.5 per 1,000 live births in 1978 to 9.2 per 1,000 in 1984. This exceeded the 30% reduction that was expected (Figure 22-6). In 1998 a National Program of Follow Up of Preterm Babies was established and documented that neonatal mortality had decreased even more, to a rate of

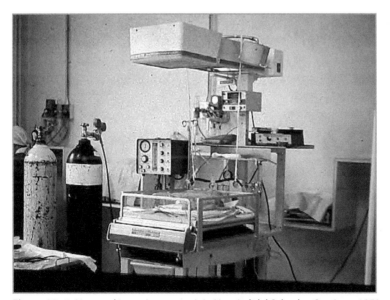

Figure 22- 5. Neonatal intensive care unit in Hospital del Salvador, Santiago, 1978.

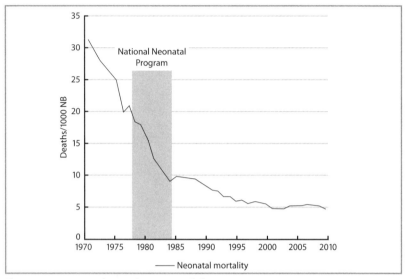

Figure 22-6. Neonatal mortality rates in Chile, 1970 to 2010.

5.9 per 1,000 live births in 2000.[6] The former MOH recently analyzed these results in a book of the history of Chilean public health policies during the 20th century.[7]

The number of babies with neurologic damage could not be measured on a national scale. Nevertheless, follow-up programs of high-risk newborns showed that the percentage of severe sequelae in babies weighing less than 1,500 g was 7%,[8] far below previous estimations. It also appeared that the number of patients with cerebral palsy in pediatric outpatient clinics was progressively reduced.

From Neonatal Care to Bioethics

Access to neonatal intensive care and prevention of neurologic damage are important ethical issues. While primarily we advocated for a better quality of life for all children, after the regionalization of neonatal care was achieved, new questions arose: how far should we go in the treatment of extremely ill newborns? What are the limits of extreme prematurity? How small is too small? These questions, bearing in mind the risk of neurologic damage and reality that neuro-rehabilitation resources in our country were extremely scarce, had no obvious answers.

I was asked by the rector of the University of Chile to work with a new international program with the PAHO called the Regional Program on Bioethics for Latin America and the Caribbean. Under the direction of the former MOH, Julio Montt, MD, we were able to promote, from 1994 to 1999, the development of bioethics in all the region's countries, focused on clinical and public health ethics. Many local programs were developed and a series of publications under the title "Cuadernos del Programa Regional de Bioética" were published and distributed. The first master's program in bioethics was organized with an agreement with Universidad Complutense of Madrid under the direction of Professor Diego Gracia. Four courses were given, 2 in Chile, 1 in the Dominican Republic, and 1 in Peru, and 120 professionals attained a master's degree in bioethics. Most of them have developed different bioethics committees and courses in their countries. I then went back to academic work in bioethics at the University of Chile in its Department of Bioethics and Humanities, and later moved into a new faculty of medicine at Clínica Alemana–Universidad del Desarrollo, where we established a new Centre for Bioethics in 2002.

Final Reflections

Although neonatal care and bioethics are different fields, they share a common ground. Both have an individual patient service perspective as well as a larger social dimension. Ethical dimensions, values, and principles are inherent in clinical situations. We must also recognize that many issues we confront are systemic, and therefore our society needs to give them high priority. If pediatricians approach their clinical and ethical problems in an analytic way, study them, and offer solutions, creative programs will be designed that will contribute to a better life for children, their families, and society.

References

1. Szot J. Reseña de la salud pública materno-infantil chilena durante los últimos 40 años: 1960-2000. *Rev Chil Obstet Ginecol.* 2002;67(2):129–135
2. Castañeda T. Contexto socioeconómico y causas del descenso de la mortalidad infantil en Chile. *Estudios Públicos.* 1996;64:1–50
3. Ferreiro M, Beca JP, Maler R, et al. Implementación de la atención neonatal en Chile. *Pediatría.* 1976;19:282–284
4. Davies PA, Tizard JP. Very low birthweight and subsequent neurological defect (with special reference to spastic diplegia). *Dev Med Child Neurol.* 1975;17(1):3–17
5. Lubchenco LO, Delivoria-Papadopoulos M, Searls D. Long-term follow-up studies of prematurely born infants. II. Influence of birth weight and gestational age on sequelae. *J Pediatr.* 1972;80(3):509–512
6. Beca JP. El desarrollo de la Neonatología en Chile. Una visión desde la ética clínica. Anibal Ariztía Conference, Hosptilal L Calvo Mackenna, November 1999
7. Jiménez de la Jara J. *Angelitos Salvados.* Santiago, Chile: Uqbar Editors; 2009:166–170
8. Morgues M. Sobrevida del niño menor de 1500 gr en Chile. *Rev Chil Obstet Ginecol.* 2002;67:100–105

Health Promotion and Child Development

Chapter 23

Campaign Against Tobacco in the World Health Organization Western Pacific Region

James Rarick, MPH
Jonathan Klein, MD, MPH, FAAP
Susan Mercado, MD, MPH
Cherry Chun-Yiu Li, MSc
Emmalita M. Manalac, MD, MPH, FPPS

Child and Adolescent Health and Tobacco Use in the Western Pacific Region

Tobacco use is the world's leading cause of preventable death, killing nearly 6 million people each year. Around 600,000 of these deaths are due to exposure to secondhand tobacco smoke (SHS); this includes approximately 170,000 innocent children who die from SHS each year, or approximately 20 children each hour of every day.[1] One-third of the world's smokers reside in the World Health Organization (WHO) Western Pacific Region (WPR), where it is also estimated that half of all women and children are regularly exposed to SHS at home and in public places.[2]

Tobacco use is now gaining more attention as a pediatric disease. Initiation to smoking, chewing, and habitual use of tobacco usually starts before the age of 18 years when the capacity to control impulsive behavior is not yet developed.[3] In addition, evidence has shown that around 50% of those who begin smoking in their adolescent years continue to smoke for at least 15 to 20 years.[4] Results from Global Youth Tobacco Surveys (GYTS) conducted in 26 countries and areas in the WHO WPR show an average rate of 13.8% of current smoking among students aged 13 to 15 years (WHO Tobacco Free Initiative, WPR, unpublished data, 2012). The use of smokeless tobacco products is also a serious concern in some Pacific Islands, which exhibit very high rates of tobacco chewing with the areca (betel) nut among adolescents.[5]

Factors such as misinformation about smoking, social acceptability of smoking, smoking history within the family, and poor self-image of young people have all been identified as playing a potential role in a young person's initiation into tobacco use.[6] Another important factor is an estimated US $12 billion that the tobacco industry spends each year on advertising and promotion to recruit young smokers.[7] These new products and colorful packaging play a significant role in attracting children and adolescents to smoke. Furthermore, when young people can afford to purchase cigarettes or other tobacco products, they are more likely to take up smoking.

As implementation of comprehensive tobacco control measures have reduced demand for tobacco products in high-income countries, tobacco companies have moved aggressively to enter and establish new markets in low- and middle-income countries.[8] In many of these countries, tobacco industry influence on policy decisions on taxation of tobacco products has been successful in keeping the price of tobacco products low and therefore affordable even to young people; this can be seen in large price differences between countries.[1] Internal documents from the industry have shown that tobacco companies are very much aware that raising cigarette prices is one of the most effective ways to reduce and prevent tobacco use among children and adolescents.[1] These disparities in cigarette prices result from lack of policies and regulations that are needed to reduced youth smoking rates in many low- and middle-income countries.

Reducing exposure to SHS is another key issue in tobacco control for child and adolescent health. Results from the 26 countries that conducted the GYTS show that slightly more than half of students (51%) reported being exposed to SHS from others at home, and the average rate of exposure to SHS in public places during the week preceding the survey was 66% (WHO WPR, unpublished data). Exposure to SHS leads to a range of serious and fatal diseases such as heart disease, respiratory illness, and lung cancer. Secondhand tobacco smoke contains up to 7,000 chemicals[9] and is especially hazardous to child health because children may have longer exposure to SHS at home throughout the different stages of their development. This increases the risk of morbidity and mortality from respiratory diseases such as asthma, chronic sinusitis, bronchitis, pneumonia, and others which are preventable. Long-term exposure to SHS can have adverse effects on children's growth, metabolism, and development.

Engaging Child and Adolescent Health Partners to Take Action on Tobacco Control

The WHO Framework Convention on Tobacco Control contains comprehensive measures to reduce supply of and demand for tobacco. Health care providers, as clinicians and influential members of the communities in which they live, can play a key role in the implementation of several of these measures. However, evidence indicates that there is a relatively high smoking prevalence and low awareness about the harms of tobacco use—and tobacco control in general—among health care providers in some WPR countries, which diminishes their effect in getting patients to quit using tobacco and as potential tobacco control advocates in their communities.

A recent survey covering more than 390,248 physicians from 977 Chinese hospitals found that 38.7% of male doctors were regular smokers and the smoking rate among Chinese physicians was only one-third lower than in the general population.[10] As 1 of 4 standardized surveys in the Global Tobacco Surveillance System,[11] the Global Health Professions Student Survey (GHPSS) has been conducted in health professional training institutions in several countries of the WHO WPR over the past decade, including medical, nursing, dental, and pharmacy schools. In Mongolia, 58% of male dental students, 62% of male pharmacy students, and 20% of male nursing students in their third year reported current cigarette smoking. In the Philippines, 29.5% of male and 16% of female medical students currently smoked cigarettes in the third year of their professional training. In Vietnam, 20.7% of third-year male medical students were current smokers.

The GHPSS results also revealed that most health professional students are not being provided with the skills to assist their patients to quit smoking. Fewer that 40% of health professional students trained in the Philippines, Mongolia, South Korea, and Vietnam reported that they had received any formal training on smoking cessation techniques. The GHPSS findings showed that many health professional training institutions did not have smoke-free policies for their campuses or did not enforce existing policies.[12] These findings point to the critical need to integrate tobacco control into health professional training curriculum, increase the number of smoke-free policies at training institutions (and ensure enforcement of policies), and engage with health professional associations and organizations to create greater awareness of tobacco control among practicing health professionals.

In some countries pediatricians have demonstrated leadership that has influenced clinician practice and affected tobacco control policies for children's health. Professional organizations have been able to create opportunities for engagement of their members in advocacy for tobacco control and have shared information on good practices in developing policies for protection from SHS. Until recently, however, this important sector has not been actively engaged in tobacco control in WPR countries.

Working with national pediatric associations and training institutions has become a strategic focus for intervention for child and adolescent tobacco control in the WPR at the clinical health care provider and community levels. This work began as a collaboration among the WHO WPR office, International Pediatric Association, and Julius B. Richmond Center of Excellence (Figure 23-1) at the American Academy of Pediatrics (AAP). The first meeting on a training network for child and adolescent health and tobacco control in the Western Pacific, held in Manila, Philippines, in December 2010, brought together child and adolescent care providers and advocates from China, Fiji, Japan, Malaysia, Mongolia, Philippines, Vietnam, and the United States. Participants reviewed training gaps and needs and mapped regional assets for training, and developed country-specific action plans for improvement. Participants also agreed to work to establish a network of professional organizations and institutions to improve curriculum in health professional training and more actively engage pediatricians and child health care providers as advocates for tobacco control.

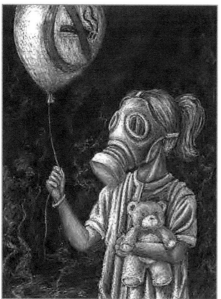

Figure 23-1. Courtesy of American Academy of Pediatrics Julius B. Richmond Center of Excellence. Children's Art Contest 2010. Minh-Tri V. 1st place; grade 9-12. http://www2.aap.org/richmondcenter/Gallery/2010/Grade9-12/THB-Minh-TriV.jpg.

Long-range goals that were identified included the development of national policies to require integration of tobacco control within health professional training curriculum, including offering cessation treatments to smokers who are addicted to nicotine, enforcing smoking bans in all health professional training institutions, providing training for health professional students on the treatment of tobacco dependence, and establishing national guidelines for the treatment of tobacco dependence.

Preparing for Action: Analyzing and Selecting Appropriate Interventions

Case Studies: Country Interventions

During the meeting on the presentation of project results on child and adolescent health and tobacco control in the WPR, held at the WHO WPR office in Manila in January 2012, ongoing activities in countries to support this strategic direction were presented. These are briefly summarized as follows:

China

China faces huge obstacles to change perception and practices related to smoking cessation and avoidance of SHS. Among these are the state monopoly of the Chinese National Tobacco Corporation; high smoking prevalence among male doctors; aggressive media advertising; slow enforcement of smoke ban; custom of offering cigarettes linked with politeness and friendship; and most of the people being unaware of the dangers of smoking and not willing to quit.

China embarked on a pilot project to build the capacity of pediatricians and other child health staff in advising parents on the harmful effects of tobacco and SHS and supporting tobacco cessation at the International Conference on Developmental Disorders, held at the Sixth Child Health Summit and Annual Meeting of the Chongqing Paediatric Society; the second training for pediatric health care professionals in Chaoyang District was held in the lecture hall of Dr Xie Xiaohua from Capital Institute of Pediatrics, October 26, 2011.

Hong Kong

Child health can be improved by adult cessation. Through clinicians' counseling advice on quitting smoking in adults and effects of SHS, parents and other adult smokers will be motivated by the goal of protecting others.

Furthermore, evidence shows that parents' unhealthy behavior models have direct effects on their children. Therefore, helping parents quit has a powerful message for youth to not start smoking. With regard to smoking cessation services, the University of Hong Kong schools of Nursing and Public Health have established the first series of programs on educating nurses and other health care professionals on smoking cessation in Hong Kong and China. More than 400 nurses, 200 social workers, 200 volunteers and students, 70 pharmacists, and 100 doctors in Hong Kong and China were trained to become smoking cessation counselors. A new role for nurses and other health professionals in Hong Kong and China was successfully developed to promote smoking cessation among patients. Smoking cessation counselors are now providing services in smoking cessation clinics in the Hospital Authority.

Japan

Three associations of child care providers, including the Japan Pediatric Society (20,735 members), Japanese Society of Child Health Nursing (4,962 members), and Japan Pediatric Association (6,319 members), united to form the Joint Committee to Protect Children from Tobacco Hazards in 2005, believing that this move was more powerful and effective in dealing with policy makers and corporations that support the tobacco industry. The joint committee issued a firm declaration that pediatricians involved in the well-being of children will remain nonsmokers themselves and will advocate for smoking cessation among future health care and welfare specialists.

The joint committee has supported the promotion of a smoke-free society backed up by no-smoking policies in academic and research institutions, public places, schools, and communities and is working to establish quit clinics in all children's hospitals. It has also developed a symbolic logo of a baby touching a no-smoking sign as a strong statement that smoking is not allowed in front of children. Through the joint committee efforts, the removal of automatic vending machines in school zones and other locations that are easily accessed by minors is being attained. The number of vending machines dropped by nearly 60% in 2011 compared with 2000 to 2005, and the sales from vending machines also dropped by nearly one-third in the same period. Alongside joint committee activity, there are several regional activities to protect children against the tobacco hazard. For example, a health promotion program in Tajimi City has a simple formula for health:

tobacco control, healthy food, and good exercise; and in Kyoto, a Tobacco-Free Caravan, undertaken as a cooperative activity among health professionals, educators, and students, was operated under the principle of learning by doing.

One problem facing Japan is that many authorities are still very insensitive concerning their influence on children. For example, following the earthquake and tsunami in 2011, a famous Japanese alpinist, Ken Noguchi, who had talked about experiences as an alpinist in front of the public under the support of the tobacco industry, distributed sleeping bags to disaster victims—along with free tobacco products. The official journal of the Science Council of Japan carried a smoking portrait of Toshitaka Hidaka, a world famous zoologist, on its front cover.

The strong presence of the tobacco industry in Japan remains a major obstacle. Corporate social responsibility activities are routinely conducted by Japan Tobacco International (JTI) and other tobacco companies in WPR countries to enhance their public image. Japan Tobacco supported many kinds of youth activities in Japan. For example, it supported afforestation all over Japan to make JTI's forest. Advertisement of JTI is more ingenious. For example, a large newspaper, Asahi, devoted a lot of space to an advertisement of a photographic exhibition of a famous photographer, which was held at the Tobacco & Salt Museum, with portraits of several Japanese master writers smoking while writing.

Philippines

The Philippine Ambulatory Pediatric Association (PAPA) has been involved in tobacco control since 2010 with the first visiting lecture of Jonathan Klein, MD, MPH, FAAP, executive director of the AAP Julius B. Richmond Center of Excellence. In collaboration with WHO and Health-Care Partners LLC, PAPA developed a manual on brief tobacco intervention skills that health care professionals could use in their clinical practices to encourage their adolescent and pediatric patients to quit smoking—and to advise parents and guardians on the dangers of exposure to SHS. This training has evolved into a 6-hour course called "Brief Advice on Smoking Cessation" that was conducted in several sites around the Philippines from November 2010 to February 2011. A total of 447 health care professionals from the public and private sectors were trained.

A Tobacco Resource Center was established in the University of the Philippines, Philippine General Hospital, for the purpose of intensifying tobacco control in 4 areas—research, training, service, and advocacy—to inform public policy. Inspired by this development, the Silliman University in Dumaguete City, Negros Oriental, established a second Tobacco Resource Center to further strengthen the local multi-sectoral response to smoking and prevention of exposure to SHS. The challenge is to devise approaches for the centers to become sustainable.

With support of the Department of Health, tobacco control may soon be integrated into government programs like the Tuberculosis Directly Observed Treatment Short Course and Integrated Management of Childhood Illness. As more advocates from national and local arenas become involved in tobacco control, PAPA may soon realize its vision to formalize a local coalition of medical organizations, local government units, media, and civic organizations to expand the reach of its advocacy and training initiatives.

Vietnam

The Vietnam Steering Committee on Smoking and Health (VINACOSH) teamed up with the Vietnam Paediatric Association in working for the inclusion of tobacco control in pediatric training. It is envisioned to build capacity of provincial-based pediatricians to address the harmful effects of smoking and SHS and cascade such trainings more widely in the province and down to the district levels. This will be integrated with the national neonatal program to better establish the link between tobacco control and reproductive health.

As part of a broad-based communication campaign, hospitals have employed all possible venues to deliver strong messages on tobacco control, such as providing information via leaflets, posters, television monitors, and hospital speaker systems; incorporating tobacco control into patient health education sessions; updating hospital Web sites with articles and research on tobacco and child and adolescent health; adding a page with tobacco control messages in the patient medical record book; and inserting a message on tobacco control in the prescription pad. Opportunities exist for conveying tobacco-control messages in the health care channel and in particular the television talk show hosted by pediatricians.

Future plans include establishing a quit line and smoking cessation clinic. The development of a standardized tool to monitor and evaluate the project will be undertaken in consultation with WHO and the Asia Pacific Alliance for Child and Family Health for Tobacco Control (CFTC).

Sustaining Action by Child and Adolescent Health Advocates in the Western Pacific Region

The implementation of tobacco control measures is crucial for protection of child and adolescent health in countries in the WPR. These measures extend far beyond clinical practice (eg, offering help to patients who are interested in quitting tobacco use) and require community-wide mobilization of support for evidence-based tobacco control policies such as complete indoor smoking bans; bans on tobacco advertising, promotion, and sponsorship; requiring graphic health warnings; and raising taxes on all tobacco products. These measures are proven to be effective in preventing young people from starting and encouraging them to quit.

While the work being carried out in countries is an important step toward integration of tobacco control into health professional training programs and greater engagement of child and adolescent health care providers in advocacy for tobacco control, more needs to be done to raise awareness and advocacy by pediatricians and other health care providers. The positive outcomes from the projects highlighted herein would be better appreciated if there was a mechanism to document and share information among countries within and outside the WPR and to support in-country work. Representatives of WHO member states, organizations, and institutions that participated in the 2 WHO-convened meetings on child and adolescent health and tobacco recognized the need to establish a network to share best practices and resources being developed regionally and internationally.

The CFTC was formally launched during the 14th Asian Pacific Congress of Pediatrics and the fourth Asian Pacific Congress of Pediatric Nursing in September 2012. A leadership training program was organized by the AAP Julius B. Richmond Center of Excellence as part of the preconvention program, helping to set the stage for the official launch of the alliance. The launch included adoption of bylaws and statements of solidarity from founding members, which included the countries and areas that participated in the first WHO-convened meeting on child and adolescent health and tobacco control in December 2010.

The founding members of the CFTC include Beijing Children's Hospital, the WHO Collaborating Center for Tobacco or Health, and the Beijing Institute of Respiratory Medicine; the Hong Kong Council on Smoking and Health, the WHO Collaborating Center for Smoking Cessation and Treatment of Tobacco Dependence (Hong Kong), and the Youth Quitline Center, School of Nursing, University of Hong Kong; the Joint Committee to Protect Children from Tobacco Hazards (Japan); the Malaysian Health

Promotion Board; PAPA and Silliman University Medical School (Philippines); KK Women's and Children's Hospital (Singapore); the standing office of VINACOSH; and SEAMEO-TROPMED Network (Thailand). Associate members include the National Hospital of Pediatrics (Vietnam) and Affiliated Centers for SEAMEO-TROPMED in Thailand, Philippines, and Malaysia. The World Health Organization will continue to provide support and technical advice to the secretariat of the alliance toward organization of the first general assembly and to sit as ex officio member of the advisory board, providing feedback to relevant WHO country offices and exploring how members of the alliance can contribute to child health as well as tobacco-control initiatives within country plans of action. The World Health Organization will also share alliance advocacy materials with other technical units of the WPR office. The first meeting of the general assembly of the CFTC is scheduled to be held in May 2013 at Kuching, Sarawak, Malaysia.

An overarching goal of CFTC will be to increase child health care provider participation in advocacy for tobacco control. This will be a long-term process in the WPR where many countries are still in the early stages of "denormalizing" tobacco use. In many cases, health care providers themselves may need to go through stages of change described in the Prochaska transtheoretical model, which has been widely applied in the treatment of tobacco dependence. Figure 23-2 show how these stages of readiness to change model might be applied to child health care providers.

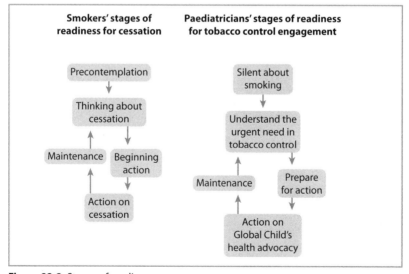

Figure 23-2. Stages of readiness.

References

1. World Health Organization. *WHO Report on the Global Tobacco Epidemic, 2011: Warning About the Dangers of Tobacco.* Geneva, Switzerland: World Health Organization; 2011. http://whqlibdoc.who.int/publications/2011/9789240687813_eng.pdf. Accessed May 13, 2013

2. World Health Organization Western Pacific Region. Tobacco Free Initiative. http://www.wpro.who.int/tobacco/en. Accessed May 13, 2013

3. Preventing tobacco use among young people. A report of the Surgeon General. Executive summary. *MMWR Recomm Rep.* 1994;43(RR-4):1–10. http://www.cdc.gov/mmwr/PDF/rr/rr4304.pdf. Accessed May 13, 2013

4. World Health Organization Western Pacific Region. Smoking statistics. http://www.wpro.who.int/mediacentre/factsheets/fs_20020528/en/index.html. Accessed May 13, 2013

5. World Health Organization Western Pacific Region. *Review of Areca (Betel) Nut and Tobacco Use in the Pacific: A Technical Report.* Geneva, Switzerland: World Health Organization; 2012. http://www.wpro.who.int/tobacco/documents/betelnut.pdf. Accessed May 13, 2013

6. World Health Organization. *Tobacco Use and Its Impact on Health. 3. Prevalence of Tobacco Use and Factors Influencing Initiation and Maintenance Among Women.* Geneva, Switzerland: World Health Organization; 2010. http://www.who.int/tobacco/publications/gender/en_tfi_gender_women_prevalence_tobacco_use.pdf. Accessed May 13, 2013

7. Campaign for Tobacco-Free Kids. Warning to parents: how big tobacco targets kids today. http://www.tobaccofreekids.org/what_we_do/industry_watch/warning_to_parents. Published March 21, 2012. Accessed May 13, 2013

8. World Health Organization. *Confronting the Tobacco Epidemic in a New Era of Trade and Investment Liberalization.* Geneva, Switzerland: World Health Organization; 2012. http://apps.who.int/iris/bitstream/10665/70918/1/9789241503723_eng.pdf. Accessed May 13, 2013

9. US Department of Health and Human Services. *A Report of the Surgeon General: How Tobacco Smoke Causes Disease—The Biology and Behavioral Basis for Smoking-Attributable Disease Fact Sheet.* http://www.surgeongeneral.gov/library/reports/tobaccosmoke/factsheet.html. Accessed May 13, 2013

10. Jiang Y, Li XH, Wu X. Smoking behavior of Chinese physicians. *Chinese J Prevent Control Chronic Dis.* 2009;13:224–227

11. Warren CW, Asma S, Lee J, Lea V, Mackay J. *Global Tobacco Surveillance System: The GTSS Atlas.* Atlanta, GA: CDC Foundation; 2009. http://www.cdc.gov/tobacco/global/gtss/tobacco_atlas/pdfs/tobacco_atlas.pdf. Accessed May 13, 2013

12. Centers for Disease Control and Prevention. Global Tobacco Surveillance System Data (GTSSData). http://nccd.cdc.gov/GTSSData/default/default.aspx. Accessed May 13, 2013

Chapter 24

Obesity: Response to a Global Epidemic

Louise A. Baur, AM, MBBS(Hons), Bsc(Med), PhD, FRACP

Obesity: A Major 21st-Century Public Health Challenge

The World Health Organization (WHO) has termed childhood obesity "one of the most serious public health challenges of the 21st century."[1] Others describe obesity as "the public health equivalent of climate change,"[2] while the International Obesity TaskForce calls it the "Millennium Disease."[3] These strong and emotive words highlight the importance of the problem and the ongoing difficulties in tackling it.

Why are we concerned about obesity in childhood and adolescence? It is in part because of the increased risk of immediate morbidities, including psychosocial distress, various orthopedic complications, insulin resistance, type 2 diabetes, fatty liver disease, and obstructive sleep apnea.[4,5] These complications are more likely in those with severe obesity and in older children and adolescents. In high-income countries there are well-documented increases in health service use and health care costs associated with obesity and obesity-associated complications even in childhood,[6,7] although no such data are available from developing countries. However, childhood obesity is also associated with a range of longer-term complications, including the emergence of risk factors for various chronic diseases, as well as the high risk of persistence of obesity into adulthood, in turn associated with further morbidity and premature mortality, such as heart disease, type 2 diabetes, and some cancers.[8,9]

Childhood Obesity in Developed and Developing Countries

So, how prevalent a problem is it? Once recognized as a problem only in westernized countries, overweight and obesity are now major health issues in many low- and middle-income countries, affecting children and adolescents as well as adults. The Web site of the International Association for the

Study of Obesity is a useful source of recent data on the prevalence of overweight and obesity in different countries and WHO regions, sourced from an amalgam of published and unpublished data.[10] As seen in Table 24-1, the prevalence of childhood obesity is highest in the Americas, Eastern Mediterranean, Western Pacific, and European regions. However, prevalence rates have risen rapidly in many countries within the Asian region (Table 24-2).

Table 24-1. Percentage of Childhood Overweight and Obesity by World Health Organization Region[a]

	Boys		Girls	
WHO Region	% Overweight or Obese	% Obese	% Overweight or Obese	% Obese
Africa	1.9	0.5	2.6	0.7
Americas	27.3	9.1	26.3	8.5
Eastern Mediterranean	15.2	6.4	16.6	6.8
European	22.1	5.3	20.3	4.4
South-East Asia	14.2	2.5	7.0	0
Western Pacific	17.7	7.0	12.7	5.9

Abbreviation: WHO, World Health Organization.
[a]Based on measured data, using International Obesity TaskForce body mass index for age cut points. Reproduced from the International Association for the Study of Obesity, with permission.[10]

Table 24-2. Childhood Overweight Percentage (Including Obesity) in Selected Asian Countries[a]

Country	Year of Survey	Age Range	Boys	Girls	Definition
India	2007–2008	2–17 y	20.6	18.3	IOTF
Thailand	1997	5–15 y	21.1	12.6	85th percentile NHANES
China	2002	7–17 y	5.9	4.5	IOTF
Singapore	1993	10 y	25.5	17.6	IOTF
Taiwan	2001	6–18 y	26.8	16.6	IOTF

Abbreviations: IOTF, International Obesity TaskForce; NHANES, US National Health and Nutrition Examination Survey.
[a]Not all data are based on nationally representative studies. Reproduced from the International Association for the Study of Obesity, with permission.[10]

Obesity is not just an issue of school-aged children and adolescents—younger children are also affected. A WHO study estimated that worldwide, 43 million preschool-aged children were overweight or obese in 2010, with prevalence having increased from 4.2% in 1990 to 6.7% in 2010.[11] Although the prevalence of overweight and obesity in this age group in developed countries is about double that in developing countries (11.7% and 6.1%, respectively), the great majority of affected children (35 million) live in developing countries. Furthermore, there has been a greater relative increase in overweight and obesity prevalence rates in developing countries (+65%) than in developed countries (+48%) in the past 2 decades.

Childhood Obesity: Increasing Prevalence in Asian Countries

A 2011 review of overweight and obesity in children and adolescents in a range of Asian countries showed that there has been a rapid increase in prevalence in recent years, especially in younger age groups.[12] Prevalence rates have tended to be highest in younger boys, in urban rather than rural children, and amongst children from households with higher economic status. Possible explanations for the higher prevalence in Asian boys, a finding not generally seen in developed countries, is the persistence of a traditional cultural belief that a plump child symbolizes family prosperity[13] and a societal view that favors boys over girls.[14] The urban/rural differences and positive socioeconomic gradient in obesity prevalence are different from patterns observed in developed countries, where obesity is more common in children from rural families and families of lower socioeconomic status.[15]

Another important issue in many low- and middle-income countries, including those in Asia, is that they are facing a double burden of undernutrition and obesity and related noncommunicable diseases.[11,16] As income rises, however, the problem of obesity becomes progressively more important, and this is what is being observed in several Asian countries.

These findings suggest that changes in the broader food and physical activity environments in those countries that are undergoing rapid nutrition and economic transition are in turn having a profound effect on the lifestyle and resultant health and well-being of children.

Preventing Child and Adolescent Obesity

Since the late 1990s, governments in many developed countries and international agencies have produced numerous plans for preventing obesity,[17–20] although the conversion of these plans to action remains largely unrealized. Unsurprisingly, there are parallels in many of the recommendations contained in these documents, given that they are based on core health promotion principles and a similar evidence base.

The common principle in these different obesity intervention plans, some of which are discussed further in this chapter, is the enabling of healthy personal choices around eating and physical activity through modifying the broader environment. Other important elements include multilevel, multifaceted interventions that influence different aspects of the food and physical activity environments; engaging national and local governments, the media, different industries, local communities, and individuals; and the need for political leadership, supporting a coordinated, inter-sectoral approach.

At the same time, the following approaches, which are examples of what has been termed "the futility of isolated initiatives,"[21] are extremely unlikely to modify obesity prevalence: focusing on one setting, such as sole school-based interventions, without engaging the family or broader community; using a single approach, such as social marketing, in the absence of any other community-level change; and cherry-picking very few interventions without using the underpinning principles noted previously.

Regulation of Food Marketing and Obesity Prevention

Comprehensive obesity prevention plans include a range of strategies to address broader food and physical activity environments. One of these is regulating food marketing directed to children. The commercially led promotion of energy-dense, nutrient-poor foods and beverages toward children is a widespread global phenomenon. Food advertising influences nutrition knowledge, food preferences, and consumption patterns of children, with subsequent implications for weight gain and obesity.[22] Cost-effectiveness modeling has shown that a reduction in the advertising of high-fat and high-sugar foods and beverages directed to children (up to 14 years of age) would be of low cost to government and have a high reach, although such a policy would be likely to meet marked resistance from parts of the food and advertising industries.[23]

The following sections focus on the issue of food marketing directed toward children in the context of obesity prevention. Of course, effective obesity prevention requires inclusion of many other targets and strategies.

World Health Organization and United Nations Recognition of Issues of Childhood Obesity and Regulation of Food Marketing

In the past decade, WHO and the United Nations have developed a range of strategies and declarations relevant to obesity and food marketing, some of which are briefly highlighted herein. These provide a sense of the *potential* policy background for obesity prevention initiatives, including those related to the regulation of food marketing directed toward children.

The WHO Global Strategy on Diet, Physical Activity and Health[18] was endorsed in 2004. That document, and the subsequent *2008-2013 Action Plan for the Global Strategy for the Prevention and Control of Noncommunicable Diseases,*[24] provided an action plan to treat these diseases. Both emphasized the need for the plan to address the marketing of foods to children. In 2010, WHO member states endorsed the set of 12 recommendations on the marketing of foods and nonalcoholic beverages to children, for which a framework for implementation was provided in 2012.[25]

The United Nations held a High-level Meeting on Non-communicable Diseases in September 2011, a landmark event that highlighted the political, economic, and social challenges of noncommunicable diseases in the 21st century. The political declaration from that meeting had a primary focus on cardiovascular diseases, cancers, chronic respiratory diseases, and diabetes, although "the rising levels of obesity in different regions, particularly among youth" and the link between obesity and the 4 main noncommunicable diseases were noted "with concern."[26] Among the many recommendations made, one highlighted the need for multi-sectoral action "in order to reverse, stop and decrease the rising trends of obesity in child, youth and adult populations, respectively." The declaration also committed the United Nations to the implementation of WHO recommendations on the marketing of foods and nonalcoholic beverages to children.[25]

Subsequent to this, WHO has worked on the development of a comprehensive global monitoring framework of noncommunicable diseases.[27] Such a framework is important because it, in turn, influences national and local policies—what gets measured is viewed as important, and what is not measured may be ignored. As has been commented on, the targets are vital because it is likely that "any health issue not covered will receive little or no attention."[28] One of the 9 voluntary global targets of the framework, announced in November 2012, is to "halt the rise in diabetes and obesity" by 2025.[27] And 1 of the 3 recommended indicators of this particular target is the prevalence of overweight and obesity in adolescents; the other 2 relate to diabetes and adult overweight and obesity.

While recognition of the need for a comprehensive monitoring framework is welcome, it would appear to have a number of limitations, at least concerning the issue of obesity. For example, the monitoring framework does not include any measure of overweight or obesity in early and mid-childhood, an age group in which obesity prevalence has been changing rapidly.[10] It also focuses on downstream health outcomes and behavioral risk factors and does not include any measure of the broader, more upstream environments that influence these, such as food marketing, food composition, walkability, and public transport access.

Regulating Food Marketing: What Is Happening Globally?

The policy environment is changing. In a review conducted in 2009 involving policy informants from 59 countries, 26 countries had made explicit statements on food marketing in strategy documents, with 20 having made or planning to make explicit policies such as statutory measures, official guidelines, or approved forms of self-regulation.[29] However, only 2 Asian countries, South Korea and Malaysia, were among those countries with policies, and the report suggested there was resistance to implementation of these policies in those countries as well as others.

Monitoring Food Marketing in Asia and Beyond

In general, the research on childhood obesity and government policy responses to obesity in many developing countries within Asia are at an earlier stage than in some more developed countries. Thus, in 2011, academics in the School of Public Health at the University of Sydney held a regional collaboration for childhood obesity prevention research program at the university, with more than 20 participants from China, Vietnam, Indonesia, and Thailand. This was funded by AusAID (the Australian government overseas aid program) and built on existing links that the academics had with researchers and policy makers in the countries. In the course of the 3-week residential workshop, participants explored a range of strategies for monitoring obesity and the factors influencing obesity, as well as obesity prevention. It became apparent in formal and informal discussions that much of the focus of academic and government work to date in many of these and other developing Asian countries has been on describing the prevalence of obesity, with much less focus on developing the evidence base for advocacy and interventions. One of the prominent issues that emerged repeatedly over the course of the workshop was the need for information, ideally collected in a systematic way, on the exposure of children to unhealthy food marketing in most Asian countries. The apparent widespread extent of food marketing in each of these countries was of clear concern to all participants. As a result, the participants agreed to work cooperatively on a multi-country television food marketing study.

Subsequently, in March 2012, a memorandum of understanding was established between the project team at the University of Sydney and researchers from a range of Asian countries. The memorandum covered such issues as intellectual property, writing and authorship, and timelines. One of the advantages of the agreement is that individual research groups can publish their own data, but all agree on pooling a minimum agreed set of data to allow intercountry and intercity comparisons to be made. A detailed protocol was given to each group to provide guidance in collecting and coding data; this was based on that used in a previous multi-country study of television food advertising led by one of the project team.[30] Further information and discussion were provided by the project team as needed. Data collection occurred from April through September 2012, and draft reports were due in February 2013. When data are finally available, it is anticipated that they will be used to advocate for consideration of regulations to limit the amount of television advertising to children in these countries. This cooperative research study is also helping to further build links between and develop the capacity of childhood obesity researchers and obesity policy makers in different parts of Asia.

The specific approach to monitoring the exposure of children to television marketing is being incorporated into the development of a framework for monitoring the effect of food and nonalcoholic beverage promotions to children. This in turn is one part of a fairly recent initiative, the International Network for Food and Obesity/Non-communicable Diseases Research, Monitoring and Action Support, which was launched by the International Obesity TaskForce in 2012.[31] The international network aims to develop and promote benchmarks for measuring the progress of governments and the food industry and develop tools for monitoring their actions in relation to unhealthy food environments. The monitoring framework covers such topics as food marketing, food composition, food pricing, and food labeling as well as public and private sector policies and actions. However, it is as yet too early to determine the effectiveness of this approach in supporting development and implementation of obesity policies.

Final Reflections on a Complex and "Wicked" Problem

This overview of the context of work being undertaken in several Asian countries on the exposure of children to television food advertising can only touch lightly on a few of the many issues pertinent to the prevention of obesity, which is a complex and intractable, or "wicked," problem. Policy responses to obesity in most developed countries have generally been slow, and the conversion of policies to action is largely unfulfilled.[32] And now most countries in Asia are confronting a rising prevalence of childhood obesity. As yet there is no successful example of an obesity prevention initiative in developing countries of Asia, reflecting the relative newness of the epidemic.

A 2011 *Lancet* series on the issue of obesity commented that obesity epidemics throughout the world "are driven by complex forces that require systems thinking to conceptualize the causes and to organize evidence needed for action."[32] The solutions to the obesity epidemic were seen to be "multi-faceted with initiatives throughout governments and across several sectors."[32] Food marketing is one of the elements contributing to changes in dietary intake in populations, so the regulation of food marketing can only be one part of a comprehensive approach to obesity prevention. The work being undertaken on monitoring the exposure of children to food market-ing in a range of Asian countries is an initial step in understanding the drivers of obesity in different countries and providing the sort of evidence that can be used for advocacy and in developing policy.

The strategies outlined in the WHO Global Strategy on Diet, Physical Activity and Health[18] and the UN high-level summit documents[26] provide a framework for action on child and adult obesity prevention. However, "the test will be how well Member States match their declarations with supportive funding and policies to support global actions."[32]

References

1. World Health Organization. Global Strategy on Diet, Physical Activity and Health. Childhood overweight and obesity. http://www.who.int/dietphysicalactivity/childhood/en. Accessed May 13, 2013

2. Lang T, Rayner G. Overcoming policy cacophony on obesity: an ecological public health framework for policymakers. *Obes Rev.* 2007;8(Suppl 1):165–181

3. International Obesity TaskForce. What is IOTF? http://www.iaso.org/iotf/aboutiotf. Accessed May 13, 2013

4. Trasande L, Chatterjee S. The impact of obesity on health service utilization and costs in childhood. *Obesity (Silver Spring).* 2009;17(9):1749–1754

5. Cretikos MA, Valenti L, Britt HC, Baur LA. General practice management of overweight and obesity in children and adolescents in Australia. *Med Care.* 2008;46(11):1163–1169

6. Reilly JJ, Methven E, McDowell ZC, et al. Health consequences of obesity. *Arch Dis Child.* 2003;88(9):748–752

7. Daniels SR. Complications of obesity in children and adolescents. *Int J Obes (Lond).* 2009;33(Suppl 1):S60–S65

8. Park MH, Falconer C, Viner RM, Kinra S. The impact of childhood obesity on morbidity and mortality in adulthood: a systematic review. *Obes Rev.* 2012;13(11):985–1000

9. Reilly JJ, Kelly J. Long-term impact of overweight and obesity in childhood and adolescence on morbidity and premature mortality in adulthood: systematic review. *Int J Obes (Lond).* 2011;35(7):891–898

10. International Association for the Study of Obesity. Obesity data portal. http://www.iaso.org/resources/obesity-data-portal. Accessed May 13, 2013

11. de Onis M, Blössner M, Borghi E. Global prevalence and trends of overweight and obesity among preschool children. *Am J Clin Nutr.* 2010;92(5):1257–1264

12. Li M, Dibley MJ. Child and adolescent obesity in Asia. In: Baur LA, Twigg SM, Magnusson RS, eds. *A Modern Epidemic: Expert Perspectives on Obesity and Diabetes.* Sydney, Australia: Sydney University Press; 2012:171–188

13. Cui Z, Huxley R, Wu Y, Dibley MJ. Temporal trends in overweight and obesity of children and adolescents from nine Provinces in China from 1991-2006. *Int J Pediatr Obes.* 2010;5(5):365–374

14. Hong TK, Dibley MJ, Sibbritt D, Binh PN, Trang NH, Hanh TT. Overweight and obesity are rapidly emerging among adolescents in Ho Chi Minh City, Vietnam, 2002-2004. *Int J Pediatr Obes.* 2007;2(4):194–201

15. Li M, Dibley MJ, Sibbritt D, Yan H. Factors associated with adolescents' overweight and obesity at community, school and household levels in Xi'an City, China: results of hierarchical analysis. *Eur J Clin Nutr.* 2008;62(5):635–643

16. Bygbjerg IC. Double burden of noncommunicable and infectious diseases in developing countries. *Science.* 2012;337(6101):1499–1501

17. Lobstein T, Baur L, Uauy R; IASO International Obesity TaskForce. Obesity in children and young people: a crisis in public health. *Obes Rev.* 2004;5(Suppl 1):4–104

18. World Health Organization. *Global Strategy on Diet, Physical Activity and Health.* Geneva, Switzerland: World Health Organization; 2004. http://www.who.int/dietphysicalactivity/strategy/eb11344/strategy_english_web.pdf. Accessed May 13, 2013

19. World Health Organization. *Set of Recommendations on the Marketing of Foods and Non-alcoholic Beverages to Children.* Geneva, Switzerland: World Health Organization; 2010. http://whqlibdoc.who.int/publications/2010/9789241500210_eng.pdf. Accessed May 13, 2013

20. Commission of the European Communities. White paper on a strategy for Europe on nutrition, overweight and obesity related health issues. http://eur-lex.europa.eu/LexUriServ/LexUriServ.do?uri=COM:2007:0279:FIN:EN:PDF. Accessed May 13, 2013

21. Butland B, Jebb S, Kopelman P, et al. *Foresight. Tackling Obesities: Future Choices—Project Report.* London, United Kingdom: Government Office for Science; 2007. http://www.bis.gov.uk/assets/foresight/docs/obesity/17.pdf. Accessed May 13, 2013

22. Hastings G, McDermott L, Angus K, Stead M, Thomson S. *The Extent, Nature and Effects of Food Promotion to Children: A Review of the Evidence. Technical Paper Prepared for the World Health Organization.* Geneva, Switzerland: World Health Organization; 2007. http://www.who.int/dietphysicalactivity/publications/Hastings_paper_marketing.pdf. Accessed May 13, 2013

23. Haby MM, Vos T, Carter R, et al. A new approach to assessing the health benefit from obesity interventions in children and adolescents: the assessing cost-effectiveness in obesity project. *Int J Obes (Lond).* 2006;30(10):1463–1475

24. World Health Organization. *2008-2013 Action Plan for the Global Strategy for the Prevention and Control of Noncommunicable Diseases.* Geneva, Switzerland: World Health Organization; 2008. http://whqlibdoc.who.int/publications/2009/9789241597418_eng.pdf. Accessed May 13, 2013

25. World Health Organization. *A Framework for Implementing the Set of Recommendations on the Marketing of Foods and Non-alcoholic Beverages to Children.* Geneva, Switzerland: World Health Organization; 2012. http://www.who.int/dietphysicalactivity/MarketingFramework2012.pdf. Accessed May 13, 2013

26. World Health Organization. Prevention and control of noncommunicable diseases. Outcomes of the high-level meeting of the general assembly on the prevention and control of non-communicable diseases and the First Global Ministerial Conference on Healthy Lifestyles and Noncommunicable Disease Control. April 20, 2012. http://apps.who.int/gb/ebwha/pdf_files/WHA65/A65_6-en.pdf. Accessed May 13, 2013

27. World Health Organization. Report of the formal meeting of member states to conclude the work on the comprehensive global monitoring framework, including indicators, and a set of voluntary global targets for the prevention and control of noncommunicable diseases. November 21, 2012. http://apps.who.int/gb/ncds/pdf/A_NCD_2-en.pdf. Accessed May 13, 2013

28. NCDs and the UN: danger of a missed opportunity. *Lancet.* 2012;380(9847):1032

29. Hawkes C, Lobstein T. Regulating the commercial promotion of food to children: a survey of actions worldwide. *Int J Pediatr Obes.* 2011;6(2):83–94

30. Kelly B, Halford JC, Boyland EJ, et al. Television food advertising to children: a global perspective. *Am J Public Health.* 2010;100(9):1730–1736

31. World Public Health Nutrition Association. Bellagio workshop. INFORMAS. How not to prevent obesity and chronic non-communicable diseases. www.wphna.org/2013_jan_hp1_informas.htm. Accessed May 13, 2013

32. Gortmaker SL, Swinburn BA, Levy D, et al. Changing the future of obesity: science, policy, and action. *Lancet.* 2011;378(9793):838–847

Chapter 25

Obesity: Engaging the Community

Juliana Kain, MPH
Boyd Swinburn, MBChB, MD(Otago), FRACP
Ricardo Uauy, MD, PhD

Introduction

Childhood obesity has increased markedly over the past decades in virtually all countries; presently it constitutes an epidemic in high- and low-income countries alike. The rise in obesity in less-developed countries has been faster over the past decade than ever before, especially among children living in urban areas, probably due to a greater exposure to what has been termed the *obesogenic environment*. The rise in obesity prevalence in developing countries is characterized by a greater prevalence in higher-income groups; however, as gross domestic product (GDP) increases, obesity progressively shifts to lower-income children.[1,2] There is a direct relationship between family income and prevalence of obesity: mean body mass index (BMI) rises in a linear fashion with GDP, up to approximately US $5,000 per capita yearly; at higher GDPs, the slope drops and becomes almost flat after reaching about US $15,000. Evidence shows that in low-income countries, obesity is higher among the wealthy population, but with increasing national income, obesity becomes more prevalent among the poorer populations, especially in women.[3]

De Onis et al[4] reported worldwide prevalence and trends of obesity among preschool children younger than 6 years based on World Health Organization (WHO) standards. A total of 450 nationally representative surveys from 144 countries were analyzed. Results show that 43 million preschool-aged children were classified as obese (>2 SD), of which 35 million live in developing countries. Worldwide prevalence of childhood obesity increased from 4.2% in 1990 to 6.7% in 2010; if this trend continues, it will reach 9.1% or approximately 60 million by 2020. The estimated prevalence of childhood obesity in Africa in 2010 was 8.5%; it is expected to reach 12.7% by 2020. Prevalence is lower in Asia than Africa (4.9% in 2010), but the number of affected children (18 million) is highest in Asia.

The US National Health and Nutrition Examination Survey (NHANES) databases show significant increases in childhood obesity over the past decades. Survey 1 and 2 studies of preschool-aged children show a 2-fold rise in prevalence of overweight for girls over a period of 20 years, compared with about 25% for boys. However, among older children, the increase has been greater among boys. Clear ethnic differences are seen, in that Mexican Americans have the highest rates. Increasing trends in the 1990s relative to the 1980s were demonstrated in the Bogalusa Heart Study, which also confirmed that children from families of low socioeconomic status have a higher prevalence of obesity independent of ethnicity. In Japan, obesity in children 6 to 14 years of age increased from 5% to 10% between 1974 and 1993. In 12 European countries, recent cross-sectional data from 6- to 9-year-olds (n=168,832) showed that obesity prevalence ranged from 6% to 27% among boys and 4.6% to 17% in girls. Multi-country comparisons suggest the presence of a north-south gradient with the highest level of overweight children found in southern European countries.[5,6] Body adiposity in children does not regress as children grow older; rather, it tends to increase progressively, serving as a predictor for the development of metabolic syndrome (insulin resistance, diabetes, hypertension, and hypercholesterolemia) in later life.[7]

The increasing prevalence of childhood obesity in most developing countries explains rising trends in the prevalence of metabolic syndrome in older children and adolescents. This is typified by clustering of cardio-vascular risk factors, which include altered blood lipids (high low-density lipoprotein, low high-density lipoprotein, and elevated triglycerides), high fasting insulin, abnormal glucose tolerance, and elevated blood pressure. The adult correlates of this phenomenon are rising rates of diabetes, cardiovascular disease, and cancer at younger ages, leading to the epidemic of chronic diseases and premature adult death and disability. Excess abdominal fatness, generally assessed by waist circumference (WC) and not by a high BMI, correlates best with the appearance of metabolic syndrome. Research shows that over the last decades, WC in children and adolescents has increased to a greater extent than overall fatness, assessed by BMI. There are ethnic differences in children's fat distribution; those from Asian origin having a greater WC at a given BMI consequently have an increased risk of metabolic syndrome, leading to adult-onset (type 2) diabetes at younger ages. The increasing prevalence and severity of obesity in children have resulted in higher rates of related comorbid conditions, including high blood pressure, early development of atherosclerosis, and type 2 diabetes. The rate of increase in adiposity in childhood has been strongly associated with the development of cardiovascular risk in young adults. Body mass index accounts for only 60% of the variance of insulin resistance in adults; WC is now considered a better predictor of metabolic syndrome because of its association with visceral adiposity. Thus, the distribution of body fat in childhood is an important early marker of risk of adult chronic disease.[8-10] As shown in Table 25-1, a substantial proportion of children are affected by one or more concurrent diseases.[11]

Genetics

The rise of obesity prevalence during the past decades cannot be accounted for by population genetic changes. The heritability of BMI is often cited as 40% to 70%, yet large genome-wide association studies to identify common single nucleotide polymorphisms associated with BMI have been unable to explain more than a small proportion (<2%) of BMI variability. Heritability is often misinterpreted as being the proportion of BMI variance caused by genetics, whereas heritability studies, rather than estimating cause,

Table 25-1. Estimated Prevalence of Disease Indicators Among Obese Children

Indicator	Mean (%)	95% CI
Raised blood triglycerides	25.7	21.5–30.5
Raised total blood cholesterol	26.7	22.1–31.8
High LDL cholesterol	22.3	18.9–26.3
Low HDL cholesterol	22.6	18.7–27.0
Hypertension	25.8	21.8–30.2
Impaired glucose tolerance	11.9	8.4–17.0
Hyperinsulinemia	39.8	33.9–45.9
Type 2 diabetes	1.5	0.5–4.5
Metabolic syndrome, 3 factors	29.2	23.9–35.3
Metabolic syndrome, 4 factors	7.6	4.6–12.2
Hepatic steatosis	33.7	27.9–41.8
Raised serum aminotransferase	16.9	12.8–22.0

Abbreviations: CI, confidence interval; HDL, high-density lipoprotein; LDL, low-density lipoprotein. Note: Definitions of obesity and the indicators differ among source surveys. Mean and confidence intervals based on weighted averages of survey findings.
Lobstein T, Baur LA, Jackson-Leach R. The childhood obesity epidemic. In: Waters E, Swinburn B, Seidell J, Uauy R, eds. *Preventing Childhood Obesity: Evidence Policy and Practices*. West Sussex, United Kingdom: Blackwell Publishing Ltd; 2010:3–14, with permission from Wiley-Blackwell.

estimate the proportion of genetic and nongenetic variance that explains BMI variance in a given study population. There is evidence that gene expression can be modified by diet and can also be programmed by epigenetic mechanisms that occur in utero or even before conception, triggered by elevated maternal blood sugar and hyperinsulinemia or by lack (folate and vitamin B_{12}) or other specific nutrients affecting DNA methylation, modifying transcription, and changing gene expression. Recent evidence supports the view that obesity in adolescents and adults is related to nutritional programming that occurs in utero, particularly in light of rising trends in maternal obesity and fetal macrosomia related to high glucose and insulin concentrations in embryonic and fetal life. However, the real driver of increasing body weight observed at all ages in virtually all countries is not a change in genetic predisposition but rather the results of the greater obesogenicity of the environment, especially exposure to amounts and type of foods.[12]

Recent studies point to the important role of maternal obesity, excessive weight gain in pregnancy, and gestational diabetes as factors that influence obesity and chronic disease risks in the next generation. Early epidemiologic data show a U-shaped relationship between birth weight and later chronic disease risk—that is, the effect of low and high birth weight is a greater risk of obesity and related chronic diseases. Recent epidemiologic evidence supports the view that fetal overnutrition can affect offspring phenotype just as well as undernutrition. For example, maternal BMI has been positively correlated with total and abdominal adiposity and with liver fat content in infancy, across the entire range of maternal BMI. Exposure to a diabetic intrauterine milieu is an important risk factor of type 2 diabetes in later life and is also associated with greater adiposity in infancy. The developmental disruption can be subtle and often can go undetected; maternal nutritional status can even affect offspring epigenetic status and body composition independent of birth weight.[13,14]

Our Experience in School-Based Obesity Prevention Programs in Chile

Obesity in Chilean children has risen markedly over the last decades. The Ministry of Health, generally guided by pediatricians, nutritionists, and other health professionals, has grown progressively motivated to tackle this condition, launching diverse efforts mainly addressing school-based preventive actions. We first called the attention of health authorities in 1990 by including reversing the rise in childhood obesity as part of the United

Nations Children's Fund Goals for 2000; we suggested that obesity prevalence should drop from 5% to 3% over the decade. Unfortunately, we were
ignored, and it rose from 5% to 9%. In 2002, we undertook a 2-year controlled intervention including close to 2,000 6- to 12-year-old children in
the city of Casablanca (located 80 km west of capital city Santiago) and a
similar-duration controlled intervention that also included teachers and
their respective 4- to 9-year-old students in a district of urban Santiago
called Macul.[15]

The Casablanca study included 1,759 children from 3 schools (intervention
group) and 671 from 1 school (control group). The intervention included
activities in nutrition and physical activity, fully applied the first year and
partially the second due to limitation of resources. Primary outcomes were
standardized BMI *(z)* and obesity prevalence; secondary outcomes, WC
and triceps skinfold. Time effects were assessed by changes in BMI-related
variables by gender and period, while intervention effects were determined
by comparing changes in obesity prevalence by gender and period and BMI
z according to gender, age, and period. Results showed that over the 2 years,
obesity declined significantly in the intervention group, from 17% to 12.3%
(boys) and 14.1% to 10.3% (girls), and mean BMI *z* dropped from 0.62 to
0.53 (boys) and 0.64 to 0.58 (girls). In the control group, obesity remained
stable at around 21% (boys) and 15% (girls), while BMI *z* increased significantly the second year. Figure 25-1 shows that BMI *z* scores declined in
all age categories for boys in intervention schools during period 1; however, the decline was significant only in the youngest. No differences were
observed in controls during that period. During summer recess, there was
practically no change in BMI *z* scores. During period 3, BMI *z* scores increased in intervention and control groups; however, this increase was only
significant among controls in the youngest category. In girls (Figure 25-2),
BMI *z* scores followed a similar trend as in boys, but none of the changes
were significant. In conclusion, this study showed that effectiveness was
greater in the first school year, and the effect was stronger in younger boys.

The intervention implemented in Macul, apart from training teachers
to deliver contents on healthy eating and increasing physical education
classes, encouraged teachers to participate in a wellness program themselves. Effectiveness was determined by comparing BMI *z* scores and
obesity prevalence between children in intervention and control schools
by year and between students of intervened and control teachers. Results
showed that although teachers in the intervention group exhibited improvements in anthropometry and blood chemistries, the effect on children was

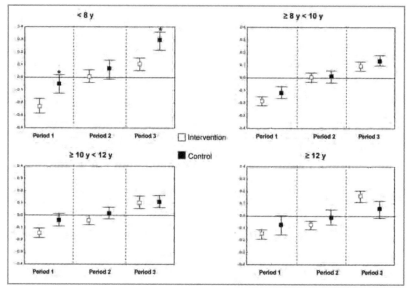

Figure 25-1. Change in mean body mass index z scores in boys (95% confidence interval) relative to baseline, in intervention and control schools according to age and period of study. Period 1: March to November 2003; period 2: November 2003 to March 2004; period 3: March to November 2004. Proc Mixed and Tukey tests were used to compare intervention versus control groups and time effects. Significant difference between intervention and control (P <0.05) is marked with an asterisk (*).

unrelated to teacher results. With the experience gained by our group in school-based obesity prevention programs over the years, and considering other studies in different places around the world, we are able to recognize some pitfalls in the overall process involving design, implementation, and evaluation of these interventions and also acknowledge lessons learned.

Recognizing Pitfalls

- *Resources.* Interventions need to be fully resourced at the outset (human and material resources need to be in place and fully trained) because changes in strength of interventions detract from securing a measurable effect.
- *Incentives.* Teacher apathy and failure to comply with requested participation cannot be overcome with persuasion alone. Authorization to work in the school and even expressed interest of school authorities were clearly not enough to secure genuine participation. Incentives, monetary or otherwise, are necessary to operate changes; verbal persuasion is unlikely to succeed, at least in Chile.

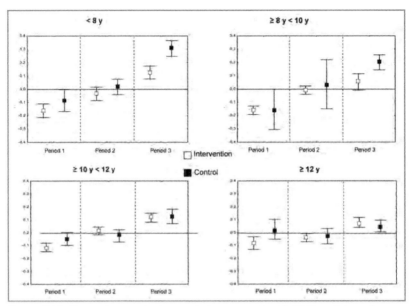

Figure 25-2. Change in mean body mass index *z* scores in girls (95% confidence interval) relative to baseline, in intervention and control schools according to age and period of study. Period 1: March to November 2003; period 2: November 2003 to March 2004; period 3: March to November 2004. Proc Mixed and Tukey tests were used to compare intervention versus control groups and time effects. Significant difference between intervention and control ($P < 0.05$) is marked with an asterisk (*).

- *Profits.* Commercial interests are commonly at odds with obesity prevention. The incentive for school kiosks is to sell what is more profitable; thus, unhealthy choices are by far most sold. Effective interventions need to fully control what is sold in kiosks and dispensing machines; unhealthy choices should be removed before the study is implemented.

Lessons Learned

- *Experimental design.* Experimental designs using random allocation of schools to one or more interventions are nearly impossible to implement within an educational system that is not accustomed to controlled evaluations and even less to random allocation to more than one treatment. Local school administration sees no real value or is not even concerned with potential consequences derived from the result of an evaluation process. We were most successful in implementing interventions in schools where children had higher obesity prevalence. However, these children were less likely to comply with the program.

- *Environmental influences.* There is a need to create an enabling environment and actively sensitize multiple stakeholders to have the potential for success. Intervention in the school setting without modifying home or social environment will hardly ever succeed.
- *Process.* Clearly defined processes, targets, and measures of success are needed at the outset. Ideally, consequences of success and failure for school administrators, teachers, and other parties involved should be in place before starting the intervention.
- *Engaging families.* Contribution of parents in the process of change is grossly underestimated and is in fact a key factor in determining success or failure. In the urban setting, it is very difficult to engage parents in their children's obesity prevention program. Possible explanations for this are that they do not acknowledge obesity as a problem, they do not have time to participate, grandmothers or other adults are in direct care of the children, or they may have the perception that cost of healthy foods is beyond their means.
- *Physical activity.* Increasing physical activity at school is difficult because academic curriculum is inflexible and uses most potential free time for additional language and math classes, subjects included in the annual evaluation and accreditation of schools. In addition, teachers report to be heavily burdened by the need to implement various programs during the school year; extra work is not welcome. Unless initiatives are integrated into school curricula, they are not sustainable and unlikely to produce sustained effects. Although extracurricular physical activity options are a possibility, these are not sustainable unless parents and communities are fully committed.

Other potential contributory factors for failure include school infrastructure being poorly suited, and possibility of training teachers to address obesity is very limited because they are committed to multiple tasks, of which obesity prevention is not a priority. In brief, culture of *change for the better* is weak at best. Also, the wider obesogenic environment outside school (heavy marketing of highly processed, energy-dense foods) is powerful and runs contrary to school goals.

Key Points in the Prevention of Childhood Obesity

- The childhood obesity epidemic demands a concerted prevention effort from governments, international organizations, the private sector, and civil society.

- A life-course approach to preventing childhood obesity provides multiple opportunities for intervention, and many childhood settings offer opportunities for access to children and parents.
- Government policies are needed to provide the backbone for health promotion activities.
- International agencies and multinational food companies have critical supporting roles in this process. Public health interests are poorly supported by regulatory approaches and policies that affect food consumption patterns and access to active living.
- Marketing of unhealthy foods to children is a multibillion-dollar commercial enterprise; present business and marketing practices severely undermine efforts of parents, governments, and health and education professionals to provide a healthy food and physical activity environment for children.[11]

The life-course approach, which considers health as a continuous process starting from conception, has been useful in identifying risk factors of development of childhood obesity. Critical periods have been described in the development and persistence of overweight in children; these are the prenatal period, pregnancy, infancy, and adolescence. In the prenatal period, prepregnancy weight, gestational weight gain, birth weight, smoking during pregnancy, and maternal diabetes appear to be the most important risk factors, while after birth, postnatal infant feeding practices, rapid weight gain, firstborn child, and sleeping patterns are the most important ones.

Prevention of disease should be based on creating healthy environments during every stage potentially associated with the development of obesity. The main options are educational and health service approaches. Education itself is usually weak, and action needs to be more inclusive than focusing just on the health sector. The rational approach is to "make the healthy choices the easy choice"; preferably, the healthy choice should be the default option supported by environmental changes, education, and social marketing. Environmental change means policies and regulations.[16]

Although praiseworthy, there is no evidence that governmental measures such as applying taxes to high-energy foods, calorie labeling in fast-food restaurants, and limiting the sale of junk foods in schools are effective by themselves.[3,11]

There is now overwhelming evidence that factors related to weight, smoking, and glucose tolerance occurring to women of childbearing age before and after pregnancy have the greatest probability of determining future obesity. The greatest risk has been shown in large-for-gestational-age (LGA) babies born to overweight mothers. The odds ratio of developing childhood obesity can be as high as 15:1 for LGA compared with normal-weight babies. Because this phenomena crosses generations, mothers who themselves were LGA are at higher risk of being overweight or obese when they become pregnant. Therefore, public health efforts should be focused on the fetal/infant period—this is clearly an important time but should not be the only basket in which to put the eggs. We should also focus on limiting weight gain in women before they become pregnant, preventing excessive weight gain and high glucose levels during pregnancy, and promoting and supporting the practice of exclusive breastfeeding for the first 6 months of life as the preferred mode of feeding.[14]

Policy for Preventing Childhood Obesity

Competing views exist about the importance and role of policy in preventing childhood obesity. Certain stakeholders claim that there is little need for government policy because the food marketplace and physical activity environment are managed democratically, with people being able to demand the food and physical activity choices they want to consume or adopt and the market efficiently providing for them. Conversely, others (including ourselves) argue that government policy is very important because it has a role in protecting and promoting the food system and physical activity environments as public goods.

There are 3 particular reasons why policy is important for preventing childhood obesity.

1. *System failures.* Food system failure may include large wastage and subsidize unhealthy foods, and most of the time healthy foods are more expensive. The modern food system does not have sufficient checks and balances in place to ensure that detrimental overconsumption and environmental effects do not happen. Indeed, the warning signs of food system failure are amply illustrated by increasing environmental damage, staple food shortages, rising food prices, and increasing obesity prevalence. This assessment is consistent with the observation that obesity is a sign of commercial success (increasing food sales) but a market failure because the market is failing to deliver the best outcomes for people. Policy provides a statement and intentions about the food system structure and operation that can help avert or correct system failure.

2. *Food choice.* Generally, it is an illusion that people have free choice and are able to demand what food they want to consume or what physical activity in which they wish to participate. In other words, our choices are not really determined by individual free will. People are rarely actively involved in how the food system operates and what food products are made available or marketed to them. Policy can be used to build a more engaged and informed citizenship in relation to the food system and the way it operates.

3. *Food democracy.* Nutrition and obesity prevalence data consistently reveal that it is the most vulnerable in society and those least able to engage with the food system that are most at risk of food insecurity and obesity. Engagement with the food system needs to be considered alongside democratic principles and rights such as participation and transparency in the decision-making process. These principles and attainment of food democracy can only be pursued within a food policy framework and cannot be left to market forces or solely to consumer demand.[16–19]

Policy Instruments

There are a number of instruments or tools that governments have available for implementing policy. Primary policy instruments are regulations and laws (rules); taxation and funding (for programs, research, monitoring and evaluation, social marketing, and capacity building); services and service delivery (providing hospitals, workforce); and advocacy (to the public, private sector, and other jurisdictions). Within the contemporary political environment of many developed countries there exists a dominant ideology of neoliberalism characterized by the use of policy instruments that place greater emphasis on individual responsibility for dietary and physical activity choices and less reliance on government intervention in the environments where those choices are made.

Results show that strong regulatory measures such as bans on food marketing to children are considered less politically feasible but more likely to be effective in obesity prevention. Conversely, policies that focus on education and information dissemination were considered politically feasible but unlikely to have an effect on obesity prevention. Making policies for the prevention of childhood obesity, as with any policy, is not a linear, rational, evidence-based process. The obesity research community has been collecting large amounts of evidence that should be informing policies for obesity prevention, but very little of it actually comes to bear on the decision-making process. Researchers and policy makers still do not have a sufficient dialogue to shape effective policies, evaluate progress, and create an enabling environment for policies that have a chance of achieving a public health effect if taken to scale.

Human judgment also is involved in translating available evidence into policies and programs. Usually, experts, panels, committees, and task forces are needed to make judgments in relation to the quantity and quality of available evidence and how it might be debated; the legitimacy of evidence derived from studies using so-called less rigorous epidemiologic methods, such as cohort studies, to inform obesity prevention policy should also be considered. A recently published WHO document[20] is very useful in providing tools to determine and identify priority areas for action in the field of population-based prevention of childhood obesity. The objectives of the suggested tools are to facilitate a prioritization process that is systematic and locally relevant. Common steps to most policy development approaches are

A. Problem identification and needs analysis
B. Identification of potential solutions
C. Assessment and prioritization of potential solutions
D. Strategy development

While these priority-setting approaches all contain common elements, the contexts in which they are used, processes they involve, and technical analyses differ. Selection of the most appropriate tool depends on the purpose, desired outcomes, criteria to be used for assessment (eg, population effectiveness, costs, cost-effectiveness, feasibility, relevance, strength of evidence base, effects on equity, sustainability, acceptability to stakeholders), level of resources (including financial and technical expertise and time), and data available.

The WHO STEPwise framework for preventing chronic diseases considers feasibility, effect, and affordability and has been developed for use mainly in low- and middle-income countries with limited resources and funding. One of the processes is called Analysis Grid for Elements Linked to Obesity and has been used to develop community action plans, taking into account importance (which incorporates relevance and impact) and feasibility as part of the prioritization process.[21]

Due consideration should be given to local, regional, or country-specific factors when analyzing potential areas for action. It is also essential to take into account all relevant sectors and settings to identify areas for comprehensive action. Finally, identifying key stakeholders and outlining their potential roles and responsibilities is critical for prioritization. Each priority-setting approach requires facilitation expertise to manage the process of working with relevant stakeholders so that the recommended priority actions are realized.

References

1. Gupta N, Goel K, Shah P, Misra A. Childhood obesity in developing countries: epidemiology, determinants, and prevention. *Endocr Rev.* 2012;33(1):48–70
2. Shih M, Dumke KA, Goran MI, Simon PA. The association between community-level economic hardship and childhood obesity prevalence in Los Angeles. *Pediatr Obes.* 2012
3. Swinburn BA, Sacks G, Hall KD, et al. The global epidemic pandemic: shaped by global drivers and local environments. *Lancet.* 2011;378(9793):804–814
4. de Onis M, Blössner M, Borghi E. Global prevalence and trends of overweight and obesity among preschool children. *Am J Clin Nutr.* 2010;92(5):1257–1264
5. Lobstein T, Baur L, Uauy R; IASO International Obesity TaskForce. Obesity in children and young people: a crisis in public health. *Obes Rev.* 2004;5(Suppl 1):4–104
6. Wijnhoven TM, van Raaij JM, Spinelli A, et al. WHO European Childhood Obesity Surveillance Initiative 2008: weight, height and body mass index in 6-9-year-old children. *Pediatr Obes.* 2012
7. Lee JM, Pilli S, Gebremariam A, et al. Getting heavier, younger: trajectories of obesity over the life course. *Int J Obes (Lond).* 2010;34(4):614–623
8. Daniels SR, Jacobson MS, McCrindle BW, Eckel RH, Sanner BM. American Heart Association Childhood Obesity Research Summit: executive summary. *Circulation.* 2009;119(15):2114–2123
9. Barlow SE; Expert Committee. Expert committee recommendations regarding the prevention, assessment, and treatment of child and adolescent overweight and obesity: summary report. *Pediatrics.* 2007;120(Suppl 4):S164–S192
10. Han JC, Lawlor DA, Kimm SY. Childhood obesity. *Lancet.* 2010;375(9727):1737–1748
11. Waters E, Swinburn B, Seidell J, Uauy R, eds. *Preventing Childhood Obesity: Evidence Policy and Practice.* West Sussex, United Kingdom: Blackwell Publishing Ltd; 2010
12. Brisbois TD, Farmer AP, McCargar LJ. Early markers of adult obesity: a review. *Obes Rev.* 2012;13(4):347–367
13. Uauy R, Kain J, Corvalan C. How can the Developmental Origins of Health and Disease (DOHaD) hypothesis contribute to improving health in developing countries? *Am J Clin Nutr.* 2011;94(6 Supp):1759S–1764S
14. Atkinson RL, Pietrobelli A, Uauy R, Macdonald IA. Are we attacking the wrong targets in the fight against obesity? The importance of intervention in women of childbearing age. *Int J Obes (Lond).* 2012;36(10):1259–1260
15. Kain J, Uauy R, Concha F, et al. School-based obesity prevention interventions for Chilean children during the past decades: lessons learned. *Adv Nutr.* 2012;3(4):616S–621S
16. Gortmaker SL, Swinburn BA, Levy D, et al. Changing the future of obesity: science, policy, and action. *Lancet.* 2011;378(9793):838–847

17. Blanck HM, Kim SA. Creating supportive nutrition environments for population health impact and health equity: an overview of the Nutrition and Obesity Policy Research and Evaluation Network's efforts. *Am J Prev Med.* 2012;43(3 Supp 2):S85–S90

18. Wang Y, Lim H. The global childhood obesity epidemic and the association between socio-economic status and childhood obesity. *Int Rev Psychiatry.* 2012;24(3):176–188

19. Swinburn B, Gill T, Kumanyika S. Obesity prevention: a proposed framework for translating evidence into action. *Obes Rev.* 2005;6(1):23–33

20. World Health Organization. *Prioritizing Areas for Action in the Field of Population-Based Prevention of Childhood Obesity: A Set of Tools for Member States to Determine and Identify Priority Areas for Action.* Geneva, Switzerland: World Health Organization; 2012. http://www.who.int/dietphysicalactivity/childhood/Childhood_obesity_modified_4june_web.pdf. Accessed May 13, 2013

21. Simmons A, Mavoa HM, Bell AC, et al. Creating community action plans for obesity prevention using the ANGELO (Analysis Grid for Elements Linked to Obesity) Framework. *Health Promot Int.* 2009;24(4):311–324

Chapter 26

Early Child Development: Health Equity From the Start in Chile

Helia Molina, MD, MPH
Miguel Cordero Vega, MS
Judith S. Palfrey, MD, FAAP
Paula Bedregal, MD, MPH, PhD
MaryCatherine Arbour, MD, MPH

Understanding the Problem

In its definition of *health,* the World Health Organization (WHO) includes development and function, emotion, and behavior.[1] A healthy child is one whose world opens up each day to new experiences, cognitive exploration, capacities, productivity, and ultimately a kind of societal belonging and citizenship. Health and development are tightly linked, with clearly established biologic explanations for the relationship. During early childhood more than 100 billion neurons are developed and connect to configure neural pathways and brain networks through the interaction of genetics, environment, and experience.[2,3] Children who experience toxic stress—prolonged exposure to stressful experiences not mitigated by relationships with supportive, loving adults—are at risk for long-term deficits in cognition and function.[4] Birth-related injuries, chronic disease, malnutrition, and infectious disease can all contribute to poor cognitive development, as can lack of stimulation, maternal depression, and exposure to violence.

As with infant and child mortality and morbidity, the developmental status of children is highly determined by the social, economic, environmental, and cultural conditions to which the child is exposed. As a result, around the world, developmental status among children is highly variable, and disparities between and within regions are great. Globally, public health practitioners and pediatricians have become committed to finding ways to ensure that children not only survive physically but also thrive developmentally, emotionally, socially, and spiritually—as whole, thoroughly healthy human beings.[5] Increasingly, health professionals are forming alliances with partners in educational, social service, and governmental sectors to sponsor programs in early childhood development.

In this chapter, we describe emerging global approaches to early childhood development and offer our experience in Chile as an example of early childhood programming in a middle-income Latin American country, analyzing factors that contributed to the success of early childhood policies, including the advocacy role of pediatricians and other key actors.

The Early Childhood Movement in the Developing World

In 2007, *The Lancet* published a series of articles on child development in developing countries that served as a call to public health practitioners worldwide to move beyond a single focus on child survival to a more inclusive child health agenda that included child development.[6] In addition to estimating that 200 million children younger than 5 years in low- and middle-income countries are not reaching their full developmental potential, the International Child Development Steering Group summarized evidence on risk and protective factors for healthy development and conducted a systematic review of randomized, controlled trials of interventions to promote child development that were conducted in the developing world—Bangladesh, China, India, South Africa, and elsewhere.

In 2008, WHO highlighted early childhood development in its landmark report on social determinants of health. In 2011, the International Child Development Steering Group updated its *Lancet* review to identify effective strategies for the reduction of inequalities and improvement of child development outcomes.[7] Among the 10 effectiveness studies and 5 program assessments reviewed, all had substantial positive effects on child cognitive or social-emotional development, parent knowledge, home stimulation, and learning activities with children. All 15 interventions had defined curricula or key messages that were delivered through a variety of mechanisms, including home visits, primary health care visits, nutrition support services, group sessions with caregivers, or combinations of these. Seven interventions worked primarily with parents or caregivers, and 8 worked with parents or caregivers and children together.

Interventions that included parent and child programs had larger effects (median 0.46, range 0.04–0.97) than parent-only programs (0.12, 0.03–0.34).

In some cases, effects were greater for younger children compared with older children and for poorer children compared with richer children. Effects by some information-based, parent-only interventions were small. The authors concluded that the most effective programs are those with systematic training methods for workers, a structured and evidence-based curriculum, and opportunities for parental practice with children with feedback.[7]

Figure 26-1 summarizes a variety of approaches that policy makers, educators, and public health and pediatric providers have tested.[8]

The Chilean Case

Chile is a middle-income Latin American nation with more than 17 million inhabitants and a gross domestic product per capita of US $12,431 in 2010. The extraordinary economic growth of the past several decades has greatly benefited the health of children. Chile has made significant investment in public health and health interventions. Since the 1950s, visionary Chilean public health professionals and pediatricians have played key roles in advancing the goal of reducing infant and child mortality. Jorge Rosselot Vicuña, Francisco Mardones Restat, Fernando Mönkeberg, and Julio Meneghello designed maternal and child health policy to progressively affect morbidity and nutrition. Their plans were implemented throughout the nation, and Chile witnessed a dramatic reduction in infant mortality from 132.6 per 1,000 live births in the 1950s to 8.9 per 1,000 in 2000. Moreover, a highly functional public primary care network with nationwide coverage was developed and structured around the mother-child dyad.

The pioneering child health advocates succeeded in putting children's issues on the public agenda and sustained their policies over time. This was all the more remarkable in that these health advances occurred during turbulent political times and across multiple changes in government. Jorge Jimenez de la Jara, a pediatrician and former health minister, masterfully recounts the advocacy process that accomplished so much for the health of children in his book, *Angelitos Salvados* (The Saved Angels).[9,10] Juan Pablo Beca, MD, and Jaime Burrows, MD, PhD, recount the clinical advocacy in Chapter 22 in this volume.

Adding Child Developmental Attainment to Local and Global Aspirations

From 2000 to 2004, as the Pan American Health Organization and WHO began to make strategic alliances with leaders of pediatrics in Latin America

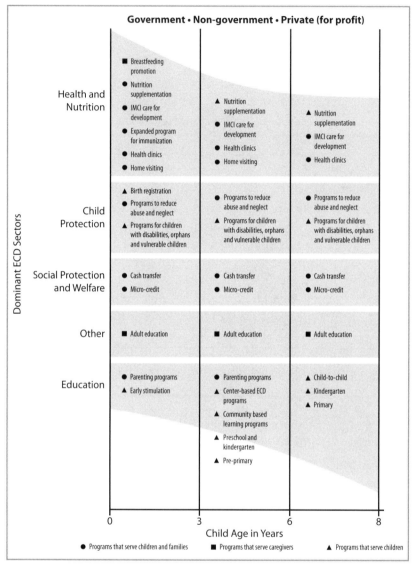

Figure 26-1. Effective strategies for reducing inequalities and improving child development outcomes. Source: Britto PR, Boller P, Yoshikawa H. Quality of early childhood development programs in global contexts: rationale for investment, conceptual framework and implications for equity. *Soc Policy Rep.* 2011;25(2):1–24. http://mathematica-mpr.com/publications/pdfs/earlychildhood/ECD_Global.pdf. Accessed May 13, 2013.

and the American Academy of Pediatrics, the topic of child development began to achieve a level of prominence. During regional events, the group carried out systematic reviews of child development literature, developed conceptual frameworks, and created a shared strategy. The child development movement grew with involvement of national scientific societies. The Latin American Association of Pediatric Societies provided spaces to discuss child development to sensitize and train pediatricians. The Chilean Society of Pediatrics strengthened the notion of integrality in pediatric care and the role given to pediatricians and parents in optimizing the developmental trajectory of boys and girls.

The Measurement of Child Development as an Advocacy Tool for Children

The need to measure child development emerged as a priority in Chile, out of the education sector. While there had been enormous strides in health, there were serious concerns that children's development had stood still. In 2000, the United Nations Educational, Scientific and Cultural Organization reported that education results in Chile were poor and gaps between the rich and poor groups were alarming.[11] For the health sector at the time, while the development issue was relevant, the absence of national data on child development made it difficult to argue about the importance of the topic and advocate for resources to address it.

In 2005, when the Ministry of Health began designing the Second National Survey of Health-Related Quality of Life, a group of researchers at the Catholic University, in collaboration with the Inter-American Development Bank, proposed to expand the first survey's child module (which focused on chronic diseases in children younger than 15 years) to integrate questions about child care and parent-reported development of children aged 3 months to 5 years. The objective of this module was to estimate the magnitude of developmental problems so that the information could be used for advocacy as well as informing the design and monitoring of early childhood policies.

The Ministry of Health granted the request, and investigators created and validated a development measurement instrument[12,13] that asks 6 to 8 questions about developmental achievement by age ranges. Its application is simple and low cost, allowing its incorporation in household surveys that collect large amounts of information.

In 2006, the instrument was applied with a nationally representative sample of 6,210 households as part of the Second National Survey of Health-Related Quality of Life. For the first time, the level of developmental deficiency and delay among Chilean children between 6 months and 5 years of age could be accurately estimated and disaggregated by sex, region, and socioeconomic situation.[14]

The national survey showed that 30% of Chilean children younger than 5 years did not reach all of their expected developmental milestones.[14] Rates of developmental risk are higher among the poorest quintile of the population (Figure 26-2). In Chile, 21.5% of children (570,000) live in poverty, compared with 14.5% of the total population.

Accurate estimates of children's developmental risk proved crucial in 2007 when the Chilean government decided to institute an integrated early child policy, Chile Grows with You (Chile Crece Contigo) (ChCC), and again in 2011 to delineate one of the health objectives of Decade 2011–2020: reduce by 15% the developmental lag in children younger than 5 years in Chile.[15]

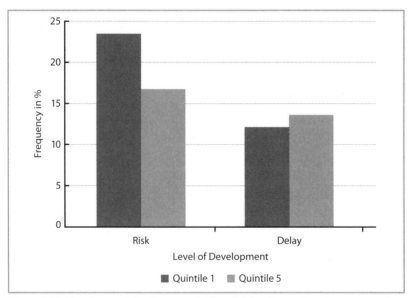

Figure 26-2. Prevalence of developmental risk and delays in a nationally representative sample of children between 1 and 5 years old, Chile 2006. Comparison of quintiles 1 (poorest) and 5 (richest) of socioeconomic status.

The Birth of Chile Grows with You

In 2006, Michelle Bachelet, a pediatrician, became the first female president of Chile. On assuming office, she established early childhood development as one of the top policy priorities of her government. She created the Presidential Advisory Board for Early Childhood Policy Reform composed of 14 people, including 3 pediatricians (Paula Bedregal, Helia Molina, and Concha, former health minister) and a wide range of professionals from across the political spectrum. She charged the advisory board with preparing an integrated child policy focused on early childhood development under the social protection system. The aim was to ensure all children's optimal development, whatever their social origin, gender, place of birth, or family situation, thereby breaking the intergenerational cycle of poverty and reducing inequity in Chile.

Based on recommendations from the advisory board, President Bachelet committed to protecting and promoting children's development from birth. Together with the team at the Ministry of Health, she conceived of a rights-based program that would ensure that young children had access to high-quality health and developmental services, first by taking advantage of every encounter that families had with health professionals, and second by coordinating services for young children across public service sectors. The resulting cross-sectoral system of integrated support services, ChCC, coordinates activities across 9 ministries, from the prenatal period through 4 years, 11 months of age.

Chile Grows with You offers a defined set of universal interventions for all Chileans that are intended to create the proper environment for healthy development, including mass education programs through television and radio programs, a Web site, and the promotion of development-friendly legislative initiatives around maternity/paternity leave and adoption. For all families who receive their health care through the free public health system (approximately 85% of Chileans), ChCC provides free routine well-child care, anticipatory guidance, and biopsychosocial support.

Chile Grows with You offers additional targeted supports for families with fewer resources or greater risk (including home visits, financial support, free nurseries and preschool, preferential access to public programs, comprehensive care, and technical aids for children with developmental delay or disability) (Figure 26-3).

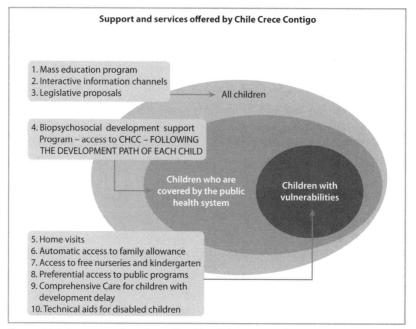

Figure 26-3. Support and services offered by Chile Grows With You (Chile Crece Contigo).

Services begin when families present for the first prenatal visit and enroll in ChCC and continue through the child's fifth birthday. Pregnant women learn the importance of good nutrition and maintenance of healthy habits (eg, refraining from tobacco, drugs, and alcohol). They learn relaxation techniques and how to anticipate the changes that a young baby will bring in their life. Once the baby is born, ChCC supports families in fully welcoming their new baby with joy and a full appreciation of the growth in physical, cognitive, and emotional abilities. Chile Grows with You materials include videos and music CDs and other appropriate child development tools.

The optimal execution of ChCC policy and opportune delivery of ChCC services require coordination, articulation, and strengthening of cross-sectoral integration structures at the municipal, provincial, regional, and national levels. To achieve this, each municipality has created a municipal ChCC network to coordinate all of the public and private institutional, human, and financial resources. After an initial period of local evaluation and review of existing services, these municipal networks elaborate work plans to generate inter-sectoral coordination and a plan for accessing and investing nationally available resources. The networks ultimately have functioned as referral mechanisms, connecting children and families with available services, as well as creating opportunities for community engagement in themes of early childhood.

Municipal networks are supported by the preexisting provincial coordinator for social protection, a ChCC manager within the National Health Service, and regional heads of ChCC from the regional offices of each participating ministry (Health, Education, Planning). At the national level, the Minister of Planning chairs a committee of ministers, with participation of the ministers of Health, Education, Work, Justice, Housing and Urbanization, Finance, Women, and Secretary General of the Presidency. This national, regional, and provincial organizational structure provides support, technical assistance, and financing to local municipalities to support optimal implementation of ChCC.

The leadership of President Bachelet and the trajectories of the professionals involved in the advisory board gave credibility and power to the initial proposal for an integrated system of services to protect and support early childhood development. Implementation began in 2007, and ChCC was scaled up to the entire country by the end of 2008. In 2009, congress passed legislation that ratified ChCC into law; CHCC is now a right and the state must guarantee all the interventions for children from 0 to 4 years. By 2009, 345 of Chile's 346 municipalities were participating in ChCC. That year, 204,935 mothers were enrolled during their pregnancies and more than 800,000 babies from birth to 4 received ChCC services.[16] Evaluation of the program implementation, users' satisfaction, results, and impact is ongoing.

Support for Child Development Through High-quality Early Education: The Birth of Un Buen Comienzo

In parallel with the creation of ChCC for children 0 to 4 years of age, President Bachelet committed to increasing the number of nurseries, child care centers, and preschools for the poorest 40% of the population. The Bachelet government made the strategic decision to begin providing early education for 4- to 6-year-olds through the public schools. Many policy makers, public officials, and families raised questions about whether the government could expand early childhood and at the same time maintain a high standard of quality. Would there be adequately trained staff, knowledgeable in child development and early childhood education? How well would schools articulate with the health system? How would the public know if children were indeed benefitting from early education in schools?

Policy makers from the ministries of Education and Planning who were interested in advancing the quality of expanded early educational services reached out to colleagues in the United States and Australia for advice. Steve Reifenberg, then director of the Santiago office of the David Rockefeller Center for Latin American Studies of Harvard University (DRCLAS), was aware of the Chilean government's interest in expanding and improving early childhood education. In 2006, DRCLAS sponsored a large meeting at the Catholic University including Chilean and American child development and public policy experts.

The Catholic University meeting led to the convening of a Mesa Técnica Interinstitucional composed of Harvard faculty, Chilean policy makers and leaders in early childhood, representatives of 3 major organizations that provide early childhood care and education (Junta Nacional de Jardines Infantiles, Integra, and Hogar de Cristo), and local stakeholders from one municipality (municipal administrators, school principals, preschool teachers). Over 18 months, the Mesa Técnica Interinstitucional worked to craft a meaningful endeavor to promote quality in the early education expansion process. With the clear intention of complementing the emerging ChCC, the Mesa specified the goal of a new program, Un Buen Comienzo (UBC): to support children's healthy development by improving the quality of early educational experiences and coordinating health services for 4- to 6-year-olds enrolled in the public school system.

Modeled roughly on Project Head Start in the United States and a successful teacher training program in Costa Rica (Amigos del Aprendizaje),[17] UBC provides public school prekindergarten and kindergarten teachers and aides with 2 years of training and in-classroom coaching in the following 4 domains:

1. *Oral language and early literacy.* Training included book-reading strategies, using extended discourse, and developing children's vocabulary and emergent writing skills.
2. *Coordination of early childhood education with health services.* Teachers were equipped with skills and materials to address health problems affecting young children in Chile, including respiratory illnesses and lack of well-child visits.
3. *Socio-emotional development.* Training focused on behavior management strategies, establishing a positive classroom climate, and individual case management.
4. *Family involvement.* Training involved strategies to get parents involved in their children's learning.

Un Buen Comienzo professional development is delivered through 12 modules (6 per year) with 4 weekly activities: a didactic workshop to introduce a topic and corresponding instructional strategies. Coaches provide in-classroom sessions and reflection opportunities for teachers. After pilot testing in 5 schools in Santiago in 2007, the intervention was revised and implemented in 64 high-need schools in 6 municipalities of Santiago from 2008 to 2011.

Schools within participating municipalities were randomized to UBC intervention (2-year intensive teacher training plus 100 books per classroom) or a comparison condition, which consisted of 10 books per classroom and one workshop on self-care for teachers and aides. Results from a cluster-randomized evaluation show that UBC has had statistically significant, moderately sized positive effects on 2 of 4 indicators of classroom quality—emotional support and classroom organization. The UBC intervention has substantially improved teachers' abilities to support children's social and emotional functioning and to organize and manage children's behavior, time, and attention in the classroom, with more time spent in meaningful language exchange, better social interactions among the children, and fewer disruptive behaviors. The full impact evaluation results will be available within the next several years, while longer-term effects require longitudinal assessment.

Together, ChCC and UBC have opened the door to a serious exploration in Chile of the essential elements to ensure that young children develop to their full potential and have increased opportunities to grow into productive citizens as their country grows in its overall maturity, prosperity, and international prominence and responsibility.

References

1. World Health Organization. Constitution of the World Health Organization. http://www.who.int/governance/eb/who_constitution_en.pdf. Accessed May 13, 2013
2. Couperus JW, Nelson CA. Early brain development and plasticity. In: McCartney K, Phillips D, eds. *The Blackwell Handbook of Early Childhood Development.* Malden, MA: Blackwell Publishing; 2006:85–105. http://onlinelibrary.wiley.com/book/10.1002/9780470757703. Accessed May 13, 2013
3. National Research Council, Institute of Medicine. *From Neurons to Neighborhoods: The Science of Early Childhood Development.* Washington, DC: National Academies Press; 2000

4. Garner AS, Shonkoff JP; American Academy of Pediatrics Committee on Psychosocial Aspects of Child and Family Health; Committee on Early Childhood, Adoption, and Dependent Care; Section on Developmental and Behavioral Pediatrics. Early childhood adversity, toxic stress, and the role of the pediatrician: translating developmental science into lifelong health. *Pediatrics.* 2012;129(1):e224–e231

5. Molina H, Cordero M, Silva V. De la sobrevida al desarrollo integral en la infancia. *Rev Chil de Pediatr.* 2008;79:11–17

6. Engle PL, Black MM, Behrman JR, et al. Strategies to avoid the loss of developmental potential in more than 200 million children in the developing world. *Lancet.* 2007;369(9557):229–242

7. Engle PL, Fernald LC, Alderman H, et al. Strategies for reducing inequalities and improving developmental outcomes for young children in low-income and middle-income countries. *Lancet.* 2011;378(9799):1339–1353

8. Britto PR, Boller P, Yoshikawa H. Quality of early childhood development programs in global contexts: rationale for investment, conceptual framework and implications for equity. *Soc Policy Rep.* 2011;25(2):1–24. http://mathematica-mpr.com/publications/pdfs/earlychildhood/ECD_Global.pdf. Accessed May 13, 2013

9. Jimenez de la Jara J. *Angelitos Salvados.* Santiago, Chile: Uqbar Editors; 2009:166–170

10. Jiménez J, Romero MI. Reducing infant mortality in Chile: success in two phases. *Health Aff (Millwood).* 2007;26(2):458–465

11. International Office of Education, United Nations Educational, Scientific and Cultural Organization. *La educación Chilena en el cambio de siglo: políticas, resultados y desafíos. Informe Nacional de Chile.* Santiago, Chile: Ministerio de Educación; 2004. http://www.ibe.unesco.org/International/ICE47/English/Natreps/reports/chile_part_1.pdf. Accessed May 13, 2013

12. Bedregal P, Scharager J, Breinbahuer C, Solari J, Molina H. Validación de un instrumento de tamizaje de población para evaluar rezagos del desarrollo en población chilena de 0 a 6 años. *Revista Médica de Chile.* 2007;135:403–405

13. Bedregal P, Hernández V, Yeomans H, Molina H. Validez concurrente de una prueba de tamiz poblacional para niños entre 6 y 59 meses de edad. Congreso Latinoamericano ALAPE, 2012

14. Segunda Encuesta Calidad de Vida, Ministerio de Salud, Gobierno de Chile, 2006

15. Ministerio de Salud de Chile. ESTRATEGIA NACIONAL DE SALUD Para el cumplimiento de los Objetivos Sanitarios de la Década. 2011-2020. http://www.minsal.gob.cl/portal/url/item/b89e911085a830ace0400101650115af.pdf. Accessed May 13, 2013

16. Molina H, Silva V. Four years growing together: memories from the early childhood protection system 2006–2010. Ministry of Health Chile. 2010. http://www.oei.es/inicialbbva/programas_infancia/Chile.pdf. Accessed May 31, 2013

17. Rolla San Francisco A, Carlo M, August D, Snow CE. The role of language or literary instruction and volcabulary in the English phonological awareness of Spanish-English bilingual children. *Appl Psycholinguistics.* 2006;229–246

Chapter 27

Child Maltreatment: A Global Perspective

Desmond K. Runyan, MD, DrPH, FAAP

Introduction

Child abuse and neglect are acts of omission or commission by a parent or adult caregiver. A World Health Organization (WHO) consultation in 1999 defined the problem as follows: "Child abuse or maltreatment constitutes all forms of physical and/or emotional ill-treatment, sexual abuse, neglect or negligent treatment or commercial or other exploitation, resulting in actual or potential harm to the child's health, survival, development or dignity in the context of a relationship of responsibility, trust or power."[1] A 2002 WHO report[2] and the 2006 UN *World Report on Violence Against Children*[3] cite numerous studies in all sectors of the globe. Professional attention was first drawn to this topic in Europe by an 1866 publication by Tardieu in France.[4] Professional recognition in South America was evidenced as early as a 1929 publication in Colombia.[5] The medical recognition of child abuse by Kempe and colleagues in the United States in 1962 antedated and helped spawn public recognition and development of governmental policies and agencies to investigate and intervene in child abuse and neglect in the United States.[6] A cascade of research from the United States and Europe followed, but laws and policies have been slow to develop in other parts of the world.[7]

Many nations of the world have no mandatory reporting or organized public systems responding to child abuse.[7] Perhaps because the most attention paid to child abuse and neglect in the medical literature has been in Europe and the United States, there is the perception that child abuse and neglect are conditions whose occurrence is greatest in these countries.[8,9] The 2002 WHO *World Report on Violence and Health*[2] and the 2006 UN *World Report on Violence Against Children*[3] cite a number of studies that report high rates of child abuse in other areas of the world. International comparisons of these data are complicated because there are definitional or methodologic differences among studies. Some studies include violence against children in schools by teachers.[10] Many international studies simply present case series.[11,12] Some studies have examined child reports,[13,14] while others use information from parents.[15,16] Very few studies estimate population-based rates, and official or police statistics are collected in relatively few countries. There is accumulating evidence that public recognition and development of treatment and prevention efforts may be reducing the incidence of child physical and sexual abuse in the United States and Europe.[17] Serious efforts to prevent or minimize the effect of child abuse around the world will require involvement of all sectors of society, including health care professionals.

Recognizing Child Abuse

Despite legal and public recognition of child abuse in the United States, the skills required to identify and respond to child physical and sexual abuse are not well-taught in medical schools there.[18] Experience suggests that lack of training in child abuse and family violence may be an even greater problem outside the United States.[19] If physicians are to help children be free of abuse, their education will need to include the recognition of and response to abuse. Medical education priorities are increasingly being directed by public health data.[20] Medical education in the area of child abuse and neglect may be prompted by population-based epidemiologic data on the occurrence and consequences of abuse and neglect to add child abuse and neglect recognition to curricula. Abuse and neglect have at their origins social, cultural, and interpersonal factors; cross-cultural comparative studies may provide important clues to causes and new strategies for prevention. For pedagogic and scientific reasons, cross-cultural examinations of child abuse are likely to be helpful in understanding and responding to child abuse.

WorldSAFE International Survey of Child Discipline

Study Design

With colleagues in 6 countries, we undertook a groundbreaking population-based study of the patterns and nature of child discipline in 19 communities around the globe.[9] The investigators named this study World Studies of Abuse in the Family Environment (WorldSAFE), and it was supported by the International Clinical Epidemiology Network. We used this study as an opportunity to ascertain from professionals and focus groups what forms of discipline were used in different countries and how discipline was influenced by culture. We were particularly interested in ascertaining patterns of the harshest forms of discipline but included in our survey verbal and psychological forms of discipline as well. Culture helps define acceptable behaviors in a community, including how children are raised. We developed a common instrument by asking parents in each country about child discipline and going over the Parent-Child Conflict Tactics Scale.[16] Focus groups in the different countries felt that we were missing several important forms of discipline, so 6 additional items should be added to the instrument. We also queried parental alcohol and substance use, intimate partner violence, and maternal mental health. The survey was designed to be completed in 30 minutes and was administered to mothers only, in their homes or a neutral community setting in complete privacy by female interviewers. We found support to survey 14 communities across India and single communities in the Philippines, Egypt, Brazil, and Chile. We shortened the questionnaire slightly and administered it using an anonymous telephone approach in 2 states of the United States.

Survey Results

We noted dramatic differences in maternal education by community. The most and least educated mothers were in the same country. Mothers in the city of Chennai averaged 15.3 years of education, while 2 communities, the slums of Delhi and rural Bhopal, had mothers with an average of less than 2 years of education (Figure 27-1).

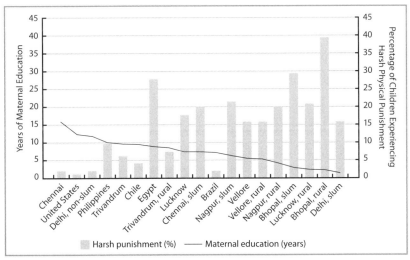

Figure 27-1. Maternal report of the percent use of harsh discipline compared with years of maternal education.

Yelling and spanking were frequent in all of the countries. Rates of the use of spanking ranged from a low of 18% in upper-income Delhi to greater than 75% in the Philippines. Yelling was greater than 80% in all of the communities except Egypt, Brazil, and rural and non-rural communities of Vellore, India. Threats of abandonment ranged from about 2% in the United States to nearly 45% of children in the Philippines and Brazil. Hitting with an object on the body other than on the buttocks ranged from 3.6% in the 2 US states to more than 50% of children in rural Trivandrum. Threats of evil spirits were used as discipline of greater than 25% of children in the Philippines and 6 of the 14 communities sampled in India.

Shaking children younger than 2 years and a combined variable of "harsh punishment," defined as shaking, choking, beating up, knocking down, or hitting with an object other than on the buttocks a child younger than 2 were dramatically related to maternal education. In 2 rural communities of India, more than 60% of children were reported to be shaken for discipline. This was not reported in Chennai, India, and was reported at a rate of 2.6% in the US states. Rates of harsh punishment overall ranged from less than 5% in the 2 most educated communities, Chennai and the United States, to 40% in rural Bhopal. The median percentage of children being harshly punished in all of the 19 communities was 16%.

A Call to Action

The WorldSAFE surveys reveal that quantitative study of parental behavior in a variety of cultures is possible and useful. The use of a parental survey of disciplinary behaviors avoids the need for a standard definition of abuse or neglect and allows the reader to determine what forms of discipline are not acceptable in a specific region or culture. There are limitations to this approach. Stigmatized behavior might not be revealed by parents, and the amount of stigma—and hence underreporting—may vary by country and culture. We used focus groups at the outset in each country to confirm the utility of a standard survey of parent discipline developed in the United States. We added 6 items to the survey because they were suggested frequently by focus groups in more than one country. We may have missed important forms of child discipline, but our survey teams of local investigators and graduate students and our focus groups felt that we captured the patterns and types of discipline used most commonly in each country.

Very harsh forms of discipline were not reported frequently in any country, except that "beaten up" in the past year was described as a form of discipline used by 25% of mothers in Egypt. Further work will be needed there to understand what was meant by this behavior, as this community stood out in this form of discipline.

Our data, with caveats about sampling specific communities and thus lacking the ability to generalize to entire countries, describe a remarkable universal pattern with interesting cultural variations. Rates for the harshest forms of punishment are low, yelling is frequent, and one form of corporal punishment, such as slapping on the face or head, are more common than spanking in 8 of the 14 Indian communities surveyed. The strongest impression from the data is that maternal education is strikingly inversely correlated with the use of harsh discipline. A global strategy of educating girls may well be the single most effective population-based approach to reducing or eliminating child abuse. We thought it remarkable that one country, India, has the safest and the most hazardous communities with respect to child discipline. We note that shaking of young children is reported frequently by poorly educated mothers and speculate that this may be an important observation related to other observations that intellectual disability is frequent among poor families in low-income countries around the world.

We remain convinced that local and national data on the use of harsh punishment are important and should inform pediatricians in every country and motivate serious national efforts to reduce child abuse and neglect.

References

1. Report of the Consultation on Child Abuse Prevention, 29–31 March 1999, WHO, Geneva. Geneva, Switzerland: World Health Organization; 1999. http://apps.who.int/iris/handle/10665/65900. Accessed May 13, 2013

2. Krug EG, Dahlberg LL, Mercy JA, Zwi AB, Lozano R, eds. *World Report on Violence and Health*. Geneva, Switzerland: World Health Organization; 2002. http://www.who.int/violence_injury_prevention/violence/world_report/en. Accessed May 13, 2013

3. Pinheiro PS. *World Report on Violence Against Children*. New York, NY: United Nations; 2006. http://www.unviolencestudy.org. Accessed May 13, 2013

4. Labbé J. Ambroise Tardieu: the man and his work on child maltreatment a century before Kempe. *Child Abuse Negl.* 2005;29(4):311–324

5. Villaveces A, Deroo LA. Child delinquency and the prophylaxis of crime in early 20th-century Latin America. *Rev Panam Salud Publica.* 2008;24(6):449–454

6. Ten Bensel RW, Rheinberger MM, Radbill SX. Children in a world of violence: the roots of child maltreatment. In: Helfer ME, Kempe RS, Krugman RD, eds. *The Battered Child.* 5th ed. Chicago, IL: University of Chicago Press; 1997:3–28

7. Dubowitz H, ed. *World Perspectives on Child Abuse,* Tenth Edition Executive Summary. http://c.ymcdn.com/sites/www.ispcan.org/resource/resmgr/world_perspectives/ wp_exec_summary_2012_final.pdf. Accessed May 13, 2013

8. Finkelhor D. The international epidemiology of child sexual abuse. *Child Abuse Negl.* 1994;18(5):409–417

9. Runyan DK, Shankar V, Hassan F, et al. International variations in harsh child discipline. *Pediatrics.* 2010;126(3):e701–e711

10. African Network for the Prevention and Protection Against Child Abuse and Neglect Regional Office. *Awareness and Views Regarding Child Abuse and Child Rights in Selected Communities in Kenya.* Nairobi, Kenya: African Network for the Prevention and Protection Against Child Abuse and Neglect; 2000

11. Sumba RO, Bwibo NO. Child battering in Nairobi, Kenya. *East Afr Med J.* 1993;70(11): 688–692

12. Kassim K, Kasim MS. Child sexual abuse: psychosocial aspects of 101 cases seen in an urban Malaysian setting. *Child Abuse Negl.* 1995;19(7):793–799

13. Kim DH, Kim KI, Park YC, Zhang LD, Lu MK, Li D. Children's experience of violence in China and Korea: a transcultural study. *Child Abuse Negl.* 2000;24(9):1163–1173

14. Choquet M, Darves-Bornoz JM, Ledoux S, Manfredi R, Hassler C. Self-reported health and behavioral problems among adolescent victims of rape in France: results of a cross-sectional survey. *Child Abuse Negl.* 1997;21(9):823–832

15. Youssef RM, Attia MS, Kamel MI. Children experiencing violence. I: parental use of corporal punishment. *Child Abuse Negl.* 1998;22(10):959–973

16. Straus MA, Hamby SL, Finkelhor D, Moore DW, Runyan D. Identification of child maltreatment with the Parent-Child Conflict Tactics Scales: development and psychometric data for a national sample of American parents. *Child Abuse Negl.* 1998;22(4):249–270

17. Jones LM, Finkelhor D, Halter S. Child maltreatment trends in the 1990s: why does neglect differ from sexual and physical abuse? *Child Maltreat.* 2006;11(2):107–120

18. Institute of Medicine Committee on the Training Needs of Health Professionals to Respond to Family Violence. *Confronting Chronic Neglect: The Education and Training of Health Professionals on Family Violence.* Cohn F, Salmon ME, Stobo JD, eds. Washington, DC: National Academy of *Sciences*; 2002

19. Oral R, Can D, Kaplan S, et al. Child abuse in Turkey: an experience in overcoming denial and a description of 50 cases. *Child Abuse Negl.* 2001;25(2):279–290

20. Evans JR. The "health of the public" approach to medical education. *Acad Med.* 1992;67(11):719–723

Section 7

A Call to Action

Chapter 28

Advocacy in All Arenas

Judith S. Palfrey, MD, FAAP
Stephen Berman, MD, FAAP

This book has pointed to a number of ways that child health professionals are engaged globally in advocacy. We could not touch on all 21st-century disease entities and functional states, all environmental exposures, or all social determinants that affect children. We would consider it amiss to publish this book without sharing a short perspective on some of the topics that we were unable to explore.

Armed Conflict and Civil Unrest

Interstate and civil war profoundly affect children. The rate at which noncombatants such as women and children are targeted seems to be on the rise. Moreover, children are often conscripted into formal and informal armies with massive exposure to danger and violence. The global advocacy voice has resulted in high-level rhetoric against such exploitation of children, but much more is needed to prevent its occurrence and provide care when it has occurred.

Cancer

Childhood cancers are increasingly amenable to treatment and cure. Across the world, oncologists are striving to use child health advocacy to raise clinical awareness about the detection of cancer and availability of protocol-based interventions. Drug procurement remains a giant challenge.

Climate Change

Only recently are child health professionals beginning to understand the health effects of climate change and the ways in which human industrial and developmental projects are altering plant, animal, and microbial ecology. New scientific understanding about climate change affords new opportunities for global child health advocacy.

Disabilities

Advocacy for children and youth with disabilities is just emerging in many countries around the world. Such advocacy is most effective when child health professionals partner with the families of children and youth with disabilities. It is critical that the advocacy address prevention, medical care, early intervention, and educational, recreational, and vocational opportunities, with an emphasis on community inclusion in all aspects of the individual's life.

Environmental Hazards

Children are exposed to heavy metals, organophosphates, hydrocarbons, and newly developed artificial compounds. The more environmental specialists unearth about the health effects of these exposures, the greater the child health advocacy role in prevention and treatment will be.

Infections

We have addressed many issues related to infectious diseases but could not cover every microbial agent. Child health advocacy continues to be particularly salient in the fight against diseases such as malaria and tuberculosis. Also, emerging diseases pose significant threats of worldwide epidemic proportion because of globalization and rapid travel around the world. Recent experiences with severe acute respiratory syndrome (SARS) and H1N1 influenza have illustrated the importance of child health advocacy in containing the spread of deadly infectious agents.

Injuries

Childhood injuries are a major source of morbidity and mortality around the world. Increasing access to automobiles and motorized bicycles has led to increasing rates of motor vehicle injuries on a global scale. Access to firearms presents acute threats in many countries, most prominently the United States. Advocacy for injury prevention has proven highly successful in many instances, and the models are readily adaptable around the world.

Natural Disasters

Hurricanes, earthquakes, tsunamis, floods, droughts, fires, and other natural disasters affect children physically and emotionally. Child health advocacy is needed to keep children's issues in the minds of governmental disaster preparedness teams. Child advocates also have direct roles to play acutely at the time of the natural disaster and throughout the recovery phase, which may last for years.

Surgically Correctable Conditions

Global child health advocacy includes identification of surgically correctable conditions and mounting of surgical teams in low-resource settings to provide interventions for children with congenital anomalies, injuries, cancer, and other conditions.

We applaud all the child health advocates who are taking on these and many other challenges. We encourage others to follow their lead. There is much to be done.

Chapter 29

ICATCH:
Become a Change Agent

Burris Duncan, MD, FAAP
Anna Maria Mandalakas, MD, FAAP
Donna M. Staton, MD, MPH, FAAP
Bronwen Anders, MD, FAAP
Ann Behrmann, MD, FAAP
Mirzada Kurbasic, MD, MSCR, FAAP

Introduction

Pediatricians are in a unique position to learn stories of the injustices inflicted on those who have no voice, the children. We cannot remain silent. Our conscience demands that we speak out, that we become the voice to help those who cannot help themselves. In the United States there are organizations that we can join and lend our voice to others to right the wrong, to protect the children. The American Academy of Pediatrics (AAP) is one such organization that advocates for children at every level of government and society. Regrettably, such organizations do not exist in many developing countries where it can be dangerous to speak out. Those who do risk loss of freedom or even loss of life. Yet in these settings, the injustices faced by children are often the most severe. What is the pediatrician to do? How can the child care provider bring such problems to the attention of those who are in a position to make a difference?

Those of us who have worked in countries where resources are limited have been impressed time and again by not just seeing but feeling the dedication and commitment that our colleagues have to the children under their care. Many work at 2 or even 3 jobs. One job may be in the university where they receive minimal pay but are recognized for their expertise and rewarded by teaching those entering the profession. Another job may be in a government post that also provides little compensation yet affords the great satisfaction of helping impoverished and marginalized patient populations. The third job is frequently in a private practice, a stark contrast to the public clinic, but where the income pays the bills. Their lives are consumed by a sea of patients, a never-ending line of children and families waiting patiently to be seen.

These very pediatricians are the ones best situated to address these challenges, and often they have ideas for creative and innovative solutions to the problems of limited resources in their community. They have ideas for projects that if implemented, would clearly improve the lives of the children they serve. But the barriers to implementing these ideas are real: too little time, a lack of resources, and an absence of support and encouragement. The will is there, but the means are not. Yet when provided with the means, even modest support, these pediatricians can and do make a significant difference.

This is the backdrop that germinated International Community Access to Child Health (ICATCH), the international grant program modeled after the domestic AAP Community Access to Child Health (ICATCH) program. The central tenets of ICATCH were born: to enable these child health care providers to implement their ideas to improve health care and decrease health disparities, and to create networks with colleagues in resource-limited settings by giving them the support they crave and helping them fulfill their desire to advocate on behalf of the children under their care.

ICATCH gives small 3-year grants of $2,000 per year to health care practitioners whose proposal meets 3 criteria: the idea must originate from a provider in the resource-limited area, the project must include collaboration with a community group or agency, and the goal must be to improve the health of children. Networking comes by providing the colleague with a mentor to help write the grant and implement funded projects. Since the first cycle of grants began in 2006, ICATCH has funded 41 projects in 25 different countries on 5 continents.

Examples From 5 Different Regions: It's Amazing What $2,000 Can Do

Elsie Locson received a grant in 2007 to increase tuberculosis (TB) awareness and demonstrate the importance of TB directly observed treatment, short-course (DOTS), in the community of Sitio Gulayan, Philippines. The government was not providing recommended prophylactic treatment to children younger than 15 years who were living with someone with active

TB. Prior to the project, many contacts refused screening and infected patients refused treatment due to shame and perceived stigma. Eighty-nine percent of targeted families were reached and given the appropriate education. Perceptions were changed. The detection rate of TB infection in adults increased 6-fold and all received treatment, as did all the infected children. Partners included local health clinics, local government, and the pediatric department of the medical center. Most importantly, the program has continued beyond the 3-year grant period.

Xiaoming Shen, chairman of the Shanghai Pediatric Society, director of the World Health Organization (WHO) Collaborative Center for Neonatal Health Care, and director general of Shanghai Municipal Education Commission, has been instrumental in decreasing childhood lead exposure and introducing newborn hearing screening in China. In his ICATCH application, Dr Shen pointed out that motor vehicle accidents were the second leading cause of death in children in Shanghai, where the number of deaths had skyrocketed from 42 in 2000 to 7,077 in 2004. He attributed this tremendous increase to the rapid transportation switch from bicycle to automobile coupled with a lack of safety education, infrequent use of car seats, and no laws mandating their use. An observation study he conducted of 1,055 vehicles carrying 1,121 child passengers revealed that only 23 of the children were riding in car seats and 30% of the child passengers were sitting in the front seat while on Shanghai freeways.

His project, "Parenting Education of Child Passengers," instituted a model safety education program in kindergartens that focused on child passenger safety and included a demonstration of the appropriate use of child passenger restraints. Following the training, the rate of parents holding a child in the front seat decreased from 12.82% to 2.71%. Nearly 73% of guardians said they wished to purchase a car seat, and 99.2% approved of legislation requiring car seat use. Future plans for the project involve convincing governmental officials to develop policies and laws to prohibit children riding in the front seat and increase the use of car seats in Shanghai.

In Bosnia and Herzegovina, Mirjana Remetic led the ICATCH-funded project "Autism Education and Early Screening." In Bosnia and Herzegovina, the diagnosis of and early intervention in autism were rare. Dr Remetic and her colleagues instituted a screening program for 18- to 24-month-olds that referred suspected children for a full evaluation and treatment. The goals were to determine the prevalence of autism and use the data to create awareness, include autism screening as a basic part of office visits, and advocate for these vulnerable children and obtain a commitment of help from governmental agencies. Working with the Ministry of Education, posters that explained autism were distributed to schools and child care centers in the entire northeast region of Bosnia. Dr Remetic and colleagues have screened more than 658 children for autism and found 28 who needed follow-up evaluations, 6 of whom were referred for treatment. The increased awareness, screening, and child identification has initiated a drive to establish the country's first autism center.

The ICATCH proposal of Ed Nignpense noted that in his country of Ghana, poisoning is among the top 5 causes of death from injury in childhood. ICATCH awarded funds to his project, entitled "Strengthening Community Awareness of Pediatric Poisoning," which was developed to advocate for children through augmenting the outreach activities of the national Ghana poison center. Two graphic posters, one promoting the poison control center in Accra and the other targeting kerosene safety in Ghana, were distributed to 76 community nurses who used them at talks they gave on child poisonings. A wallet-sized card was developed that provided contact information and basic poisoning prevention messages. Calls to the center have doubled.

Naeem Zafar is an ICATCH grant recipient who has committed his life to the recognition and prevention of child abuse in his country and is considered the "father" of defending children against that injustice in Pakistan. He was facing not only political hurdles but also significant cultural obstacles, with corporal punishment an accepted practice and an ingrained belief that "my home is my castle." However, Dr Zafar succeeded in introducing the concept of child protection and created an advocacy organization to alert politicians, educate the people, and protect the children. The idea for the ICATCH project originated from a request by the Children's Hospital Nursing School. He developed a curriculum that has been adopted by nursing schools and includes a 2-day hands-on training module and training kit. Over the grant period, his goal is to train more than 300 student nurses with the ultimate goal of convincing legislators to pass laws addressing this prevalent problem in Pakistan.

Conclusion

Nigel Crisp, who directed England's National Health Service for 5 years and who has worked in many resource-limited countries as an advisor to Tony Blair and a consultant to WHO, has published 2 influential reports: *Global Health Partnerships: The UK Contribution to Health in Developing Countries* and *Scaling Up, Saving Lives.* The common theme in his most recent book, *Turning the World Upside Down: The Search for Global Health in the 21st Century,* is the essence of ICATCH. He recognized that there are creative, passionate local people in resource-limited communities who somehow are "…finding solutions and working out how to use the materials at hand to provide the best deal they could for their patients." Moreover, "…they were training people differently, creating new types of organizations, involving families and communities, and concentrating much more on promoting health and independence rather than on just tackling disease."

ICATCH has demonstrated that if these talented, committed health care advocates are provided with even a small amount of financial resources coupled with collegial professional support and encouragement, they will do amazing things. If we observe keenly and listen astutely we can learn much from them, for they have much to teach us. And most importantly, the children will be the greatest beneficiaries.

For additional information about ICATCH and to access an application, visit http://www2.aap.org/sections/ich/i_catch.htm.

Chapter 30

Global Networks

Judith S. Palfrey, MD, FAAP

The chapters in this book point to the importance of collaboration and network generation. Following are Web resources that steer the reader to many of the large groups working toward improving global child health:

Child Development
United Nations Children's Fund and World Health Organization:
Care for Child Development: Improving the Care for Young Children
www.who.int/maternal_child_adolescent/documents/care_child_
development/en/index.html

Disasters
American Academy of Pediatrics: *Pediatric Education in Disasters Manual*
www.aap.org/en-us/advocacy-and-policy/aap-health-initiatives/Children-
and-Disasters/Pages/Pediatric-Education-in-Disasters-Manual.aspx

HIV/AIDS
World Health Organization: HIV/AIDS
www.who.int/hiv

Immunizations
GAVI Alliance
www.gavialliance.org

Bill & Melinda Gates Foundation: What we do: vaccine delivery:
strategy overview
www.gatesfoundation.org/What-We-Do/Global-Development/
Vaccine-Delivery

Integrated Management of Childhood Illnesses

World Health Organization: Integrated Management of Childhood Illness (IMCI)
www.who.int/maternal_child_adolescent/topics/child/imci/en/index.html

International Organization

Pan American Health Organization
www.paho.org

Maternal and Infant Health

Save the Children
www.savethechildren.org

American Academy of Pediatrics: Helping Babies Breathe
www.helpingbabiesbreathe.org

Millennium Development Goals

United Nations Development Programme: The Millennium Development Goals: Eight Goals for 2015
www.undp.org/content/undp/en/home/mdgoverview.html

Countdown to 2015: Maternal, Newborn & Child Survival
www.countdown2015mnch.org

Nutrition

World Health Organization: Nutrition: Global targets 2025: To improve maternal, infant and young child nutrition
www.who.int/nutrition

Pneumonia and Diarrhea

United Nations Children's Fund: *Pneumonia and Diarrhoea: Tackling the Deadliest Diseases for the World's Poorest Children*
www.unicef.org/media/files/UNICEF_P_D_complete_0604.pdf

Professional Organizations

American Academy of Pediatrics: AAP Global
www.aap.org/international

American Academy of Pediatrics Section on International Child Health:
International Community Access to Child Health (ICATCH)
www2.aap.org/sections/ich/i_catch.htm

International Pediatric Association
www.ipa-world.org

Sickle Cell Anemia

World Health Organization Regional Office for Africa: Sickle cell
disease: a strategy for the WHO African region: Report of the
Regional Director
www.afro.who.int/index.php?option=com_docman&task=
doc_download&gid=6638

Tobacco

World Health Organization: *WHO Report on the Global Tobacco Epidemic,
2011: Warning About the Dangers of Tobacco*
www.who.int/tobacco/global_report/2011/en

Index